Health Promotion in Medical Education

Health Promotion in Medical Education

FROM RHETORIC TO ACTION

Edited by
ANN WYLIE
Senior Teaching Fellow and Health Promotion Lead
Department of General Practice and Primary Care
King's College London School of Medicine at Guy's, King's College and
St Thomas' Hospital London

and

TANGERINE HOLT
Director, International Education and Research, Office of International Engagement
Senior Lecturer, Centre for Medical and Health Sciences Education, Faculty of
Medicine, Nursing and Health Sciences, Monash University
Former Academic Convenor, MBBS Community Based Practice Program

Foreword by
AMANDA HOWE
Professor of Primary Care
University of East Anglia, Norwich

Radcliffe Publishing
Oxford • New York

Radcliffe Publishing Ltd
18 Marcham Road
Abingdon
Oxon OX14 1AA
United Kingdom

www.radcliffe-oxford.com

Electronic catalogue and worldwide online ordering facility.

British Library Cataloguing in Publication Data
A catalogue record for this book is available from the British Library.

ISBN-13: 978 184619 292 0

The paper used for the text pages of this book
is FSC certified. FSC (The Forest Stewardship
Council) is an international network to promote
responsible management of the world's forests.

Mixed Sources
Product group from well-managed
forests and other controlled sources
www.fsc.org Cert no. SGS-COC-2482
© 1996 Forest Stewardship Council

FSC

Typeset by Pindar NZ, Auckland, New Zealand
Printed and bound by TJI Digital, Padstow, Cornwall, UK

Contents

Foreword

Health promotion, like most aspects of healthcare, is a contested area. It is a relatively recent aspect of clinical training – often included in medical discourse for the sake of political correctness, but without the weight of history, authority or orthodox bioscientific evidence base to permit it a central place in the canon. Indeed, even the definition adopted by the authors – *'the study of, and the study of the response to, the modifiable determinants of health'* – may appear unfamiliar to the jobbing health professional. This book will humanise this context, while informing many who do not understand the bigger picture.

It sets out to explain how health promotion has developed, and its current international context; focuses on both its principles and practice within educational settings; and pays novel attention to the complexities of learning and assessing health promotion in basic clinical training. Do not fear another dry discussion of how to stop patients smoking! This book takes a stimulatingly lateral view of the scope of the subject – tackling international examples of health promotion from Camden to Cuba, and raising the uncomfortable subject of unhealthy behaviours in medical students and practitioners as an overt and overdue challenge to the conventional tendency to treat health promotion as something patients need but doctors do not.

Whenever the going gets tough in medical education, subject champions have to fight to hold on to their place in the curriculum and the resources for their teachers, and to win ideological commitment from the medical school, which will enthuse rather than disengage the learners. Health promotion is in a hard place because of its interdisciplinary nature, and its person-centred and population-based approaches, which sit at odds with the traditional disease- and system-based curricular models: it is neither led by a specific discipline, nor does it have a powerful political profile. This book goes a very long way to showing why it nevertheless is essential to medical education, and gives good advice on how to support and develop both the subject and its tutors in today's medical schools. Finally it gives both chapter and verse to those who are committed to health promotion but do not have either theory or practice examples to hand. It will be particularly valuable to those who have to deliver health promotion training in medical education, and to those who host and assess that training. Students, doctors and patients need health promotion – this book gives more how than why, which is a welcome shift of gear and should be read by many.

Amanda Howe
Professor of Primary Care
University of East Anglia, Norwich
November 2009

Preface

The aims of this book were originally to share with the medical education community our experiences of developing and implementing health promotion curricula. It became clear however that the task needed to be more comprehensive, that health promotion had been the neglected newcomer to modern curricula of both medical and other health professional vocational courses. At the same time, directives from regulating bodies and the changing healthcare needs were anticipating a skilled professional workforce able to apply health promotion intervention as relevant to patient care, to promote the health of the community and contribute to wider population health issues in an informed and authoritative way.

This book aims to be informative, in a practical way, to medical educators and curriculum developers about the background to health promotion, its own development and emerging epistemology, how curricular structures could accommodate this eclectic discipline, examples of health promotion teaching sessions and how this can be assessed within integrated curricula.

We have gathered together a number of experienced and enthusiastic writers, some with expertise in health promotion, some with expertise in public health and most with expertise in medical education. Many are actively involved in both research and implementation of health promotion curricula and willingly share the experiences and lesson learned thus far. Both the editors and writers have made two assumptions:

➤ that few faculties will have specialist and experts in health promotion who are also educationalists

➤ that health promotion needs to be integrated into existing curricula without major disruption or change and be relevant to the learner's context, the patient's or clinical context and the teacher's context.

As such we are not seeking to provide a definitive health promotion textbook but a medical education textbook to enable health promotion to be a more visible, integrated and less fragmented curricular component, with an aspiration to having some agreed principles of what constitutes quality in health promotion teaching across various faculties.

The book is set out in five parts and although each chapter and each part is intended to be comprehensive as an entity we also see the book as having overall cohesion, although we realise few readers will read it in linear fashion.

There will, however, be some repetition as each chapter has to place itself in a wider context, taking into consideration the development, integration and implementation of health promotion within medical and health professional education at international levels. We are particularly aware of the frequent reference to the Ottawa Charter. This is essentially to assert how important this Charter is for the discipline of health promotion rather than an oversight of the editorial process.

What can be taught, learnt, experienced and assessed with regard to health promotion may at first seem vast given the multiple determinants of health. However this book has hopefully set out some parameters to guide and direct the health promotion teaching in medical and health professional education.

Ann Wylie and Tangerine Holt
November 2009

About the editors

Dr Ann Wylie

Ann, although starting her professional life in the field of medical microbiology, has been involved in health promotion as a senior specialist for more than 20 years and completed a Masters at Southampton University. She then moved to medical education and focused on the epistemology of health promotion, the challenges to medical curriculum development and was awarded her PhD at King's College London. During the last 14 years she has conducted many small-scale projects, run workshops, presented findings and published papers related to the development of health promotion as a discipline within medical education, conducting longitudinal research regarding the impact of health promotion teaching with Monash Medical School and currently supervises a number of medical students, researching health promotion issues such as obesity prevention and child health promotion.

Dr Tangerine Holt

Tangerine has recently been appointed as Director, International Education in the Office of the Deputy Vice Chancellor International at Monash University. As a Senior Lecturer at the Centre for Medical and Health Sciences Education Monash University, her academic leadership has focused on developing excellence in medical and health professional education with an international focus through innovative educational developments of teaching and learning, community engagement with allied health professionals through the Bachelor of Medicine and Bachelor of Surgery (MBBS) Community-Based Practice Program, fairness, social justice and best practice. In 2007, as Academic Convenor of the Community Based Practice programme, Tangerine received the Australian Business and Higher Education Research and Training (BHERT) *Award for Outstanding Achievement in Collaboration in Research and Development and Education and Training* for the (MBBS) Community Partnerships. Previously, as Assistant Professor at the Kent School of Social Work at the University of Louisville, Kentucky, USA, Tangerine developed the Master of Social Work program on Advanced Macro Practice and served as the Director of the federally funded Kentucky Interdisciplinary Community Screenings Programs (KICS) across medicine, nursing, social work, dentistry and public health disciplines. In 2003 the KICS received the American *National Academies of Practice Group Interdisciplinary Award*, being highly recognised for its interprofessional health education within a community.

List of contributors

Dr Amin Azzam
Amin is Assistant Clinical Professor and Director of the Contextually Integrated Case-Based Curriculum for the University of California Berkeley-University of California San Francisco Joint Medical Program. His teaching and research interests are focused on teaching and learning styles in medical education, the role of 'near-peers' in teaching, problem-based learning and small group instruction.

Dr Richard Bordowitz
Richard is Deputy Director, General Preventive Medicine Residency and Assistant Professor of Community and Preventive Medicine at Mount Sinai School of Medicine, New York. He is also Assistant Professor of Medical Education, Pediatrics and Preventive Medicine. Richard's research interest is in clinical preventive medicine. He is particularly interested in the use of the electronic health record for preventive medicine and public health.

Dr Kathy Boursicot
Kathy is Reader in Medical Education at St George's School of Medicine, London, and is current Treasurer for the Association for the Study of Medical Education (ASME). She has specialised is aspects of assessment research in medical education and is part of the Education Research Group within ASME.

Dr Bev Daily
Bev qualified at Charing Cross Hospital in 1960. In 1961 he went into general practice in Burnham, Bucks where he worked as an NHS GP until 1999. Since then he has been a subject teacher at the Burnham Health Centre and Chairman of the Burnham Health Promotion Trust. He has had his own columns in, and written numerous articles for, a number of medical publications here and in the USA, devised a series of books for GPs, *What Shall I Do?*, has written a novel and about 30 short films of a medical nature. He is married with two children.

Professor Alan Maryon Davis
Alan is Honorary Professor of Public Health at King's College London. After hospital medicine and general practice, he switched to health education, health policy and public health. He was Head of Health Sciences and Chief Medical Officer at the Health Education Council, and more recently Director of Public Health for Southwark in south London. His academic career includes over 20 years' experience as Honorary Senior Lecturer and Professor of Public Health at Guy's, King's and St Thomas' Medical School

(now part of King's College London) where he has taught students from a range of disciplines at undergraduate and postgraduate level.

Dr Max de Courten
Max currently holds the position of Associate Professor Clinical Epidemiology, at the Department of Epidemiology and Preventive Medicine, Monash University, Melbourne. His medical education started in Switzerland where he undertook clinical research in the area of hypertension and insulin resistance. In the USA he worked at the National Institutes of Health on diabetes. His international experience was enhanced through positions at the World Health Organization as scientist at HQ and as Medical Officer Chronic Disease Control for the South Pacific.

Dr Ann Deehan
Ann is a National Institute for Health Research faculty manager at the Department of Health in London. She has worked in health and public health research for 15 years at the Addictions Research Unit and the Institute of Psychiatry and several government departments including Communities and Local Government and the Home Office. She has published widely on alcohol research and policy.

Dr Peter Duncan
Peter is Programme Director of the Postgraduate Programmes in Health Promotion and Health and Society at the Centre for Public Policy Research, King's College London. He is the author of *Critical Perspectives on Health* (Palgrave Macmillan, 2007), *Values, Ethics and Health Care: frameworks for reasoning, reflection and debate* (Sage, forthcoming) and (with Alan Cribb) *Health Promotion and Professional Ethics* (Blackwell Science, 2002).

Dr Erica Friedman
Erica is Associate Dean for Undergraduate Medical Education and oversees curriculum and assessment for the Mount Sinai School of Medicine, New York. She is also the Medical Director of the Morchand Center for Clinical Competence, which is a state-of-the-art Standardized Patient (SP) Center that assesses clinical skills including history taking, physical examination, communication and cultural competency. In addition, she is an Internist and Rheumatologist who runs the Mount Sinai Arthritis Clinic and teaches medical students, Internal Medicine residents and Rheumatology fellows. Her interests include enhancing physician-patient communication, promoting effective healthcare teamwork and educating people about osteoporosis and chronic illness management.

Dr Elizabeth Garland
Elizabeth is Director, General Preventive Medicine Residency and Associate Professor of Community and Preventive Medicine at Mount Sinai School of Medicine, New York. Since 2002 she has served as Chief of the Division of Preventive Medicine. She has been the Director of the Student Health Center at Mount Sinai School of Medicine since 1997. She has worked in the East Harlem community since 1981, and is the Co-Chair of the Pediatric/Child Health Sub-committee of the East Harlem Community Health Committee. Her research interests have centred on health disparities: pediatric asthma, reducing risk factors for diabetes in adolescents and violence intervention and prevention.

Professor Stephen Gillam
Stephen is a GP in Luton and Director of Undergraduate Public Health Teaching at the University of Cambridge. Previously, he was Director of Primary Care at the King's Fund where he was heavily involved in charting the impact of health policy under New Labour. He began his career in general practice and trained in public health following a period overseas with the Save the Children Fund. He holds honorary positions at the Cambridgeshire Primary Care Trust and the University of Bedfordshire.

Dr Craig Hassed
Craig is a GP in Melbourne and medical educator at Monash Medical School, Melbourne, where he has led the health promotion component, including the focus, in the early years, on medical students' own health and well-being. He has shared his teaching content and approaches with the Harvard School of Medicine. He links his interest in philosophy and ethics to the approaches used in health promotion and mindfulness teaching. He has written several books on mindfulness.

Professor Markus Herrmann
Markus is based at the University of Magdeburg, Germany, in the Institute of General Practice at the Medical Faculty. He is responsible for the core curriculum in health promotion including the health issues of students.

Dr Dragan Ilic
Dragan is a senior lecturer at the Monash Institute of Health Services Research, School of Public Health and Preventive Medicine, Monash University, Melbourne. He is based at the Monash Medical Centre, Clayton and is course coordinator of the Evidence-Based Clinical Practice Unit for the Monash University MBBS degree. He is also co-coordinator for the Data in Evidence theme for the Bachelor of Health Science degree at Monash University. His research interests include medical education, male reproductive health and health services research.

Professor Brian Jolly
Brian has spent many years in medical education and has had many roles, including current Deputy Editor for *Medical Education*. His specialist areas of interest and research have been in assessment.

Dr Aliya Kassam
Aliya is a psychiatric epidemiologist from Canada and is completing her PhD at the Institute of Psychiatry, King's College London. She has worked in evaluating mental illness related stigma and discrimination training programmes with medical and nursing students. Her current research interests include mental illness related stigma in medical education, mental health promotion and evaluation of public mental health programmes.

Dr Andreas Klement
Andreas is a GP and a senior lecturer teaching General Practice and Health Promotion, Undergraduate Medical Education Team, Department of General Practice and Family Medicine, Martin-Luther-University, Halle, Germany.

xvi   LIST OF CONTRIBUTORS

Professor Albert Lee

Albert is Professor (Family Medicine) of the Department of Community and Family Medicine, and also Director of the Division of Health Improvement and Centre for Health Education and Health Promotion of the School of Public Health of the Chinese University of Hong Kong. He established the first Masters programmes in health education and health promotion, and also family medicine in Hong Kong.

He pioneered the concept of Health Promoting Schools in Hong Kong to promote child and adolescent health. On many occasions he has been invited by the World Health Organization to become a temporary advisor on school health and health promotion, to conduct international workshops and consult with other Asian and Pacific countries on health promotion.

Dr Gillian Maudsley

Gillian is a clinical senior lecturer in Public Health Medicine at the University of Liverpool. Her research interest and practical expertise are in medical education, problem-based undergraduate medical education (including its definition, tutoring and relationship to students' learning approaches and cognitive development), and public health education for medical students.

Dr Nisha Mehta

Nisha was a final-year medical student at King's College London. She studied Medicine as a second degree after reading Modern History at Oxford and then working in the Civil Service on projects including quality-of-life research in prisons and primary care policy in the Scottish Government. She is a Visiting Research Associate at the Health Services and Population Research Department, Institute of Psychiatry, King's College London, where her current interests include stigma and discrimination against people with mental illness. When she graduated as a doctor in August 2009 she commenced a two-year Academic Foundation Programme at King's College London, which will allow dedicated research and teaching time.

Dr Patricia Nolan

Pat is currently a Clinical Assistant Professor of Community Health at Brown University. She received her medical degree from McGill University, Montreal, in 1969, and her Masters in Public Health from Columbia University, New York City, in 1973. She is board certified in Public Health by the American Board of Preventive Medicine. Pat is the current president of the Association of State and Territorial Health Officials. She is actively involved in the American Public Health Association and serves on the board of the Alliance to End Childhood Lead Poisoning. She is also Director of the Rhode Island Department of Health.

Jo Reynolds

Jo is a research assistant in the Institute of Primary Care and Public Health at London South Bank University. She has worked on several funded projects including an evaluation of public health attachments as part of GP specialty training.

Dr Emily Rigby

Emily is a Foundation Year 1 House Officer at Ealing Hospital. Since medical school, she has been involved with medical education issues, as Chair of the British Medical

Association's Medical Students' Committee and European Coordinator for Medical Education within the International Federation of Medical Students' Associations. She has spoken widely in an international arena on undergraduate medical education with a particular interest in the Bologna Declaration and methods of assessment.

Dr Angela Scriven

Angela is Reader in Health Promotion at Brunel University, London, with research centred on the relationship between policy and practice in health promotion. The main thrust of her work is to assess the impact of national and international health and other related policy initiatives on the delivery of health promotion in specific contexts. She has published extensively, including six books and over 90 journal articles, chapters in books, conference papers, occasional papers and reports. Articles have appeared in leading health promotion journals and the books have international circulation.

Richard Shircore

Richard developed his health promotion skills and understanding in the NHS and voluntary sectors. He has pushed the development of health promotion theory and methods into new areas such as reduction of antisocial behaviour. He is an Honorary Member of Staff at the University of Reading, Berkshire, and a Trustee of a major children's charity dealing with adoption and family welfare. He founded www.healthpromotion.uk.com in July 2007.

Associate Professor Karen Sokal-Gutierrez

Karen is the Site Director for PRIME-US (Program for Medical Education in the Urban Underserved) for the University of California Berkeley-University of California San Francisco Joint Medical Program. Her research interests have focused on children's health in child care, parenting education, maternal–child health, health education for low-literacy populations, early childhood development, health and safety and early childhood oral health in Latin America.

Associate Professor Marc Soethout

Marc studied Medicine at the Vrije Universiteit medical centre (VUmc) in Amsterdam. He followed this with postgraduate training in public health medicine and different courses in epidemiology and medical education. At present he is Education Coordinator in the Department of Public and Occupational Health at VUmc in Amsterdam, and is actively involved in undergraduate and postgraduate education in public health. He is a referee for many medical education journals, and a member of different national and international public health education organisations.

Dr Tim Swanwick

Tim is training lead for General Practice at the London Deanery. He is also the Specialty and assessment lead.

Professor John Edward Swartzberg

John is Director of the University of California Berkeley-University of California San Francisco Joint Medical Program. He is also Chair of the Editorial Board at the University of California Berkeley Wellness Letter. His recent publications in the UC Berkeley Wellness Report have focused on achieving optimal health, women's health and men's health.

Professor Jane Wills

Jane is Professor of Health Promotion at London South Bank University. She has been involved in the health promotion education of healthcare practitioners for many years and has written several textbooks that contribute to many nursing and health curricula both in the UK and internationally. Her research interests relate to the discourse of health promotion and its practice.

Acknowledgements

This book has been possible because of the generosity of many people including our colleagues and friends, as well as our families. First we want to thank all contributors to this book, some of whom are emerging scholars and others highly regarded and well known in their fields of expertise on medical and health professional education. We have been privileged to have contributions from internationally recognised experts in the fields of health promotion, public health and medical education and we are grateful to our contributors who work enthusiastically to develop and implement health promotion core content in medical education and have generously shared their experiences.

We are especially grateful to our department colleagues at King's College London and Monash University, including a Monash University-King's College travel grant that supported this endeavour, enabling us to have the time to write and meet, and to share experiences. Dr Anne Stephenson was very generous and supportive, and given her own experiences of writing, provided good counsel at the various stages of the book's development as well as helping to map a way of managing this project, with minimum disruption to our workload. Our team in the Department of General Practice and Primary Care, King's College, managed the day-to-day work with little call on our time whilst the main writing was being carried out during August 2008. In particular, thanks to Professor Brian Jolly, Professor Ben Canny, Mr John Goodall and Ms Helen Mandeltort for their ongoing support during the development and write-up of this book.

Associate Professor Marc Soethout, from Amsterdam, not only contributed to the book but also helped us to keep the context relevant. He came over to meet with us in London, discussed the book and our related presentations at the Association of Medical Education in Europe (AMEE) conference in Prague, which he gave on our behalf. We have collaborated with related research plans and shared our materials. Marc has been generous and enthusiastic, and with his expertise in public health as well as his interest in medical education and health promotion, we have been very fortunate.

Many colleagues have generously given their time to share their materials and research, made suggestions and commented on early drafts of chapters, providing constructive feedback. Our colleagues Professor John Swartzberg, Associate Clinical Professor Karen Sokal-Gutierrez and Dr Amin Azzam at the University of California, Berkeley Campus hosted Tangerine's visit and provided input about their fascinating program known as 'PRIME-US'. Similarly, colleagues Associate Professor Elizabeth Garland, Dr Richard Bordowitz and Associate Professor Erica Friedman at Mount Sinai School of Medicine were generous in their time and provided excellent input on their unique programs.

Our families have been most supportive and we would like to thank them for their generosity. Rod, Ann's husband, endured a summer of papers, drafts and very limited free time as we worked away on the book. He was generous with hospitality as Tangerine and I much appreciated, and he never doubted this project would result in a published book. Tangerine's family had to cope without her for more than a month as she travelled to the USA and UK to prepare for this, and her husband, Fabian, took on the parenting role supported by George and Marian (Tangerine's parents), while their children, Leah and Aaron, kept in regular contact without complaint but happy that Mum was doing this important project.

There are many others who have at various stages provided valued input and good advice, some from health promotion, some from medical education and others who have had the experience of co-editing books. We are appreciative of all those who have helped in any way with this book, and we hope the finished book is worthy of the time and effort given by all.

PART ONE

The rationale and historical context to justify the inclusion of health promotion in curricula

INTRODUCTION
Ann Wylie and Alan Maryon Davis

The discipline of health promotion is relatively young compared to the more established and wider field of public health, with which it is closely aligned. Nevertheless many of the principles and practices embodied in what we now call 'health promotion' have been integral to medicine in its broadest sense since the days of Hippocrates. There are few healthcare professionals, of whatever discipline, whose work does not involve some element of health promotion, and it is therefore important that those preparing to enter the healthcare field should have a sound understanding of health promotion and its relevance to their future professional practice.

Since the World Health Organization's Ottawa Charter for Health Promotion in 1986,[1] more robust parameters have emerged, defining and shaping the discipline in terms of both its skills base for practice and its landscape for research. The discipline extends far beyond the clinical arena, and most practitioners and specialists in health promotion are working in non-clinical settings.

That said, as we face ever more complex multifactorial public health concerns such as obesity, inequalities and communicable diseases, there are ethical dilemmas as to the level and type of intervention that health professionals, including doctors, should be involved with and therefore what competencies and knowledge base they need from this discipline for best practice.

In the UK, within medical education, the General Medical Council have expressed concerns about the 'crowded' curriculum, and D'Eon and Crawford as well as others have tried to give some guidance to those charged with deciding curriculum content.[2,3] It is not exactly true that if something new goes in, something else must be deleted. Instead the discussion should be focused on how these essential topics could be integrated effectively. A well-argued rationale for the inclusion of a discipline, albeit at a basic level, that could otherwise be so easily marginalised or omitted altogether, will be helpful for curriculum planners, developers and teachers as well as students.

The following chapters in Part One explore the rationale to justify the inclusion of health promotion in health professional curricula, identifying some of the challenges facing curriculum developers and how we can learn from recent experiences.

REFERENCES
1 World Health Organization. *Ottawa Charter for Health Promotion*. Geneva: World Health Organization; 1986.
2 General Medical Council. *Tomorrow's Doctors*. 2nd ed. London: General Medical Council; 2003.
3 D'Eon M, Crawford R. The elusive content of the medical-school curriculum: a method to madness. *Med Teach*. 2005; 27(8): 699–703.

CHAPTER 1

Medical and health professional education: a call for health promotion in curricula

Ann Wylie

INTRODUCTION

This chapter reflects on the rhetoric and the trajectory of health promotion as it juxtaposes with public health and clinical practice for a place in core curricula. From aspiring ideals to actual requirements, health promotion has been fraught with difficulties, some of which are highlighted in following chapters. There is now more universal acceptance that health promotion skills need to be integral to medical and health professional curricula.

EARLY ENTHUSIASM

It is thought that the term 'health promotion' was first used in 1974 by Marc Lalonde when he was Canadian Minister of National Health and Welfare. *A New Perspective on the Health of Canadians* bravely argued that the major causes of morbidity and mortality were less to do with biomedical sciences but related to environments, individual behaviour and lifestyle.[1] This was a time when science and pharmacology were in the ascendancy, with vast amounts of investment and expectation going to medical research and development. Just over a decade later, Lalonde's ideas of health had informed the World Health Assembly and influenced the Ottawa Charter.

Following the publication of the Ottawa Charter,[2] there was a flurry of activity to examine how this new field, health promotion, discrete from public health, could be part of core medical undergraduate curricula. In 1989 a World Health Organization (WHO) consultation was held in Italy and some challenges were highlighted and also some areas for discussion.[3] The scale of the challenge at the time was considered by those likely to have to lead on change and implementation.

> The responsibility and the time and resources needed to facilitate such a development should not be underestimated. Until the importance of the subject is recognised by universities, by long-term funding of these posts, the future of health

promotion teaching in medical schools will remain uncertain and consequently in doubt.[4]

Health promotion specialists had been in posts for many years, and within the UK, mainly within the National Health Service (NHS) and associated with public health departments and in local authorities but frequently called health educationalists. Within a few years of publication of the Ottawa Charter, their status improved and most changed their professional title from health educationalist to health promoter. One of the standard textbooks, *Promoting health. A practical guide*, first published in 1985 and now with a fifth edition,[5] was the staple both for the specialists and those they trained for field-related health promotion work. The specialist health promotion journals published scientific and humanities research papers, reflecting the eclectic nature of health promotion, and there was a society and institute that professionals could join although not mandatory. Higher degrees were available within various faculties such as health, education and sociology. However, professionalism was challenged, given that this was one of the few health-related occupations that did not require registration and was not regulated.[6,7] Public health physicians may have been aware of the situation but given that most senior health promotion specialists held a master's degree or diploma, there was limited concern in the wider field of medicine and medical education. However both the lack of registration and the 'electric' nature also ensured that for another two decades the field was a contested field with an inability to define its own territory and a host of contrasting definitions appearing in well argued journal discussion papers.[8,9] Whilst this type of debate is ostensibly healthy and characteristic of an academic and practitioner community, it presented uncertainty and scepticism to those within medicine who were more familiar with scientific evidence and certainty, especially where high-stakes assessment was required for qualification and progression.

At the same time, the World Conference on Medical Education in Edinburgh made an important declaration stating that medical education should produce doctors 'who will promote the health of all people'.[10]

Two disciplines, with emerging epistemologies, medical education and health promotion, reliant on multiple research paradigms, were at the forefront of change. Whilst there was enthusiasm for modernising curricula, both content and pedagogy, there also was a perceived opportunity for integrating health promotion.

The Ottawa Charter set out three principal approaches for health promotion: advocate, enable and mediate, within five domains as follows:
➤ build health public policy
➤ create supportive environments
➤ strengthen community action
➤ develop personal skills
➤ reorient health services.

Linked to this were other WHO declarations such as the Declaration of Primary Care at Alma Ata and Health for All.[11,12] Whilst these ideals are worthy there was limited appreciation of how these would translate into learning outcomes in modern curricula already 'crowded' with science, and given that assessment drives learning,[13] what could be assessed was far from clear.

Within the UK, it was in Scotland that the first steps towards integrating health promotion into medical curricula were attempted, when the Scottish Health Education

Group (SHEG) provided funding for a dedicated lectureship post. Amos, *et al.* disseminated their work to the medical education community.[14] The other earlier example to publish was from Gillies and Ellwood from Nottingham Medical School.[15] Neither publication referred to the contested nature of health promotion; the focus was intervention associated with disease prevention and lifestyle change.

DIRECTIVES BY REGULATORY BODIES

The next milestone was the publication of *Tomorrow's Doctors* in 1993 by the General Medical Council (GMC),[16] which was a major catalyst for reform both of curriculum content and pedagogy. Examples of health promotion in nursing education were published in the same year.[17,18] The scene was set for change, and change that could potentially embed health promotion in curricula for medicine and nursing. In terms of curriculum content, *Tomorrow's Doctors* was critical of scientific overload in curricula and sought to enhance the curriculum with humanities promoting the integration of communication skills and ethics. The document frequently referred to health promotion, health education, disease prevention and public health. The introduction acknowledged that the focus of medical education had centred on disease processes at the expense of population health, pointing out that the achievements of public health had been 'temporarily lost from the vocabulary'. The goals of medical education were to include the principles of disease prevention and health promotion. Within a few years medical education journals were publishing papers about new curriculum design and implementation.[19] Some examples of new curricula and health promotion were also being published.[20–24]

By the end of the twentieth century, most medical schools in the UK, North America and Australia had modernised their curricula with significant core curriculum time given to communication skills and ethics, having moved to integrated curricula and having reformed assessment. Whereas agreed learning outcomes had emerged for communication skills and ethics content,[25] with external examiners looking specifically at these fields, health promotion was fragmented and limited to schools where interested individuals championed it. Rather than health promotion making the anticipated headway, it was marginalised or restricted to topics such as smoking cessation skills.

In the intervening years from the publication of *Tomorrow's Doctors* (1993), the field of health promotion had developed its evidence base and the public health concerns and burden of diseases, such as type 2 diabetes, had come into focus, with the role of doctors in contributing to health promotion now being more clearly argued. The second edition of *Tomorrow's Doctors* (2003) reiterates that the health and safety of the public must be an important part of the curriculum, as well as promoting health (paragraph 33, page 16).[26] Other countries have similar documentation published by regulatory bodies. For example, in North America, USA and Canada, the Association of American Medical Colleges (AAMC) states that students should be exposed to a wide variety of topics including community and population health.[27] Likewise the Australian Medical Council, which also is applicable in New Zealand, requires that medical graduates know the 'principles of health education, disease prevention and screening'.[28]

THE NEEDS OF LEARNERS

Within the field of higher education in Europe, the Bologna Declaration for Medical Education was the subject of a conference in Bristol in 2006, with the International Federation of Medical Students Association (IFMSA) and European Medical Students Association (EMSA) producing a summary of the discussions about the core curriculum. They identified 76 learning outcomes based around nine domains and asserted that medical students do have an active role in developing new approaches to medical education. Domain 4, Health in Society, describes learning outcomes for graduates that would come under the field of health promotion such as:

➤ know key factors and strategies for prevention
➤ be able to promote the health of the individual patient and of society, including active education of patients
➤ be able to understand the impact of culture, religious and social aspects on health, health behaviour and treatment process.[29]

Although evidence suggests that few medical students show an interest in a public health career,[30] Soethout, *et al.* also state that graduates should be able to contribute to shaping health policy choices during their medical career, and their curriculum, by implication, should have prepared them for this task.[31]

HEALTH PROMOTION IN CLINICAL PRACTICE: INCENTIVES AND DIRECTIVES FOR PRACTICE

One of the most remarkable approaches to medical education and practice has been in Cuba, where central to the ethos is public health and health promotion at community level, not just in Cuba itself but for the countries that have benefited from Cuba's generosity.[32] This generosity involves offering free places for medical education to 13 000 students from 17 countries in Latin America, the Caribbean and Asia. The students are exposed to population health principles and prevention with approximately 17% of curriculum time class hours dedicated to this. For a relatively poor country, Cuba's health indices are comparable with richer Western countries, testimony to its approach to healthcare and medical education possibly.

It is unlikely that such an approach and level of input for public health and health promotion would be widely adopted elsewhere. However, given that there are continuing preventable health concerns which are a burden to economies,[33] not to mention the distress to individuals and families, governments set out targets and strategies to reduce risk factors and reverse trends such as the increasing prevalence of obesity.[34,35] The role of healthcare professionals in these policy directives is usually linked to incentives such as payments or indeed, penalties. In the UK the NHS Quality Outcomes Framework (QOF) has been encouraging Primary Care Teams (PCTs) to take a more proactive role in promoting health. There are for example, in all areas of the UK, smoking cessation services available free of charge. The smoking cessation services are provided by trained advisors and payments to the service providers are linked to patients being smoke-free or quitters of a minimum four weeks' duration. The approach to these health-promoting interventions is given credence by National Institute of Clinical Excellence(NICE) which has now produced a number of guidance papers for practitioners.[36–38] But these NICE guidelines are not mandatory and inconsistencies are reported.[39,40]

While such variation in approach to behavioural and lifestyle change has been identified in general practice, no such data is readily available from other medical specialities. The reality is that many senior health practitioners, consultants and general practitioners would have had limited exposure, if any, to the relatively young discipline of health promotion and may still question whether they have a legitimate role in questioning their patients about lifestyle and providing advice. In contrast, public health would have been taught, probably focused on population health indices, communicable diseases and epidemiology. The link with clinical practice would have been limited. That said, for clinicians their public health knowledge may have informed their initial investigations and prognosis, enabled some probabilities to be considered or eliminated, and provided the rationale for notifying communicable diseases and promoting immunisation.

There is, therefore, a possible deficit of health promotion knowledge and skills in those professionals who are the core medical teachers. The lifelong learning ethos of contemporary medical practice can facilitate a process of students and teachers learning together as evidence informs about the effectiveness of health promotion interventions. The skills and knowledge base associated with applied health promotion within the clinical context can be integrated in core medical curricula, given that many of the major health concerns will benefit from such skilled, evidence-based health promotion activity and interventions. Lord Darzi, in his recent report, has highlighted that health practitioners have a role in keeping people healthy, and advocates that health professionals should have expertise in health promotion to address the rise in obesity and alcohol misuse and to respond to health inequalities, cancer prevention and heart disease reduction.[41]

In the next chapter, this increasing body of evidence to support health promotion intervention within the clinical context is explored.

REFERENCES

1 Lalonde M. *A New Perspective on the Health of Canadians.* Ottawa: Ministry of Supply and Services; 1974.

2 World Health Organization. *Ottawa Charter for Health Promotion.* Geneva: World Health Organization; 1986.

3 Weare K, Kelly P. *Health Education in Medical Education: a report of a World Health Organization consultation at the University of Perugia.* Geneva: World Health Organization; 1990.

4 Weare K. Developing health promotion in undergraduate medical education. Report of a national conference held at the University of Sheffield, March 1987. London: HEA; 1988.

5 Ewles L, Simnett I. *Promoting Health. A practical guide.* 5th ed. London: Bailliere Tindall; 2003.

6 Duncan P. *Moral Problems in the Theory and Practice of Health Promotion.* London: King's College London; 2000.

7 Cribb A, Duncan P. Making a profession of health promotion? Grounds for trust and health promotion ethics. *Int J Health Promot Educ.* 1999; 37(4): 129–34.

8 French J. Boundaries and horizons, the role of health education within health promotion. *Health Educ.* 1990; 49(1): 7–10.

9 Tones K. Richness and variety in health education. *Health Educ Res.* 1990; 5(1): 1–3.

10 World Federation for Medical Education. The Edinburgh Declaration. *Lancet.* 1988; 8068: 464.

11 World Health Organization. *Report of the International Conference on Primary Health Care.* Geneva: World Health Organization; 1978.

12 World Health Organization. *Targets for Health for All.* Copenhagen: World Health Organization; 1985.

13 Lowry S. *Medical Education.* London: BMJ Publishing Group; 1993.

14 Amos A, Church M, Forster F, *et al.* A health promotion model for undergraduate medical students. *Med Educ.* 1990; **2**: 1–8.

15 Gillies P, Ellwood JM. Health promotion in the medical curriculum. *Med Educ.* 1989; **23**: 440–6.

16 General Medical Council. *Tomorrow's Doctors.* London: General Medical Council; 1993.

17 Wilson-Barnett J, Macleod-Clark J, editors. *Research in Health Promotion and Nursing.* London: Macmillan; 1993.

18 Wilson-Barnett J. The meaning of health promotion: a personal view. In: Wilson-Barnett J, Macleod-Clark J, editors. *Research in Health Promotion and Nursing.* London: Macmillan; 1993.

19 Harden RM, Davis MH, Crosby JR. The new Dundee medical curriculum: a whole that is greater than the sum of the parts. *Med Educ.* 1997; **31**(4): 264–71.

20 Meakin RP, Lloyd MH. Disease prevention and health promotion: a study of medical students and teachers. *Med Educ.* 1996; **30**: 97–104.

21 Toon PD, Jolly B, Cowburn G. *Undergraduate Teaching in Health Promotion at Three UK Medical Schools.* [Unpublished report] 1998.

22 Pringle M, von Fragstein M, Craig B. *Health Promotion in the Medical Undergraduate Curriculum.* London: HEA; 1997.

23 Jones KV, Hsu H. Health promotion projects: skill and attitude learning for medical students. *Med Educ.* 1999; **33**(8): 585–91.

24 Taylor WC, Moore GT. Health promotion and disease prevention: integration into a medical school curriculum. *Med Educ.* 1994; **28**: 481–7.

25 Doyal L, Gillon R. Medical ethics and law as a core subject in medical education. *BMJ.* 1998 (May); **316**(7145): 1623–4.

26 General Medical Council. *Tomorrow's Doctors.* 2nd ed. London: General Medical Council; 2003.

27 Association of American Medical Colleges. *The Medical Student Education Program.* Available at: http://services.aamc.org/currdir/about.cfm (accessed 28 October 2009).

28 Australian Medical Council. *Assessment and Accreditation of Medical Schools: Standards and Procedures.* Available at: www.amc.org.au/images/Medschool/standards.pdf (accessed 28 October 2009).

29 Hilgers J, DeRoos P, Rigby E. European core curriculum: the students' perspective. *Med Teach.* 2007; **29**(2): 270–5.

30 Soethout MBM, ten Cate OJ, van der Wal G. Development of an interest in a career in public health during medical school. *Public Health.* 2008 (April); **122**(4): 361–6.

31 Ibid.

32 Huish R. Going where no doctor has gone before: the role of Cuba's Latin American School of Medicine in meeting the needs of some of the world's most vulnerable populations. *Public Health.* 2008 (June); **122**(6): 552–7.

33 Wanless D. *Securing Our Future Health: taking a long-term view: interim report.* London: HM Treasury; 2001.

34 Department of Health. *Choosing Health: making healthier choices easier* [Public Health White Paper]. London: Department of Health; 2004.

35 Department of Health. *Healthy Weight, Healthy Lives: a cross-government strategy for England.* London: Department of Health; 2008.

36 National Institute for Health and Clinical Excellence. *Brief Interventions and Referral for Smoking Cessation in Primary Care and Other Settings: public health guidance PH1.* London: NICE; 2006. http://guidance.nice.org.uk/PH1.

37 National Institute for Health and Clinical Excellence. *Smoking Cessation Services: public*

health guidance PH10 (supersedes TA39 Smoking cessation: bupropion and nicotine replacement therapy). London: NICE, 2008.

38 National Institute for Health and Clinical Excellence. *Brief Interventions and Referral for Smoking Cessation in Primary Care and Other Settings*, op. cit.

39 Kerr S, Watson H, Tolson D, *et al.* An exploration of the knowledge, attitudes and practice of members of the primary care team in relation to smoking and smoking cessation in later life. *Prim Health Care Res Dev.* 2007; **8**(1): 68–79.

40 Vogt F, Hall S, Marteau T. General practitioners' beliefs about effectiveness and intentions to recommend smoking cessation services: qualitative and quantitative studies. *BMC Family Practice.* 2007; **8**(1): 39.

41 Lord Darzi. *A High Quality Workforce: NHS next stage review.* London: Department of Health; 2008.

CHAPTER 2

Health promotion: the challenges, the questions of definition, discipline status and evidence base

Ann Deehan and Ann Wylie

THE DIFFICULTY OF DEFINING HEALTH PROMOTION – HISTORICAL AND CONTESTED ASPECTS

This chapter considers the challenge of defining health promotion, why this is an integral aspect of sourcing and exploring the evidence base and subsequently how such a challenge will impact on medical and health professional curricula.

There is a varied and vast literature around how health promotion should be defined, but no clear and widely adopted consensus of what that definition should be.[1,2] Some definitions focus on activities, others on values and aims.[3] Most of the definitional difficulties emerge from the diverse range of professional and lay notions of what health is. Complicating the definitional debate further is the fact that health promotion is not rooted in one discipline – rather it is eclectic and draws on theoretical and research paradigms from psychology, sociology, education and epidemiology for example – and that it is often performed in multidisciplinary settings.[4]

Additionally, the breadth of activity leaves health promotion specialists with an ill-defined client and target group. It is important to recognise that health promotion is considered by some as a 'process' and is directed at achieving an outcome, usually a change in lifestyle behaviours.[5] It is not a 'quick fix'; there are many components and it can take some time to achieve its broader aims, which is a contributory factor to the challenge of evaluating its impact, and as such it will be difficult to demonstrate positive change as mainly or solely attributable to a health promotion intervention.

Outcomes in 'successful' health promotion interventions are associated with aims of the intervention – both the short term and long term. These aims need to be clearly stated, demonstrable and measurable. A smoking cessation programme, for example, may be multifocused and involve short-term or proximal outcomes which:

➤ raise awareness among smokers, about cessation services
➤ increase consultations with potential service users for information about accessing services, location and times
➤ facilitate smokers to develop an action plan.

The long-term or distal outcome of such a programme would be to reduce smoking prevalence in a defined population or target group.

Contemporary health promotion as a discipline emerged with the WHO Declaration of Alma Mata in 1978, which for the first time acknowledged that improvements in health could not be determined by investments in the healthcare system alone but must take into account the impact of wider societal determinants such as economic or educational systems. Tones traces the emergence of health promotion as a major force to the 1984 publication of the World Health Organization's (WHO) discussion document on the concepts and principles of public health.[6] WHO later confirmed its commitment to health promotion in the Ottawa Charter in 1986[7] which declared health promotion to be:

> . . . the process of enabling people to increase control over and to improve their health
> . . . Health is a positive concept emphasising social and personal resources as well as physical capacities. Thereby health promotion is not just the responsibility of the health sector, but goes beyond healthy lifestyles to well-being.

This definition from the Ottawa Charter still provides the most frequently adopted definition of health promotion. The Charter identified five key strategies that have informed the development of health promotion practice and policy development:
➤ building healthy public policy
➤ creating supportive environments
➤ strengthening community action
➤ developing personal skills; and
➤ reorienting health services.

The Ottawa Charter has been built on with further WHO international conferences in Adelaide, Sundsvall, Jakarta and Bangkok aimed at lifting the health status of people and improving quality of life.[8]

The Ottawa definition however is visionary. Many theorists consider it to be too idealist and rhetorical and in need of further refinement if possible to inform frontline theory, research and practice. One commentator, Tones, provided a substantive and pragmatic approach to defining or explaining the work of health promotion:[9]

> Health promotion incorporates all measures deliberately designed to promote health and handle disease . . . A major feature of health promotion is undoubtedly the importance of 'healthy public policy' with its potential for achieving social change via legislation, fiscal, economic and other forms of environmental engineering.

He further progressed this to what has widely been adopted as a slogan: 'Healthy public policy × health education = health promotion', with the implication that both public health, through policy, and health education for individuals would mean the 'Healthy choice is the easy choice'.

This field, health promotion, not only has links with public health but also to health education, which Tones defined as:

> . . . any intentional activity which is designed to achieve health or illness-related

learning; it may facilitate the acquisition of skills; it may even effect changes in behaviour or lifestyle.

Today, information giving is still part of what is understood by health education, and French described it in 1990 as:

> ... a practical endeavour, focused on improving understanding about the determinants of health and illness and helping people to develop the skills they need to bring about change.[10]

For medical educators attempting to introduce health promotion to medical students, a more conventional body of knowledge is needed which would enable curricula to identify components for teaching and assessment.

Conceptual frameworks of health promotion for medical educators should facilitate the design of curricula. Nordenfelt presents one such conceptual framework for health promotion (*see* Figure 2.1), describing it as a part of health enhancement and offering four categories, namely environmental care, legal health protection, health education and medical disease prevention.[11]

Nordenfeldt's framework is based on the premise that health promotion does not presuppose a health problem exists. Health enhancement constitutes health promotion at one end of the continuum and healthcare at the other.

DEFINING HEALTH PROMOTION – DEVELOPING A WORKING DEFINITION

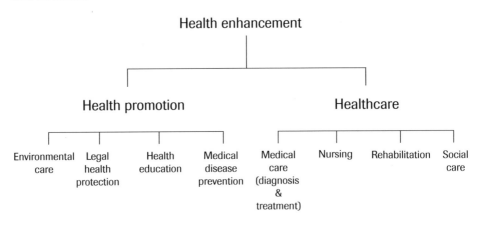

FIGURE 2.1 Conceptual framework that incorporates health promotion[11]

Although definitions abound in the literature, all present some limitations to those in medical curriculum development, which in part has led to fragmentation and variable approaches to constructing health promotion content, or in some cases omitting it from curricula entirely. Wylie's ethnographic study explored how medical educators, teachers and health promoters interpreted health promotion, how they constructed the practice, what informed practice and what they would see as a knowledge and skill base.[2] The research trajectory, adapted from Ball,[12] is illustrated in Figure 2.2. The findings cluster into three domains as illustrated in Figures 2.3 and 2.4. In Figure 2.3 they appear rigid and although linked they provide limited flexibility. For some respondents these clearly defined areas inform health promotion content, who takes responsibility and what could be assessed. In Figure 2.4 the domains are arranged in a more flexible way, are interlinked and enable a synthesis of various research paradigms to inform practice and learning.

Based on this work, Wylie constructed a working definition for health promotion for those working with curriculum development both in medical education and in other health-related fields.

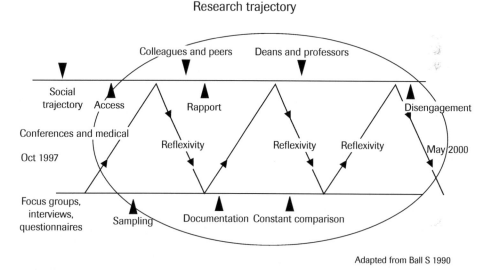

FIGURE 2.2 Research trajectory derived from Wylie's study on views of health promotion

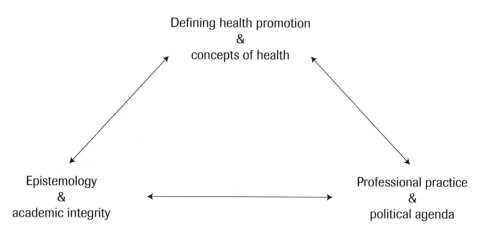

FIGURE 2.3 Wylie's research findings clustered in three domains (Model 1)

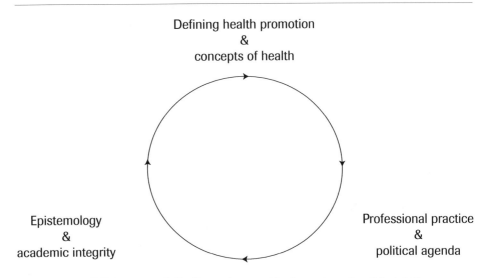

Defining health promotion
&
concepts of health

Epistemology
&
academic integrity

Professional practice
&
political agenda

FIGURE 2.4 Wylie's research findings clustered in three domains (Model 2)

> Health promotion is *the study of, and the study of the responses to, the modifiable determinants of health and disease.*

This definition is further explored in Chapters 12 and 15 but essentially has three aspects as follows:

➤ response: pertaining to intervention, action, strategy or policy and the skills and evidence needed to devise and implement health promotion

➤ determinants: pertaining to the factors influencing health or disease, both by association and causal, as determined by scientific and other rigorous methods of inquiry, including public health

➤ modifiable: pertaining to the notion of a determinant of health or disease, or a cluster of associated determinants in the context, with the resources, being modifiable, this being based on complex evidence from multiple sources to developed informed argument.

HEALTH PROMOTION EVIDENCE BASE

Any credible discipline must have a robust evidence base upon which its practitioners can make sound clinical and policy decisions. Health promotion is no different. However, as the difficulty in providing one clear definition of the discipline attests, health promotion is in many ways a special case when decisions are made of the value of its emerging evidence base.

During the 1980s public services began to expect to be able to make evidenced-based policy and clinical decisions, which led to the health promotional field desiring credible scientific evidence for their work.[13,14] Cochrane initiated evidenced-based medicine in the UK, arguing that investment should be made only in interventions that were proven to work, recommending the cause-and-effect methodologies of randomised controlled trials (RCT) as the most robust methodology[15] to assess impact. The value of RCTs to the health promotional field have been well-debated – they are expensive, suited best to single-factor interventions, are more suitable to closed environments than open ones and often raise ethical issues about informed consent.[13] Nonetheless, RCTs continue to be viewed as a robust methodology.

The growing interest in evidencing clinical and policy ideas has led to the development of the Cochrane collaboration, which provides systematic reviews of a wide range of clinical practices. The criteria for the inclusion of research in such a systematic review are rigorous, focusing on the RCT as the standard to which they aspire. Systematic reviews are controversial as they often omit research not deemed to meet defined criteria which judge it to be of a 'gold standard'.[16] RCTs, in the scientific disciplines, usually meet systematic review criteria but are not, as discussed above, atypical methodologies in evaluating health promotion initiatives. As a result, there may be many effective health promotional interventions in place that would not be included in a systematic review because of the criteria used for assessing the quality of their evaluation. Morgan comments that the reviews of such scientific studies highlight the problems faced by health promoters striving to evidence their work by searching through a limited amount of health promotion evaluations that will fit into the biomedical model of evidence.[14]

McQueen summarised the issues faced by the young health promotion discipline, identifying three 'critical and unresolved' issues in developing the research and practice evidence base.[17]

First, McQueen argues that the 'rules of evidence' are tied to disciplines and not the type of projects that usually make up health promotional projects. As a result the standards for what confirms proof of causation have developed through scientific methods such as cause-and-effect experimentation. This methodology does not work for health promotion because most projects are not rooted in a single discipline. Second, McQueen argues that the health promotion field has no consensus on a 'hierarchy' of evidence. There continues to be debate about what knowledge is and what constitutes evidence while RCTs are still viewed by many as the 'gold standard' methodology, despite their obvious limitations in understanding whether health promotional activity has its desired impact. Third, McQueen attests that the complexity of most multidisciplinary health promotion interventions means that the simple methodologies designed to demonstrate cause and effect are unsuitable for their evaluation. This is because, usually, there are many confounding factors and variables that can impact on the outcome, making measurement difficult. Experimental designs may not capture the distal impact of interventions, which are not seen for some time, or may not be sustainable, both issues requiring long-term and complex evaluation methodologies.

Nutbeam describes providing evidence in the health promotion field as a 'challenge' for many of the reasons outlined by McQueen above, citing three issues that need to be considered as the field develops its evidence base:[16]

➤ health promotion needs to clarify what it means by the effectiveness of its interventions and to judge effectiveness not only on short-term impacts
➤ evidence of effectiveness will only come from interventions that have a reasonable chance of success
➤ contemporary health promotion now has an understanding of what constitutes good practice to select suitable interventions, and practitioners need to use this developing knowledge to design appropriate services.

Finally, when evaluating health promotion interventions, the research methodology must be directed by the intervention, focusing on what is the most relevant and appropriate approach to evaluate the intervention.

To some degree the evidence for the impact of health promotion and public health activities has become more mainstream, as both the National Institute for Health and Clinical Excellence (NICE) and the Cochrane Collaboration have public health work streams.

DOES HEALTH PROMOTION WORK?

This is ostensibly a reasonable and worthy question, and one that is also proffered to medical educators about a type of teaching, the presentation of new material or a complete restructure of curricula. Yet the question as it stands is often meaningless, relying on some objective and definitive answer which is clearly not appropriate. More pertinent questions to explore may be:

➤ Is health promotion a worthwhile endeavour?
➤ Is it rational and morally sound?
➤ How well developed are the arguments and evidence to support intervention?

Additionally, questions about the underpinning theoretical principles and frameworks, whether practitioners have skills and resources to implement health promotion activities, whether there has been sufficient input and time to produce intended outcomes, and what variables have been at play, should also be part of the exploration. There is a pragmatic need to move towards a more secure and accepted health promotion evidence base, which accommodates such questions.[18]

The value of public health interventions in addressing lifestyle issues related to preventing chronic diseases has begun to be recognised. The General Medical Council's *Tomorrow's Doctors* has highlighted the need for public health and health promotion in undergraduate medical school curricula.[19,20] Likewise the Department of Health White Paper, *Choosing Better Health*, has emphasised the value of public health and health promotion.[21] Wanless, in his review of the resources needed to provide a future high-quality National Health Service (NHS), illustrated the impact of reducing health service demand through individuals' engagement with their own health. His analysis for the review suggested that low levels of the public's engagement with its own health would result in future high, possibly unsustainable, costs associated with delivering high-quality health service outcomes.[22] More recently Darzi argues that the NHS workforce needs to have the skills and competence as well as the knowledge base to be health promoters within the context of their work.[23]

For medical and healthcare professionals, much of their role with regard to health promotion will be linked to disease-related issues and either the prevention of diseases or the approach to managing and improving the patient's situation. The evidence to support health promotion from this perspective is now considerable and is frequently presented in medical journals, whether focused on individual behaviour changes or community and policy change. There is, for example, a large and growing evidence base pointing to the possibility of preventing new cardiovascular disease (CVD) events in subjects who have already experienced an event using specific pharmacological tools and by multifactorial prevention using drugs and advice to stop smoking.[24,25] More recently there is encouraging evidence about the effectiveness of approaches to managing and reducing risk factors for newly diagnosed type 2 diabetes patients.[26] It has been more difficult to detect a preventive effect of interventions directed towards populations.

There have been many community-based CVD programmes based on a community public health educational model that use social marketing techniques and community activation to change health-related behaviours in populations. The rationale behind the community health education model is that most risk is due to modest elevations in risk factors in large numbers of people rather than the extreme elevations of a few.[27] Large-scale projects to test this model on CVD began in the early 1970s with the North Karelia project in Finland and in three cities near Stanford in California. Ten-year results from the North Karelia project showed significant reductions in coronary heart disease in middle-aged men as well as reductions in smoking, hypertension and serum cholesterol levels. Early results from the Stanford study showed beneficial effects on smoking, hypertension, lipid levels and saturated fat intake.[28]

Despite the success of the Stanford and North Karelia models, strategies to cost-effectively change the behaviour of entire communities remain underdeveloped. The cost and complexity of these programmes have made them difficult to reproduce. Communities are complex entities, governed by formal and informal networks, institutions and members. The community structures both maintain and change norms by influencing the amount and type of information and services that are available to its members. Community studies emphasise the complexity of the communities because to elicit change the study must work within the formal and informal structures.

Population-level change often requires more time than is funded, with the premise being that a small immediate change can lead to bigger impacts over time. Lasting and widespread change requires alterations in the communities' 'rules for living'[29] so that new behaviours are incorporated into society. To do this often requires more time than initial interventions are funded for. North Karelia, for example, did not see changes in smoking behaviour until 10 years after the project was initiated, while the American Community Intervention Trial for Smoking Cessation (COMMIT) did not see results in smoking cessation until three years after the communities were randomised.[29] Little research has been conducted on what happens in large community projects once external funding has been withdrawn. So, these interventions rarely have quick gains and are not a quick fix for a community health issue. The 1% or less campaign focused successfully on changing only one aspect of a community's lifestyle, which may arguably be a more cost-effective approach. Consumer research has shown that many consumers feel overwhelmed by the multitude of nutritional messages they are exposed to. The 1% or less programme reasoned that a focused message might be more effective, requiring only one behaviour change at a time.

These large-scale community studies have produced evidence not just about what works in health promotion but also about how best to implement such complex projects, for example the Heartbeat Wales project.[30] More recently Davies, *et al.*[26] have presented their effectiveness evidence from 13 different geographical locations with regard to health behaviour improvements such as weight loss, smoking cessation and health beliefs.

One of the key messages from these studies is the importance of developing *strategic communications*. The media are often key institutions and modes of mass communication in community studies. Some methods of communication of public health information only reach certain populations. The Stanford Five-City Project found it difficult to engage the local media in one of the intervention sites and as a result developed multiple channels of communication that did not exaggerate the knowledge behaviour gap in certain subpopulations. Maintaining the intervention for a long period is essential, given the Stanford Five-City Project, in its six years, exposed the population to a fraction of the amount of information messages they receive from normal television viewing but worked because the messages were targeted and sustained over a long period of time.[28] The North Karelia Project found that changing lifestyles in the population is a slow and not always continuous process. They noted that changes were found to take place in stages, with plateaus in between, and new ideas for interventions were, as a result, constantly needed.[29] The *credibility of staff* and their training to deliver intervention, their medical status and their ability to work in non-medical settings were vital to programme impact.

The *context* in which the intervention takes place is incredibly important to consider when designing a community intervention. Context-level factors, which may affect intervention uptake, success and sustainability, are 'the density of interorganisational ties within which the intervention must take place, the agencies delivering the intervention, and the amount of resources contributed by the participating agencies'.[31] Although there are many checklists in common use to assess quality of evidence for a public health and health promotion intervention, few include details on how the differential effect of context can be taken into account. Public health efforts to reduce the incidence of CVD by modifying risk factors in large population groups are likely to be more effective if they are based on knowledge of the relationship between those risk factors and basic social factors such as social class and ethnicity. The Stanford study was 'carefully designed' to reach Spanish speakers and lower social class groups by factoring in how they sourced and interpreted information, hence preparing messages that both suited those media habits and were also culturally appropriate. Over the three years of the programme, all groups reported 20–40% decreases in dietary cholesterol and saturated fat. These decreases were as large in lower social class groups as in higher social class groups. Spanish-speaking groups reported significantly greater decreases in dietary saturated fats, and changes in cholesterol were marginally more favourable in Spanish-speaking groups. Had the project not taken into account the different ways the various targeted groups received and interpreted their messages it might well have failed.

Engaging with and retaining the services of local community influencers has also been found to be an important factor in the success of community-level programmes. Public health policies are the products of negotiation and compromise, often between competing political, commercial, professional and community stakeholders.[32] As such, public policies will reflect the values of those with the most influence in a community. The process of approaching community leaders can influence the whole intervention process. Time must be invested in creating relationships with community leaders and the community itself prior to intervention.

Earlier in this chapter, the problems associated with evaluating health promotion activity were briefly discussed. Large-scale studies have produced a long and significant literature which discusses the *methodological limitations* of evaluating community interventions. Insignificant or modest results in trials can be the result of poorly designed or implemented evaluations. Public health interventions tend to be complex, programmatic and context-dependent. Evidence thus must be sufficiently wide-ranging to encompass this complexity. Importantly, evaluation approaches and evidence must be capable of determining whether an intervention is not just theoretically and conceptually valid (impact evaluation) but also whether it can be delivered (process evaluation).[32] Clinical risks will occur much less frequently in normal populations than in high-risk groups, necessitating much larger study groups to achieve a sufficient statistical power explaining to some degree why community studies have not always demonstrated positive results.[33]

Evaluation of programmes in whole communities requires special considerations and approaches.[34] Programmes administered on a large scale cannot be as tightly organised as programmes administered to a small group. The fact that multiple-component programmes addressing a single health promotional issue are occurring simultaneously makes it difficult to assess the effects of one component of the programme. As participants are located throughout a community they may be difficult to identify, making evaluation data collection unwieldy, complex and expensive. In addition most projects do not occur in a vacuum, making it difficult to disentangle the program under consideration from other programs or indeed from the real-life context that people live in. Pirie identified a typology of evaluation issues for community programmes identifying eight elements of evaluation:[34]

➤ formative evaluation: includes studies evaluating programmes and messages in the development stages for appropriateness, comprehensibility and ability to capture audience interest but also pilot testing prior to their large-scale implementation and diagnostic studies of audience characteristics and informational needs.
➤ quality assurance: includes monitoring of programme delivery and participant satisfaction with programmes.
➤ assessment of delivered dose of intervention: assessment of the number of programmes or messages delivered by the intervention programme to the community – implementation monitoring, essential before outcomes can be evaluated.
➤ assessment of received doses of intervention: number of programmes or messages actually received by the communities, including the number of programmes or messages coming from sources other than the intervention programme and the number of such messages/programmes received by comparison communities.
➤ component programme impact: outcome studies of specific component programmes.
➤ intermediate outcomes: assessment of variables considered intermediate, between programme participation and risk factor change – such as knowledge attitudes and trial behaviours; their specification depends heavily on the investigators' model of how the programme is thought to achieve its success – also useful to demonstrate change in the time lag between intervention rollout and outcome.
➤ community impact: includes assessment of impacts above the level of the individual, such as impacts on organisational units and on leadership and provider groups.
➤ costs analysis: both for component programmes and the overall community programmes.

Few studies outside those that are wholly managed by health promotion specialists and reported in health promotion journals will be able to address all the elements for evaluation. Hawe provides a fuller, more comprehensive coverage of health promotion evaluation, beyond the scope of this chapter's discussion.[35]

This section started with the question 'Does health promotion work?' and undoubtedly there are successes but there are also barriers to success, which highlight slightly different challenges. Although health promotion is eclectic, the approaches to behaviour change in the clinical one-to-one setting are predominately based on theory and evidence from psychology paradigms, yet persuading professionals to use these approaches has remained challenging.[38] This may, in part, be an inability by health promotion specialists to relate the evidence base and a lack of awareness amongst clinicians as to how to interpret it.[37–39]

Conversely, those who are willing to accept the evidence but have applied it with disappointing results may also be making unreasonable claims. Tappin, *et al.*, for example, in a trial of smoking cessation techniques for midwives, found that pregnant women who were smokers did not change their behaviour after intervention.[40] Yet these women were not assessed for their motivation to change, and little or no attempt was made to improve their social circumstances, factors which are known to be an integral aspect of working with modifiable determinants in this context.

Whilst behavioural change models have value, they need to be applied with attention to the other complex and confounding factors that influence behaviour and as Graham reported, smoking for women living in disadvantage has probable multiple roles in their daily lives.[41,42]

How engaged and accepting medical and other health professional practitioners are of health promotion evidence will be a factor in what could be included in curriculum content and taught in clinical settings.

SUMMARY

Defining health promotion is a continuing challenge, especially for those with curriculum development responsibilities. However, a working definition, 'the study of, and the study of the response to, the modifiable determinants of health' offers educationalists a way of approaching curriculum content and the various evidence sources required to support this eclectic and divers discipline.

Developing the research evidence associated with intervention effectiveness will continue to be a challenge in this discipline. McQueen advises taking a broad vision of evidence that acknowledges the complexity of the field and its projects. It is a challenge for health promotion to convince its enthusiasts and detractors that there are no easy answers to complex human phenomena. What is clear from the existing evidence base is that what is regarded as 'gold standard' in the scientific disciplines will not always apply in the complex environment of community intervention and individual behaviour change. This link between defining a discipline and demonstrating its research evidence base is crucial for credibility and hence integration with high-stakes curricula.

REFERENCES

1 Ewles L, Simnett I. *Promoting Health: a practical guide.* 5th ed. London: Bailliere Tindall; 2003.
2 Wylie A. *Health Promotion and Medical Education: an exploration of the epistemology and the challenge.* London: King's College; 2003.
3 Seedhouse D. *Health Promotion: philosophy, prejudice and practice.* Chichester: Wiley; 1997.
4 Wylie A. Health promotion in general practice. In: Stephenson A, editor. *A Textbook of General Practice.* 2nd ed. London: Arnold; 2004.

5 International Union for Health Promotion and Education. *The Evidence of Health Promotion Effectiveness: sharing public health in a new Europe.* Parts I and II. Brussels: IUHPE; 1999.

6 Tones K. The empowerment imperative. In: Scriven A, Orme J, editors. *Health Promotion: professional perspectives.* Basingstoke: Palgrave; 2001. pp. 3–18.

7 World Health Organization. *Ottawa Charter for Health Promotion.* Geneva: World Health Organization; 1986.

8 World Health Organization. *Global Conferences on Health Promotion.* Available at: www. who.int/healthpromotion/conferences/en/ (accessed 2 November 2009).

9 Tones K, Tilford S. *Health Promotion Effectiveness and Efficiency.* 2nd ed. London: Chapman and Hall; 1994.

10 French J. Boundaries and horizons: the role of health education within health promotion. *Health Educ J.* 1990; **49**(1): 7–10.

11 Nordenfelt L. On medicine and health enhancement – towards a conceptual framework. *Med Healthc Philos.* 1998; **1**: 5–12.

12 Ball SJ. Self-doubt and soft data: social and technical trajectories in ethnographic field work. *Int J Qual Stud Educ.* 1990; **3**(2): 157–71.

13 Learmonth A, Watson NJ. Constructing evidence-based health promotion: perspectives in the field. *Crit Publ Health.* 1999; **9**: 317–33.

14 Morgan A. Evaluation of health promotion. In: Davies M, editor. *Health Promotion Theory.* Berkshire: Open University; 2006.

15 Cochrane A. *Effectiveness and Efficiency: random reflections on health service.* London: Nuffield Provincial Hospital Trust; 1972.

16 Nutbeam D. The challenge to provide 'evidence' in health promotion. *Health Promot Int.* 1999; **14**: 99–101.

17 McQueen D. Perspectives on health promotion: theory, evidence, practice and the emergence of complexity. *Health Promot Int.* 2000; **15**(2): 95–7.

18 Green J, Tones K. Towards a secure evidence base for health promotion. *J Publ Health Med.* 1999; **21**(2): 133–9.

19 General Medical Council. *Tomorrow's Doctors.* London: General Medical Council; 1993.

20 General Medical Council. *Tomorrow's Doctors.* 2nd ed. London: General Medical Council; 2003.

21 Department of Health. *Choosing Health: making healthier choices easier.* [Public Health White Paper]. London: Department of Health; 2004.

22 Wanless D. *Securing Our Future Health: taking a long-term view: interim report.* London: HM Treasury; 2001.

23 Lord Darzi. *A High Quality Workforce: NHS next stage review.* London: Department of Health; 2008.

24 National Institution for Clinical Evidence. Statins for the prevention of Cardiovascular Disease: Technical Appraisal 94. London: NICE; 2006. http://guidance.nice.org.uk/TA94

25 Second Joint Task Force of European and Other Societies on Coronary Prevention. Prevention of coronary risk in clinical practice: summary of recommendations. *Eur Heart J.* 1998; **19**: 1503.

26 Davies MJ, Heller S, Skinner TC, *et al.* Effectiveness of the diabetes education and self management for ongoing and newly diagnosed (DESMOND) programme for people with newly diagnosed type 2 diabetes: cluster randomised controlled trial. *BMJ.* 2008; **336**(7642): 491–5. Epub 14 February 2008.

27 Rose G, Khaw K-T, Marmot M. *Rose's Strategy of Preventive Medicine.* Oxford: Oxford University Press; 2008.

28 Fortmann SP, Flora JA, Winkleby MA, *et al.* Community intervention trials: reflections on the Stanford five-city project experience. *Am J Epidemiol.* 1995; **142**(6): 576–86.

29 COMMIT Research Group. Community intervention trial for smoking cessation

(COMMIT): 1 Cohort results from a four-year community intervention. *Am J Publ Health*. 1995; **85**: 183–92.

30 Tudor-Smith C, Nutbeam D, Moore L, *et al*. Effects of the Heartbeat Wales programme over five years on behavioural risks for cardiovascular disease: quasi-experimental comparison of results from Wales and a matched reference area. *BMJ*. 1998; **316**(7134): 818–22.

31 Hawe P, Shiell A, Riley T, *et al*. Methods for exploring implementation variation and local context within a cluster randomised community intervention trial. *J Epidemiol Commun H*. 2004; **58**(9): 788–93.

32 Rychetnik L, Wise M. Advocating evidence-based health promotion: reflections and a way forward. *Health Promot Int*. 2004; **19**(2): 247–57.

33 Thomson H, Hoskins R, Petticrew M, *et al*. Evaluating the health effects of social interventions. *BMJ*. 2004; **328**(7434): 282–5.

34 Pirie PL, Stone EJ, Assaf AR, *et al*. Program evaluation strategies for community-based health promotion programs: perspectives from the cardiovascular disease community research and demonstration studies. *Health Educ Res*. 1994; **9**(1): 23–36.

35 Hawe P. Evaluation. In: Moodie R, Hulme A, editors. *Hands-on Health Promotion*. Melbourne: IP Communications; 2004. pp. 16–28.

36 Marteau T, Dieppe P, Foy R, Kinmonth AL, Schneiderman N. Behavioural medicine: changing our behaviour. *BMJ*. 2006; **332**(7539): 437–8.

37 Kerr S, Watson H, Tolson D, *et al*. An exploration of the knowledge, attitudes and practice of members of the primary care team in relation to smoking and smoking cessation in later life. *Prim Health Care Res Dev*. 2007; **8**(1): 68–79.

38 Vogt F, Hall S, Marteau TM. General practitioners' and family physicians' negative beliefs and attitudes towards discussing smoking cessation with patients: a systematic review. *Addiction*. 2005; **100**(10): 1423–31.

39 Vogt F, Hall S, Marteau T. General practitioners' beliefs about effectiveness and intentions to recommend smoking cessation services: qualitative and quantitative studies. *BMC Fam Pract*. 2007; **8**(1): 39.

40 Tappin DM, Lumsden MA, Gilmour WH, *et al*. Randomised controlled trial of home-based motivational interviewing by midwives to help pregnant smokers quit or cut down. *BMJ*. 2005; **331**(7513): 373–7.

41 Graham H. Women and smoking in the United Kingdom: implications for health promotion. *Health Promot Int*. 1988; **3**(4): 371–82.

42 Graham H. *Hardship and Health in Women's Lives*. London: Wheatsheaf; 1993.

CHAPTER 3

Medical students learning a population perspective: a review of the resistance and experiences

Gillian Maudsley

BACKGROUND TO THE CHALLENGE

The challenge to ensure that medical students synthesise basic, behavioural, clinical and population health science in their clinical practice is longstanding, as Simon lamented in the 1960s.[1] In referring to a standard definition of public health – *'the science and art of preventing disease, prolonging life and promoting health through the organised efforts of society'* – the overlap with health promotion is evident.[2] Both require a systematic and creative approach to embedding the principles in the curriculum for medical students, who might otherwise undervalue their relevance.[3] Schön considered that the problems causing most human concern do not inhabit his 'technical rationality' high ground, but wallow down in his swampy ground, which seems a likely location for most population health concerns.[4] Schön raised the 'rigour versus relevance' issue, which also bedevils public health education for medical students:

> Public health doctors are probable inhabitants of Schön's 'swampy lowlands', be-
> cause population-relevant problems potentially challenge conventional notions of
> science.[5]

The 'it is all common sense' perception (despite one person's common sense being another person's downfall) is another likely challenge, which might lead to students' poor attendance at non-compulsory sessions.[6] Furthermore, a tendency for their social responsiveness to wane somewhat over their time at medical school is disturbing.[7]

This chapter explores the literature about facilitating medical students' population perspective learning to enhance their clinical practice and impact – challenges (including measurement tools) and possibilities. The literature search took a systematic approach[8,9] focused mostly on Web of Science (supplemented by Medline and manual searching of several core journals), with key terms approximating to 'medical student/school/undergraduate' *plus* 'public (population) health (perspective)' *plus* perception/conception/attitude/outcome (*see* Box 3.1).

BOX 3.1 Literature search strategy: What is known about medical students' population health learning?

Searched (English Language titles, all documents):
- free-text in Web of Science (Science Citation Index Expanded, 1945–; Social Sciences Citation Index, 1956–; Arts and Humanities Citation Index, 1975–), advanced search in topic field (of title, abstract, keyword lists), to September 2008, with supplementary searches
- Medline (advanced search of subject headings and keywords of title and abstract, appropriate), 1966- to September 2008
  — combining search terms:

  ~ ~ ~medical school*/student*/curricul*/education ~ ~ ~ *or* ~ ~ ~undergraduate medical ~ ~ ~ *and*
  ~ ~ ~population health/perspective ~ ~ ~ *or* ~ ~ ~public health/epidemiology ~ ~ ~ *and*
  ~ ~ ~perception*/conception*/attitud*/outcome*/performance/risk factor*/predict*/determinant* ~ ~ ~

  *=`wildcard' character(s)

  — checked (+/-abstracts) for articles reviewing theory or practice, or providing empirical data

Included:
- ad hoc `finds', personal collection, and January 2004–October 2008 `handsearching' of *Medical Education, Medical Teacher, Advances in Health Sciences Education*, and *Academic Medicine* journals plus *Journal of Public Health, Journal of Epidemiology & Community Health*, and *International Journal of Epidemiology*

THE CHALLENGE TO MAKE THIS LEARNING RELEVANT

Around the world, there have been various attempts to match population health-care needs with the type of doctor graduating,[10] and the soul-searching continues.[11] Honouring this medical school `social contract' (or `social accountability')[12] should see curricula being more community-orientated[13-15] and focused on common and important clinical presentations, while incorporating more awareness raising about health policy and health systems.[16] Students should gain sufficient experience with generalists in both the community and hospital settings.[17]

Various countries have reviewed *what* medical students should learn about population health[15,18-22] with clinical epidemiology predominating,[23] but an underpinning philosophy would help with *how* to do this, including extensive integration, not tokenism and segregation.[24,25] By the 1980s, the Edinburgh Declaration was still required. This international consensus statement focused medical education on supplying lifelong-learning, health-promoting doctors.[26-28] The response to the General Medical Council's (GMC) *Tomorrow's Doctors*[29,30] recommendation about promoting public health medicine as an integrated theme was patchy,[24,31-34] despite examples such as community stakeholder involvement,[35] and political and subject integration at whole-programme level.[24] Indeed, integration is crucial for demonstrating relevance, enhancing clinical practice,[36] and giving a holistic view of health problems:

> There is an old story in Indian folklore about how five blind men perceived the trunk, body, legs, tail and ears of an animal as a snake, wall, tree, rope and dustpan, respectively. If they had only been told in the first instance that it was an elephant they were trying to decipher, they would have appreciated the magnificent animal better. Likewise, the holistic presentation of the subjects in the curriculum as the discipline of medicine perceived from various angles may help to raise the quality of the practice of medical science.[37]

Simon considered preventive medicine and public health to resemble students' original beliefs about medicine, before they become disillusioned – such courses thus require 'much more imagination, study, planning and experimentation'[1] and a better image from staff to engage students. Indeed, given their historical tensions with clinical medicine,[38] and the potential to marginalise medical student-related issues,[39] the approach of public health professionals is also crucial. Better awareness and use of education theory and evidence would also help meet the challenge.

Medical students'[40,41] and doctors' aversion to population health learning (including specific obstacles such as 'numerophobia'[42] and innumeracy)[43] has been reported continually in recent decades. A recurrent lament is how to tackle students' indifference:[44–47]

> As teachers of preventive medicine, all of us have observed the Medical Student Myopia Syndrome (MSMS), but we have not always diagnosed or successfully treated this plague . . . MSMS is usually manifested by medical school classes in epidemiology and preventive medicine full of empty chairs . . . The epidemiology of MSMS is classically described by its own unique person, place, and time. MSMS is . . . transmitted by word-of-mouth. Words such as 'this is going to be boring' and 'I'll never use this stuff' are vectors for transmission of this intellectually crippling condition . . . [It is] found at every medical school throughout the world . . . its one pathognomonic sign – a student reading the newspaper in the middle of class . . . In terms of treatment, only one [is effective] . . . RICE therapy (relevant, innovative, clinical with exacting expectations).[44]

Determinants might include medical school selection,[48] students' apathy about self-orientated preventive medicine,[49] or students' antagonism, or tendency to be judgemental, when managing patients' risk-taking behaviours (such as substance misuse).[50] Furthermore, despite noble intentions, over-intense didactic courses disjointed from clinical practice can be counterproductive, for example, medical students' readiness to specialise in preventive/social medicine declined statistically significantly and substantially with a 'new' 294-hour course.[46] Negative role-modelling is also possible.[51] Attitudes to related behavioural science aspects, for example, might parallel this, such that staff mindsets[52] might shift the informal curriculum against this learning. Integration of a psycho-sociological perspective becomes a major challenge,[53,54] compounding problems with public health education. There is also a tendency for students to lose some of their sense of social responsiveness as they progress through the curriculum.[55]

North American literature tends to focus medical students' public health education on 'preventive medicine', that is, a more individually orientated approach (such that international health experience[56] gains importance for awareness raising,[57] as does project work,[58,59] for example, a community-orientated project to highlight community, service and advocacy).[60] In a 1998 survey about 'professional development' in 125 US medical schools, only 41% of 116 responses agreed that the curriculum did 'respond to societal needs and reflect a social contract with the communities served'.[61] Woolliscroft, *et al.*'s three-year follow-up of Michigan's 1984 entry cohort of medical students (n=73) found significant differences in how they incorporated preventive medicine into their clinical write-ups.[62] Students in Year 2 highlighted more such issues than in Years 1 and 3, and the former struggled most to translate risk factors into their problem/action list. In a randomised trial to increase Year 3 awareness, the group receiving the intervention (of using history-taking forms with subheadings as cues) improved significantly, and this effect persisted for those also receiving specific written feedback.

Focusing on evidence-based medicine (or clinical epidemiology)[63] can limit the population health horizon. Arguably,[64] it is easier to 'measure' though,[65] and it helps to demonstrate relevance, as critical appraisal (underpinned by clinical epidemiology principles) is crucial for safe clinical practice. As Chessare noted:

> Rather than perpetuating the message to those in training that senior clinicians are the depository of all relevant information and that the goal is to learn as much as they 'know', educators of evidence-based medicine should attempt to show the learner how to find information efficiently and to judge its reliability and validity. It is a model of lifelong learning.[66]

Nevertheless, senior medical students may well be less adept at it than they think.[67]

In summary, quite a dirge pervades the literature about what students should learn (to assimilate a population dimension into their clinical practice), and more empirical evidence is needed to characterise how students conceptualise and approach such requirements.

WAYS OF MEASURING AWARENESS AND ATTITUDES ABOUT POPULATION HEALTH ISSUES

Given how countries and curricula conceptualise core public health education differently, the transferability of some topic-specific measurement tools might be slightly limited.

The 63-item (in seven scales for Likert-type scoring) Attitudes to Social Issues in Medicine (ATSIM) questionnaire is one way of exploring students' awareness and attitudes about population health issues, but psychosocial and professional/personal development items overshadow population perspective items, and might not transfer so well to UK curricula.[68,69] Items include: 'I believe that at least half of all patients in general hospitals have health problems related to social factors', and 'I believe that our present method of training medical students does not take into account the frequently social nature of illness in contemporary North American Society'.

Parlow and Rothman had 750 Toronto healthcare profession students (denoting an 83% response) answer the ATSIM (with only absentees as non-responders):

> From social work, nursing (including postgraduate), medical, dental, and pharmacy students, social work and nursing scored significantly more on human relations (two

scales) and social issues (five scales) than medical students, with self-selection and admissions processes being probable explanations.[70]

The researchers noted that dental students answered similarly to medical students on all seven scales, which reminded Parlow and Rothman of Rosenberg's findings of similar personality results at entry in the two groups:[71]

> Before entering San Francisco Bay medical and dental schools, 47 male dental students and 34 male medical students (of unspecified sampling method or denominator) completed the California Personality Inventory. Over four years, Rosenberg found medical students to change on more scales than dental students, who retained a more stable profile of conformity and conventionality. Rosenberg apparently expected more personality change after four years of dental education: 'One could cite the atmosphere of indifference that surrounds most dental schools.'[71]

If taking a population perspective, like ethics, is considered a core element of medical professionalism,[72] Price, *et al.*'s study of Queensland medical students' moral dilemmas showed another way of measuring relevant attitudes. They deduced that in '1-from-4' responses to such dilemmas in 25 scenarios, Year 1 valued 'Doctors have an obligation to society which can override their duty to the patient (and to each other)' tenth highest (in a list of 23 ethical statements to which the responses mapped).[73] Year 5 and Year 6 valued this only 19th and 21st, respectively (the latter only valuing it above not 'punishing' patients and being obliged to use resources properly). Year 5 students invoked this statement (positively) significantly less than Year 1 students (6.6% versus 25.3% of possible score, respectively), but a caveat was that fewer than three of the '25×4' possible responses mapped to that statement.

Novick, *et al.* claimed a first when reporting measurement of willingness to use population-based prevention in managing clinical scenarios.[74] Their questionnaire had responders splitting 100 points between five alternatives (covering treatment, clinical prevention and population prevention) for each of nine scenarios. Piloted on public health directors (with 13/15 responding) plus family medicine doctors from Syracuse and Baltimore (n=18 and n=23, respectively, of undetermined sampling frames), only a heart disease scenario discriminated significantly between them on the population prevention, treatment, *and* population–treatment differential measures. Studying 145 medical students found significantly larger values for the population prevention scale and the population–treatment differential after a Year 2 epidemiology course. (Details of response, questionnaire distribution, the course, etc. were undisclosed.) Measuring orientation to population-based prevention like this was tricky, given that only one scenario (about maternal and child health) showed significant differences on the population scale and population–treatment differential between public health directors and one of the family medicine groups, and for medical students before and after their epidemiology course.

In summary, while there are a few instruments for measuring some elements of public health learning, a challenge is to address context specificity if evidence is to be more generalisable.

EXAMPLES FROM EDUCATIONAL EVIDENCE AND THEORY ABOUT MAKING PUBLIC HEALTH EDUCATION RELEVANT

The illustrations from education evidence and theory relate mostly to students' attitudes to their public health education, specifically about its relevance. The tendency to focus on how evidence-based medicine promotes the relevance of critical appraisal skills based on epidemiological principles is understandable.

Interest in population health matters varies by specialty. Very few medical students will see public health medicine as a likely career, with only 0.3–0.4% of UK graduates[75] citing it as first choice, and their public health tutors' skills and interests may well not appeal to them:

> The community medicine faculty members who are found in the medical school often focus on such topics as population dynamics or economics – not attractive role models for would-be healers.[76]

Although omitting the specific figures, Phillips, *et al.* reported that general surgeons scored preventive medicine significantly less relevant than did family practitioners.[77] From a random sample of 200 Kentucky doctors, 54% responded to this questionnaire survey ranking the relevance of 23 preventive medicine topics to their practice, including topics as broad as 'epidemiology'. While the doctors' age, sex or practice location did not affect the mean 'preventive' score across all topics, unsurprisingly, they ranked highest the 'diseases' or 'risk factors' (such as tobacco, cancer, diabetes, nutrition, 'coronary heart disease' and alcohol).[78] Lowest were family planning, infant health, epidemiology and oral health:

> Epidemiology and disease reporting are not felt to be as relevant by the practicing [sic] physician and perhaps might best be presented as 'how to read the medical literature' by those trying to educate future or current practitioners.[78]

In their cross-sectional study of Years 1, 2 and 3 Kentucky medical students (1990/91), Phillips, *et al.* found the mean preventive medicine score to increase successively and significantly (but did not report the scores). They used an anonymous 'in-class' 35-item questionnaire for 212 students to score agreement with preventive medicine statements about lung disease (on 5-point Likert scales).[78] For that academic year compared with the previous, the mean preventive score increased significantly in a cohort followed longitudinally (n=157; but year-group and denominator were unclear). Of Year 2 students asked to provide an identifying number, 24 responded both before and after their preventive medicine course and showed a significant increase in mean preventive score (but denominator, time between administrations and absolute or differential scores were undisclosed). They also surveyed 2544 medical students from 12 institutions about careers ('Planned specialty [one only]: medicine, surgery, paediatrics, family medicine, ob/gyn, neurology, other [specify], uncertain'), but did not report the response rate. Overall, mean preventive score differed significantly between career intentions. Those with surgery or obstetrics/gynaecology career intentions were most negative about preventive medicine compared with six other career groups.

Research about how students learn public health concepts are rare. Hmelo-Silver, *et al.* investigated how Year 4 medical students, 'novices', learnt about one aspect of critical appraisal skill, namely study design.[79] The study simulated a complex task, that is, designing a randomised controlled trial of a new drug. Compared with a group of cancer experts (n=4), novices (six groups, n=24) used a different approach but reached a similar result. Significant findings were that, while the students ran fewer 'tests', they changed more variables simultaneously, planned much less from theory (rather than using recent data), and evaluated their progress in this complex task less.

Imperato, *et al.* contributed evidence about how assessment drives learning, using population health concepts as the example.[80] Between 1978 and 1985, Year 2 New York State medical students evaluated a 'preventive medicine and community health' course five times (with good–excellent response rates of 60–94%). In 1979, despite its not being the faculty intention to make the mid-term examination difficult, students perceived it so. Akin to the negative halo effect ('horns effect'), their negativity pervaded their rating of many other aspects of the course that had previously been received positively. In 1983, problematic examinations increased students' projected negativity again by exploring required readings that lectures did not cover.

Other evidence about the effect of assessment (and again probably not specific to public health education) came from the epidemiology examination performance of Year 3 Birmingham medical students in 1985 (n=152).[81] Multiple regression showed females and students who sat their *clinical* examination the week previously rather than the same week to perform better. If their *clinical* examination at *that* time was surgery (not medicine), students apparently scored higher (but not significantly so) on epidemiology, suggesting that students probably valued medicine more and allowed more time for studying epidemiology when not preparing for that. For a female sitting the clinical examination in surgery the week before the epidemiology examination, Marshall estimated a 9% points higher mark on epidemiology than a male sitting the clinical examination in medicine in the same week as epidemiology. The closeness to other examinations affecting performance would presumably have been irrelevant if students took the same examinations simultaneously, but the females' better performance prompted the researcher to suggest that maybe females still had to outperform males to gain medical school entry, such that an educational advantage in epidemiological performance resulted.

While selection into medical school might inadvertently contribute to a more negative outlook for a population perspective on health, Ewan's work with Year 1 New South Wales medical students at entry did not support this.[82] She explored the notion that academic high achievement would mean low awareness and sensitivity to social issues. Using the ATSIM scale to compare medical students (n=121, denoting a 72% response) with entrants to other faculties with similar and lower achievement (three random samples of 100, 55–63% response rates) showed that, while they were similarly or more concerned than the other students on attitudes that did not challenge the doctor's knowledge, role or status, these attitudes related to prevention and doctor-patient relationships. At follow-up, consistent with evidence from elsewhere, Final year medical students were significantly less likely to acknowledge social determinants of disease than at entry.[83]

Reports about population perspective issues in problem-based curricula are few, despite the potential for a problem-based system to help integrate population health issues into relevant clinical context. Reports from North American curricula tend to focus more on problem-based learning (PBL) as a way of integrating basic science, not population science (or behavioural science), in an individual clinical context. Examples tend to be from undergraduate subject-based courses[84–86] or postgraduate programmes[87] that are solely for public health and/or epidemiology. Nevertheless, three examples illustrate the potential and challenges.

➤ In Newcastle's (New South Wales) problem-based curriculum, Rolfe, *et al.* used their Attitudes to Community Medicine (ATCM) questionnaire with entrants and found significantly more positive attitudes compared with Adelaide entrants (in a conventional curriculum). Newcastle final-year students retained these attitudes,[48] consistent with that curriculum having had *Population Medicine* as one of its five curriculum domains.[88] Nevertheless, the effect might not persist into preregistration house officer work though, if hectic 'internships' and assessments ignore the population perspective[88] and fritter the gains made at undergraduate level.

➤ Régo and Dick found that despite the Queensland problem-based curriculum having *Population and Preventive Health* as one of its four curriculum domains, 48.1% and 53.4% of mid-Year 2 medical students attributed knowledge and application of public health and of health promotion principles, respectively, to common sense.[89] As only 41.3% students perceived faculty to be positive about population and psychosocial matters, this suggested an 'informal curriculum' predictably undermining public health education somewhat.[89] Negative role modelling would probably reinforce students' views that time would be better spent learning to practise acute medical care safely.[89] Indeed, in 1999 and 2000, 47.9% and 60.4% of students considered that PBL tutors were not good role models for the public health domain. Of Queensland students, 42.5% were unclear how they could practise population health on graduation,[89] and only 70.0% felt that they grasped this domain.

➤ In an open item in a postal questionnaire survey (71% and 78% response rate from 279 and 204, respectively), both end-Year 1 and mid-Year 3 Liverpool medical students described the vocational utility of learning a population perspective in generally positive ways. They highlighted particularly that it would help them critically appraise evidence, give 'big picture' context for individual consultations, and give specific detail about proportions, causes and severity of diseases.[90] This was in a problem-based curriculum with *Population Perspective* as one of its four core curriculum themes.

In summary, the research about how medical students learn a population health perspective is rather lightweight. (Crucial aspects of study design or implementation are omitted from many such research reports.) Examples where public health education is integrated comprehensively throughout problem-based curricula are scarce, but illuminating.

POSSIBILITIES FOR IMPROVING PUBLIC HEALTH EDUCATION FOR MEDICAL STUDENTS

Despite recurring worldwide pleas to match medical education to public health needs and produce health-promoting doctors, the dynamics of medical students' public health education remain rather peripheral in the literature (particularly in public health journals), without much empirical study. The systems approach in problem-based curricula[91] (in which students generate diverse learning objectives across conventional subject boundaries, and learn in the simulated 'messy' context of clinical scenarios) has much potential for helping students learn to apply a population perspective to their clinical practice.

From reviewing the literature, it is noted that:

➤ more robust educational evidence and theory should inform public health education for medical students, addressing the tendency for their potentially low interest in this domain to wane further, and countering the tendency for public health educators to be distant from mainstream (medical) educationalists.

➤ more effort is needed to focus educational research on issues specific to public health education, while assimilating educational research and theory that apply as much to learning about public health as they do to other domains.

➤ more robust approaches to reporting original research about public health education are needed, let alone more interest from public health journals and public health professionals, generally.

➤ medical students should be able to grasp the relevance of a population perspective to their clinical practice, have various learning opportunities to deliberate about and use it, and encounter positive role-modelling from faculty.

REFERENCES

1 Simon HJ. The medical student: what he wants and needs versus what he gets. *J Med Educ.* 1967; **42**(8): 775–80.

2 Committee of Inquiry into the Future of Public Health Function. *Public Health in England.* London: The Stationery Office; 1988.

3 Wylie A, Thompson S. Establishing health promotion in the modern medical curriculum: a case study. *Med Teach.* 2007; **29**(8): 766–71.

4 Schon DA. From technical rationality to reflection-in-action. In: Dowie J, Elstein A, editors. *Professional Judgement: a reader in clinical decision making.* Cambridge: Cambridge University Press; 1988. pp. 60–77.

5 Maudsley G, Strivens J. 'Science', 'critical thinking' and 'competence'. *Med Educ.* 2000; **34**(1): 53–60.

6 Mattick K, Dennis I, Bligh J. Approaches to learning and studying in medical students: validation of a revised inventory and its relation to student characteristics and performance. *Med Educ.* 2004; **38**(5): 535–43.

7 Littlewood S, Ypinazar V, Margolis SA, *et al.* Early practical experience and the social responsiveness of clinical education: systematic review. *BMJ.* 2005; **331**: 387–91.

8 Haig A, Dozier M. Best Evidence Medical Education (BEME) Guide No 3: Systematic searching for evidence in medical education: Part 1, Sources of information. *Med Teach.* 2003; **25**(4): 352–63.

9 Haig A, Dozier M. Best Evidence Medical education (BEME) Guide No 3: Systematic searching for evidence in medical education: Part 2, Constructing searches. *Med Teach.* 2003; **25**(5): 463–84.

10 White KL, Connelly JE, editors. *The Medical School's Mission and the Population's Health.* New York: Springer Verlag; 1992.

11 Solyom AE. Viewpoint: Improving the health of the public requires changes in medical education. *Acad Med.* 2005; **80**(12): 1089–93.

12 Woollard RF. Caring for a common future: medical schools' social accountability. *Med Educ.* 2006; **40**(4): 301–13.

13 Wasylenki D, Byrne N, McRobb B. The social contract challenge in medical education. *Med Educ.* 1997; **31**(4): 250–8.

14 Stone DH. The Beer Sheva experiment and its lessons for community medicine. *Community Med.* 1988; **10**(3): 228–34.

15 Steering Committee on Social Responsibility of Medical Schools. *Social accountability: a vision for Canadian medical schools.* Ottawa: Health Canada; 2001.

16 Riegelman R. Health systems and health policy: a curriculum for all medical schools. *Acad Med.* 2006; **81**(4): 391–2.

17 Raik B, Fein O, Wachspress S. Measuring the use of the population perspective on internal medicine attending rounds. *Acad Med.* 1995; **70**(11): 1047–9.

18 Chappel D, Maudsley G, Bhopal RS, *et al. Public Health Education for Medical Students: a guide for medical schools.* Newcastle-upon-Tyne: University of Newcastle-upon-Tyne; 1996.

19 Gillam S, Maudsley G, editors. *Public Health Education for Medical Students: a guide for medical schools.* Rev. ed. Cambridge: Department of Public Health and Primary Care, University of Cambridge; 2008.

20 Maeshiro R. Responding to the challenge: population health education for physicians. *Acad Med.* 2008; **83**(4): 319–20.

21 Riegelman RK, Garr DR. Evidence-based public health education as preparation for medical school. *Acad Med.* 2008; **83**(4): 321–6.

22 Johnson I, Donovan D, Parboosingh J. Steps to improve the teaching of public health to undergraduate medical students in Canada. *Acad Med.* 2008; **83**(4): 414–8.

23 Jenicek M, Fletcher RH. Epidemiology for Canadian medical students: desirable attitudes, knowledge and skills. *Int J Epidemiol.* 1977; **6**(1): 69–72.

24 Maudsley G. Public health education for medical students: a problem-based curriculum and new opportunities. In: Tsouros AD, Dowding G, Thompson J, *et al.*, editors. *Health Promoting Universities: concept, experience and framework for action.* Copenhagen: World Health Organization; 1998. pp. 67–71.

25 Stone DH. Public health in the undergraduate curriculum: can we achieve integration? *J Eval Clin Pract.* 2000; **6**(1): 9–14.

26 World Federation for Medical Education. The Edinburgh Declaration. *Lancet.* 1988; **8068**: 464.

27 Warren K. World Conference on Medical Education, Edinburgh. *Lancet.* 1988; **8068**: 462.

28 Walton HJ, editor. Proceedings of the 1993 World Summit on Medical Education of the World Federation for Medical Education. *Med Educ.* 1994; **28**(Suppl 1).

29 General Medical Council. *Tomorrow's Doctors.* London: General Medical Council; 1993.

30 General Medical Council. *Tomorrow's Doctors.* 2nd ed. London: General Medical Council; 2003.

31 Edwards R, White M, Chappel D, *et al.* Teaching public health to medical students in the United Kingdom: are the General Medical Council's recommendations being implemented? *J Publ Health Med.* 1999; **21**(2): 150–7.

32 Bligh J. *Tomorrow's Doctors*: extending the role of public health medicine in medical education. *Med Educ.* 2002; **36**(3): 206–7.

33 Christopher DF, Harte K, George CF. The implementation of *Tomorrow's Doctors. Med Educ.* 2002; **36**(3): 282–8.

34 Gillam S, Bagade A. Undergraduate public health education in UK medical schools: struggling to deliver. *Med Educ.* 2006; **40**(5): 430–6.

35 Howe A, Billingham K, Walters C. Helping tomorrow's doctors to gain a population health perspective: good news for community stakeholders. *Med Educ.* 2002; **36**(4): 325–33.

36 Sawyer SM, Cooke R, Conn J, *et al.* Improving medical student performance in smoking health promotion: effect of vertically integrated curriculum. *Med Teach.* 2006; **28**(5): 135–8.

37 Hariprasad G. Holistic presentation of the undergraduate medical curriculum. *Med Educ.* 2008; **42**(8): 849.

38 Jefferys M, Lashof J. Preparation for public health practice: into the twenty-first century. In: Fee E, Acheson RM, editors. *A History of Education in Public Health: health that mocks the doctors' rules.* Oxford: Oxford University Press; 1991. pp. 314–35.

39 Woodward A. Public health has no place in undergraduate medical education. *J Publ Health Med.* 1994; **16**(4): 389–92.

40 Delnevo CD, Abatemarco DJ, Gotsch AR. Health behaviors and health promotion/disease prevention perceptions of medical students. *Am J Prev Med.* 1996; **12**(1): 38–43.

41 Moffat M, Sinclair HK, Cleland JA, *et al.* Epidemilogy teaching: student and tutor perceptions. *Med Teach.* 2004; **26**(8): 691–5.

42 Ben-Shlomo Y, Fallon U, Sterne J, *et al.* Do medical students with A-level mathematics have a better understanding of the principles behind evidence-based medicine? *Med Teach.* 2004; **26**(8): 731–3.

43 Windish DM, Huot SJ, Green ML. Medical residents' understanding of the biostatistics and results in medical literature. *JAMA.* 2007; **298**(9): 1010–22.

44 Riegelman RK. Medical student Myopia Syndrome: a recently recognized pan-epidemic. *Am J Prev Med.* 1991; **7**(4): 252.

45 McKillop JH, Oakley CA. The teaching of social medicine: an undergraduate view. *Proc Roy Soc Med.* 1971; **64**(12): 1302–4.

46 Radovanovic Z, Djordjevic-Gledovic Z. Attitudes of medical students in Belgrade, Yugoslavia, toward preventative medicine and epidemiology. *Soc Sci Med.* 1983; **17**(23): 1873–5.

47 Amos A, Forster F. Assessing personal process learning in a health promotion module for medical students. *Med Educ.* 1995; **29**(3): 211–15.

48 Rolfe IE, Pearson SA, Clearly EG, *et al.* Attitudes towards community medicine: a comparison of students from traditional and community-orientated medical schools. *Med Educ.* 1999; **33**(8): 606–11.

49 Lewis CE. Illness behavior and academic performance among medical students: implications for preventive medicine. *Arch Environ Health.* 1966; **12**(6): 776–80.

50 Landy J, Hynes J, Checinski K, *et al.* Knowledge of and attitudes to substance misuse in undergraduate British medical students. *Drugs-Educ Prev Polic.* 2005; **12**(2): 137–48.

51 Maudsley G. The limits of tutors' comfort zones with four integrated knowledge themes in a problem-based undergraduate medical curriculum. *Med Educ.* 2003; **37**(5): 417–23.

52 Gale J, Wakeford R. Medical students' perceptions of teachers' attitudes towards psychology and sociology. *Med Teach.* 1984; **6**(3): 97–100.

53 Litva A, Peters S. Exploring barriers to teaching behavioural and social sciences in medical education. *Med Educ.* 2008; **42**(3): 309–14.

54 Astin JA, Sierpina VS, Forys K, *et al.* Integration of the biopsychosocial model: perspectives of medical students and residents. *Acad Med.* 2008; **83**(1): 20–7.

55 Frank E, Modi S, Elon L, *et al.* US medical students' attitudes about patients' access to care. *Prev Med.* 2008; **47**(1): 140–5.

56 Gaaserud A, Jotkowitz A, Gidron Y, *et al.* Development and validation of a new measure of student attitudes and knowledge of international health and medicine. *Med Teach.* 2005; **27**(2): 136–9.

57 Ramsey AH, Haq C, Gjerde CL, *et al.* Career influence of an international health experience during medical school. *Fam Med.* 2004; **36**(6): 412–16.

58 Chamberlain L, Wang NE, Ho ET, *et al.* Integrating collaborative population health projects into medical student curriculum at Stanford. *Acad Med.* 2008; **83**(4): 338–44.

59 Chamberlain SE, Searle J. Assessing suitability for a problem-based learning curriculum: evaluating a new student selection instrument. *Med Educ.* 2005; **39**(3): 250–7.

60 O'Toole TP, Kathuria N, Mishra M, *et al.* Teaching professionalism within a community context: perspectives from a national demonstration project. *Acad Med.* 2005; **80**(4): 339–43.

61 Swick HM, Szenas P, Danoff D, *et al.* Teaching professionalism in undergraduate medical education. *JAMA.* 1999; **282**(9): 830–2.

62 Woolliscroft JO, Calhoun JB, Billiu GA, *et al.* Medical student attention to preventive medicine: change with time and reinforcement. *Am J Prev Med.* 1988; **4**(3): 166–71.

63 Stone DH. The clinical epidemiology ward round: can we teach public health medicine at the bedside? *J Publ Health Med.* 1998; **20**(4): 377–81.

64 Glasziou P. What is EBM and how should we teach it? *Med Teach.* 2006; **28**(4): 303–4.

65 Shaneyfelt T, Baum KD, Bell D, *et al.* Instruments for evaluating education in evidence-based practice: a systematic review. *JAMA.* 2006; **296**(9): 1116–27.

66 Chessare JB. Evidence-based medical education: the missing variable in the quality improvement equation. *Joint Comm J Qual Im.* 1996; **22**(4): 289–91.

67 Caspi O, McKnight P, Kruse L, *et al.* Evidence-based medicine: discrepancy between perceived competence and actual performance among graduating medical students. *Med Teach.* 2006; **28**(4): 318–25.

68 Parlow J, Rothman AL. ATSIM: a scale to measure attitudes toward psychosocial factors in health care. *J Med Educ.* 1974; **49**(4): 385–7.

69 Schwartz PL, Loten EG. Effects of a revised preclinical curriculum on students' perceptions of their cognitive behaviors, attitudes to social issues in medicine, and the learning environment. *Teach Learn Med.* 2008; **15**(2): 76–83.

70 Parlow J, Rothman A. Attitudes towards social issues in medicine of five health science faculties. *Soc Sci Med.* 1974; **8**(6): 351–8.

71 Rosenberg JI. Attitude changes in dental and medical students during professional education. *J Dent Educ.* 1965; **29**(4): 399–403.

72 Stephenson A, Higgs R, Sugarman J. Teaching professional development in medical schools. *Lancet.* 2001; **357**(9259): 867–70.

73 Price J, Price D, Williams G, *et al.* Changes in medical student attitudes as they progress through a medical course. *J Med Ethics.* 1998; **24**(2): 110–7.

74 Novick LF, Cibula DA, Sutphen SM, *et al.* Measuring orientation to population-based prevention. *Am J Prev Med.* 2003; **24**(4 Suppl. 1): 95–101.

75 Lambert TW, Goldacre MJ, Turner G. Career choices of United Kingdom medical graduates of 1999 and 2000: questionnaire surveys. *BMJ.* 2003; **326**: 194–5.

76 Plovnick MS. Primary care career choices and medical student learning styles. *J Med Educ.* 1975; **50**(9): 849–55.

77 Phillips B, Rubeck R, Hathway M, *et al.* Preventive medicine: what do future practitioners really need? *J Ky Med Assoc.* 1993; **91**(3): 104–11.

78 Evans P, Suzuki Y, Begg M, *et al.* Can medical students from two cultures learn effectively from a shared web-based learning environment? *Med Educ.* 2008; **42**(1): 27–33.

79 Hmelo-Silver CE, Nagarajan A, Day RS. 'It's harder than we thought it would be': a comparative case study of expert-novice experimentation strategies. *Sci Educ.* 2002; **86**(2): 219–43.

80 Imperato PJ, Feldman J, Nayeri K. Second-year medical student opinion about public health and a second-year course in preventive medicine and community health. *J Commun Health.* 1986; **11**(4): 244–58.

81 Marshall T. Influences on the examination performance of medical students: the pressure of other examinations. *Med Educ.* 1987; **21**(5): 381–5.

82 Ewan CE. Attitudes to social issues in medicine: a comparison of first-year medical students' attitudes with first-year students in non-medical faculties. *Med Educ.* 1987; **21**(1): 25–31.

83 Ewan C. Social issues in medicine: a follow-up comparison of senior medical students' attitudes with contemporaries in non-medical faculties. *Med Educ.* 1988; **22**(5): 375–80.

84 Dietrich AJ, Moore-West M, Palmateer DR, *et al.* Adapting problem-based learning to a traditional curriculum: teaching about prevention. *Fam Pract Res J.* 1990; **10**(1): 65–73.

85 Usherwood T, Joesbury H, Hannay D. Student-directed problem-based learning in general practice and public health medicine. *Med Educ*. 1991; **25**(5): 421–9.

86 Dyke P, Jamrozik K, Plant AJ. A randomized trial of problem-based learning approach for teaching epidemiology. *Acad Med*. 2001; **76**(4): 373–9.

87 Wiers RW, van de Wiel MW.J, Sa HLC, *et al*. Design of a problem-based curriculum: a general approach and a case study in the domain of public health. *Med Teach*. 2002; **24**(1): 45–51.

88 Pearson SA, Rolfe IE, Henry RL. The relationship between assessment measures at Newcastle Medical School (Australia) and performance ratings during internship. *Med Educ*. 1998; **32**(1): 40–5.

89 Rego PM, Dick M-L. Teaching and learning population health: challenges for modern medical curricula. *Med Educ*. 2005; **39**(2): 202–13.

90 Maudsley G. Medical students' expectations and experience as learners in a problem-based curriculum: A 'mixed methods' research approach [Masters dissertation]. Liverpool: University of Liverpool; 2005.

91 Dangerfield P, Dornan T, Engel C, *et al*. *A Whole System Approach to Problem-Based Learning in Dental, Medical and Veterinary Sciences: a guide to important variables*. The Centre for Excellence in Enquiry Based Learning (CEEBL): a Centre of Excellence in Teaching and Learning (CETL) University of Manchester 2007. Available at: www.campus.manchester.ac.uk/ceebl/resources/guides/pblsystemapproach_v1.pdf (accessed 30 October 2009).

CHAPTER 4

Health promotion in the medical curriculum: what are the essential competencies and who decides?

Angela Scriven and Ann Wylie

INTRODUCTION

In this chapter we explore the need to identify competencies associated with professional practice with regard to health promotion. There are two complementary issues about health promotion competencies that need to inform curricula, these being what is required for the health promotion professional and, more relevant for this book, the competencies for health professionals, many of whom will have a health promotion remit within the wider context of their professional practice. This situation occurs in many disciplines associated with health professional education such as behavioural psychology, pharmacy and epidemiology. The level of knowledge and skills needed is fluid and those involved in regulatory processes will necessarily have some input on defining these competences for the various professional groups.

The health professions occupy an interconnected world within healthcare systems, with multiprofessional action commonly regarded as a prerequisite to the goals and attainments of health improvement. One area of practice that has been significant in pulling together different professional groups under the same banner is that of health promotion.[1-3] With the emergence in the UK of the new public health agenda, building multiprofessional understanding and capabilities in the promotion of health is now seen as crucial.[4,5]

PROFESSIONAL HEALTH PROMOTION: IN SEARCH OF STABILITY

These are interesting times for those who have been working in health promotion and for academics actively engaged in the education and training of students with ambitions and requirements to incorporate health promotion into their professional roles and functions. There is little doubt that the past decade has been tumultuous in the UK in terms of health promotion as a professional field of activity, with new and often misleading professional titles superseding the term health promotion in many health trusts, but with job descriptions still incorporating the core competencies that are associated with health promotion. A review of job advertisements has shown these to include titles such as Health Development Officer Primary Prevention, Specialist in Health Improvement and Health Inequalities, Public Health Development Manager, Senior Health Promotion Specialist, Public Health Information Specialist, Public Health Development Officer, Director of Public Health, Public Health Medicine, Healthcare Information and Knowledge Manager, Chief Specialist Public Health, Health Promotion Strategic Coordinator, Health Improvement Advisor, Public Health Development Officer, Health Promotion Officer and Young People's Substance Misuse Strategy Coordinator.[6] The plethora of titles is a direct result of the dominance from the late 1990s of public health over health promotion. This has resulted not only in health promotion as a title being lost in some healthcare systems and in many universities in the UK,[6] but also in the fragmentation of health promotion as a distinct field of activity within public health.

There is evidence that things are changing rapidly. During the most recent past, politicians, through various policy forums, have articulated the urgency of incorporating health promotion competencies into healthcare systems.[7] This movement to a health-promoting health service has coincided with many countries examining the economic costs of healthcare and the role of prevention in alleviating health budgets.[8] This has happened in the past, and it was from the premise of economic expediency that health promotion was first coined as a term.[9] It is perhaps an important indicator that the Treasury rather than the Department of Health has recently led the debate in the UK. Sir Derek Wanless, the author of a major review of health spending, suggested three different scenarios for future spending in health, with the most cost-effective, the so-called 'fully engaged' scenario, relying on more investment in public health.[10,11] As Catford[8] points out, the proponent was not a group of well-meaning health promotion activists, but the ex-chief of one of the UK's biggest banks, backed by the strength of the Chancellor of the Exchequer Gordon Brown. Since taking over as prime minister, Gordon Brown has placed health high on his political agenda and at the time of writing has initiated *Putting Prevention First*[12] with a view to primary care to take on a much more significant role in the promotion of health. There is clearly a need therefore, for doctors to have developed health promotion competencies during their training so that they are able to deliver on the new policy agenda. This training is likely to be simultaneously happening with the qualified doctor as well and the medical students. What can guide and inform this training is considered below.

COMPETENCIES IN EVIDENCE-BASED HEALTH PROMOTION PRACTICE

Developing the capacity to deliver evidence-based health promotion is a key goal within Europe as demonstrated by the Getting Evidence into Practice (GEP) project, and worldwide by the Global Programme on Health Promotion Effectiveness (GPHPE). The dissemination of Phase 1 of the GEP project in the special supplement of *Promotion & Education* in 2005 was dominated by five key issues, all of which have relevance for those with a responsibility for training the health promoters and health professionals with health promotion remits. There were issues around the nature of evidence; the need for a common framework for getting evidence into practice; workforce capacity and capability; linkage between research, policy and practice; collaborative action and the need for a unified terminology.[13] The third on this list, workforce capacity and capability, has relevance to the medical education sector.

At a national level in the UK, increasing capacity and capability in evidence-based practice (EBP) is high on the public health agenda. The Health Development Agency in England had a major remit to produce and disseminate to practitioners the evidence of effectiveness of public health and health promotion. This role was transferred to the National Institute for Health and Clinical Excellence (NICE) in April 2005. Also in the UK the National Standards for Public Health Practice have EBP competencies embedded in them.

For registration on the Public Health Register, specialists need to demonstrate 'Know How' and 'Show How' competencies. Standard 3 of the National Standards for Specialist Practice in Public Health, *Developing quality and risk management within an evaluative culture*, specifically focuses on EBP and requires professionals to know how to:

> 3.2 Assess the evidence and impact of health and healthcare interventions, programmes and services and apply the assessment to practice.

For medical students, and by implication medical teachers, many of whom will be practising doctors who will work with a health promotion remit, the draft competencies published by Public Health Resource Unit, June 2005[14] have included 'know how' under Standard 3 that involve:

> 23 Critical appraisal of primary and secondary research and knowledge of the hierarchy of evidence.

> 24 Assessment of evidence of effectiveness of services, programmes and interventions, which impact on health.

These are now gradually becoming established in medical undergraduate curricula[15] and are distinguished from public health content.

At the next level of core competencies, practitioners, under core area 24, are required to be able to 'show how' they can:

> 2.1 Conduct a literature review, which includes the use of electronic databases, defining a search strategy and summarizing results.

> 2.2 Apply research evidence, evidence of effectiveness, outcome measures, evaluation and audit to influence programme interventions, services or development of clinical or practice guidelines and protocol.

> 2.3 Interpret and balance evidence and effectiveness from a range of sources to inform decision making.

These national standards provide coherent and important indicators to those with a responsibility for curriculum development in health promotion but remain a challenge.

FROM MEDICAL MODELS TO PRACTICE: RESPONDING TO RISK FACTORS, BEHAVIOURS AND SCREENING

The dominance of the medical model is not to be discredited but accepted as a legitimate approach to patient care, the doctor being an expert advice giver and having a professional opinion. That said, however, there seem to be alternatives roles that can and should be apparent in medical practice if health promotion is to have an impact. Naidoo and Orme[16] have argued that the medical profession has a central role in contributing to health promotion and that this requires doctors to contribute to planning health promotion activities for local populations. They show, through a series of vignettes, how teachers could enhance the effective delivery of health promotion for medical students, and how to integrate health promotion into medical education. They maintain that core competencies are around understanding issues of equity, and being able to engage effectively in collaborative working, with evidence from the literature, research, policy and practice used to demonstrate how these areas could be integrated appropriately into the medical curriculum.

Frankish, *et al.*[17] argue that the incorporation of the principles and practices of health promotion requires that the medical model, which has been the default model of care, is unlikely to have marked effects on health inequities or health status. They present two dimensions (values, structures) of a health promotion philosophy and approach that are relevant to the medical curriculum, with a strategy and framework to support practical and attainable action. They argue that fundamental philosophical values provide a foundation for health promotion. These values should be reflected in the structures that create a supportive environment for health.

Based on these values and structures, they conclude that subsequent strategies (interventions), processes (client- and community-centred care), and desired health promotion outcomes (intended or unintended) may be achieved by the medical practitioner.

What percentage of time does a doctor spend in health promotion? What are the essential competencies and what are the desirable competencies and who decides? How should these be woven in to the curriculum? These questions remain and are far from easy to explore or address but throughout this book there are some pointers, and consideration is given to what is seen as essential and what is desirable.

REFERENCES

1 Scriven A. *Alliances in Health Promotion: theory and practice.* Basingstoke: Palgrave; 1998.
2 Scriven A. Promoting health: policies, principles and perspectives. In: Scriven A, editor. *Health Promoting Practice: the contribution of nurses and allied health profession.* Basingstoke: Palgrave; 2005.
3 Scriven A, Orme J. *Health Promotion Professional Perspective.* 2nd ed. Basingstoke: Palgrave; 2001.
4 Department of Health. *The Report of the Chief Medical Officer's Project to Strengthen the Public Health Function.* London: The Stationery Office; 2001.
5 Department of Health. *Shifting the Balance of Power within the NHS: Securing Delivery.* London: The Stationery Office; 2001.
6 Scriven A. *Report of a Survey into the Impact of Recent National Health Policies on Specialist Health Promotion Services in England.* London: Brunel University; 2003.
7 Scriven A, Speller V. Global issues and challenges beyond Ottawa: the way forward. *Promot Educ.* 2007; **14**(4): 194–8.

8 Catford J. Creating political will: moving from the science to the art of health promotion. *Health Promot Int.* 2006; **21**(1): 1–4.

9 Lalonde M. *A New Perspective on the Health of Canadians.* Ottawa: Ministry of Supply and Services; 1974.

10 Wanless D. *Securing our Future Health: taking a long-term view: interim report.* London: HM Treasury; 2001.

11 Wanless D. *Securing our Future Health: taking a long-term view.* London: HM Treasury; 2002.

12 Department of Health. *Putting Prevention First: Vascular Checks.* Available at: www. networks.nhs.uk/news.php?nid=2156 (accessed 30 October 2009).

13 Jones C, Scriven A. Where are we headed? The next frontier for the evidence of effectiveness in the European Region. *Int J Health Promot Educ.* 2005; Special edition 1.

14 Public Health Resource Unit. *UK Voluntary Register Framework for Retrospective Portfolio Assessment of Specialists Practising in Special Areas of Public Health Practice.* London: UK Public Health Register; 2005.

15 Wylie A, Thompson S. Establishing health promotion in the modern medical curriculum: a case study. *Med Teach.* 2007; **29**(8): 766–71.

16 Naidoo J, Orme J. Health promotion in the medical curriculum: enhancing its potential. *Med Teach.* 2000; **22**(3): 282–7.

17 Frankish CJ, Moulton G, Rootman I, *et al.* Setting a foundation: underlying values and structures of health promotion in primary health care settings. *Prim Health Care Res Dev.* 2006; **7**: 172–82.

CHAPTER 5

Medical educators' experience: lessons learned

Stephen Gillam and Ann Wylie

INTRODUCTION

In recent years medical educationalists have reported on new curricular themes such as communication skills[1] and innovative teaching methodologies such as problem-based learning[2] as well as contemporary approaches to assessment. However, the teaching of health promotion and the more established field of public health have found limited representation on the pages of educational journals.[3]

This chapter looks at the barriers and challenges associated with health promotion and public health teaching. It reports on lessons learnt as well as identifying opportunities to improve the quality of teaching and learning in these areas. Based on the authors' own experiences and research, as well as a review of existing literature in the field, we identify three main challenges:

➤ strengthening the public health curriculum
➤ strengthening the resource base
➤ increasing teacher capacity and skills.

Greater integration with other clinical teaching will enable students and teachers alike to see the relevance of such teaching in a clinical context.

A HISTORICAL SCHISM

The teaching of undergraduate public health has always reflected a number of tensions. Debates about the place of public health in the teaching of medical school students go back over a century. This was reflected at an institutional level in the establishment of schools of public health and hygiene distinct from medical schools. By the early twentieth century in many countries, the field of population health had been separated from the mainstream of medical training. The influential Flexner Report of 1910 entrenched medical sciences at the core of medical training.[4] Even today, there is continuing debate over the relevance of population health-related disciplines for strictly clinical practitioners and about the latter's wider, societal role in promoting population health. There remain those who regard public health as an entirely postgraduate discipline.

However, in the developing world, medical training emphasised skills needed to promote community health. The World Health Organization continues to emphasise that public health promoting competencies, especially as they relate to the management of chronic disease, will be of increasing importance to the twenty-first century global healthcare workforce.[5] In the UK, the General Medical Council's (GMC) blueprint for medical training, *Tomorrow's Doctors*, helped to entrench the position of public health and related disciplines in undergraduate curricula.[5,6] *Choosing Health*, a recent white paper on public health, has further served to emphasise the importance of training in this area.[7]

However, government policy has been consistently ambiguous. Hospital-based, specialist services have absorbed the bulk of recent increases in health spending and the impact of frequent health service reorganisations on the public health function has been disastrously disruptive. In many parts of the country, health promotion departments bringing together expertise in this field have all but disappeared. This has affected training and recruitment. Always a 'shortage speciality', teachers of public health and health promotion have been and continue to be in short supply.

In the UK, until the 1990s, specialist public health practice was dominated by the medical health profession. However, in a review of the public health function, the Chief Medical Officer (CMO) of England described three levels of the public health promoting workforce:

- **Public health specialists**: Certified consultants in public health who work at a senior strategic level to influence the health of the population, e.g. in primary care trusts.
- **Public health practitioners**: Those who spend a major part of their time in preventive practice, e.g. health visitors, environmental health officers and community development workers.
- **The wider workforce**: Anyone with a role in health improvement and reducing inequalities: e.g. teachers, housing officers, social workers, doctors and health service managers.[8]

While the focus in this book is on medical students, many countries are seeking to maximise the contribution of a broader public health workforce. The steady diversification of primary care nursing roles is a quiet revolution with major implications for public health practice.[9] Recognition is also growing of the importance to health improvement of people in other jobs whose activities have a significant impact on population health.[10] For example, a range of occupations from local government chief executives to catering assistants can substantially influence public health but they would not traditionally have been viewed as such. The lessons gleaned from this book are therefore relevant to the training of many different groups within a broad health promoting workforce.

EXPERIENCE IN MEDICAL SCHOOLS

We undertook a literature search of Medline using the search terms 'Health Promotion' [Mesh] or 'Public Health' [Mesh] or 'Public Health Nursing' [Mesh] or 'Students, Public Health' [Mesh] or 'Schools, Public Health' [Mesh] or 'Education, Public Health Professional' [Mesh] or 'Public Health Dentistry' [Mesh]. We also searched using 'Education' [Mesh] or 'Education, Nursing, Continuing' [Mesh] or 'Health

Education'[Mesh] or 'Education, Medical, Undergraduate' [Mesh] or 'Education, Medical, Graduate' [Mesh] and 'Teaching/methods' [MAJR], and 'Public Health/education' [MAJR] or 'Health Promotion' [Mesh]. Finally, we used 'Models, Educational' [Mesh] and 'Education, Medical, Undergraduate' [Mesh] and 'Public Health/education' [MAJR] or 'Health Promotion' [Mesh].

We aimed to examine teaching inputs to medical undergraduate curricula, to identify perceived challenges in the delivery of public health teaching and strategies that may overcome them. The findings of our review are distilled under three main headings:

➤ strengthening the public health curriculum
➤ resources for teaching and learning
➤ developing the teaching faculty.

Strengthening the public health curriculum

Students' attitudes to health promotion and preventive medicine are mixed. Rego and Dick found 60% of their respondents to be positive about psychosocial and preventive health issues but many also considered these issues to involve 'no more than common sense'.[11] The fields of public health and health promotion continue to have limited appeal as a career choice for medical students.[12] Most students will be in clinical practice and tend to marginalise these aspects of curriculum with poor attendance at lectures and seminars. Some students fear that the opportunity costs of dedicating study time to population and preventive health might compromise their future clinical knowledge and skills in patient management. They may decide that study time is more judiciously spent developing clinical skills. This, in turn, discourages teachers and may influence those designing curricula. That said, students link health promotion, but not necessarily public health, with general practice. If they see general practice as a career option, they may be more concerned with patients' wider health needs and how best to meet them, for example people who are overweight, who want to stop smoking or people who are materially deprived.

The main challenge facing curriculum developers therefore is to ensure clinical relevance, for information learned in context will be more readily retrieved. The teaching of preventive health has to balance students' understanding of the principles of population health with application of a biopsychosocial model of patient care.[11,13] Gillam and Bagade found that public health and clinical teaching were integrated to some extent in three-quarters of UK medical schools but there is scope for much improvement.[13]

The link between attitudes and practice is notoriously unpredictable. However, Bellas, *et al.* found positive attitudes towards health promotion and prevention amongst first-year medical students. They stress the need for educators to consider other personal and social values held by the students and address the political aspects of these disciplines.[14]

Later on, public health is widely regarded by medical students as peripheral to the acquisition of clinical knowledge and skills. The points of convergence between public health and clinical practice are not self-evident. Practical demonstrations of the application of public health principles to clinical problem solving in acute or community settings are the most effective means of raising its profile. Stone has offered a theoretical framework of integrated public health education for curriculum development and evaluation.[15] The interrelationships between clinical practice and public health may be represented in the form of a grid (*see* Box 5.1). The vertical headings are the clinical skills that relate to the different stages of the natural history of disease – from the pre-disease state through diagnosis, treatment and follow-up. The horizontal headings describe four key public health dimensions: epidemiology, behaviour/lifestyle, environment and health policy. The text in the boxes suggests appropriate topics for discussion. The grid is also potentially useful for course documentation and content evaluation.

Students need to be equipped with basic skills, such as techniques for behavioural change in their clinical work. These must be seen as essential learning outcomes for curricula. A study of smoking cessation skills teaching in UK medical schools was highlighted.[16] The relatively new NHS smoking cessation service was being established at the time and the evidence to support these interventions was convincing. Students were generally encouraged to take a smoking history and were made aware of tobacco-related disease, but 42% of responding medical schools made no reference to smoking cessation in curriculum material. Most smoking-related teaching occurred early in the course, apart from other practical teaching. Doctors are frequently ill-equipped to deal with smoking cessation and tend not to intervene unless the presenting complaint is associated directly with smoking behaviour. This lack of self-confidence is itself a barrier to teaching these important skills.[17–19]

In line with GMC recommendations,[6] the proportion of teaching delivered as lectures is decreasing and that of self-directed learning is increasing.[20] Many of the new medical schools and graduate courses are developing problem-oriented curricula. More in-depth consideration of curricular design and problem-based learning (PBL) is presented in Part 2, Chapter 6. Where discretionary study modules are available, students selecting public health and health promotion study modules evaluate their time highly. At King's College London (KCL), students doing health promotion modules have helped modify the core curriculum in the light of their experiences. The core curricular health promotion content has greatly benefited from their involvement and feedback at the development stage with regard to the behavioural change sessions in the third year and how to approach prevention of childhood obesity.[21] In many medical schools special study modules offer opportunities to explore more exciting aspects of these disciplines such as global public health. Additionally, overseas electives often provide students with their first major insights into the relevance of population-level public health and health promotion opportunities. In preparing for these electives students need to consider the health status of the country they are visiting, the health needs and priorities as well as their own health and safety issues. Hence, indirectly, such opportunities can have significant influence on students' views of public health and health promotion. The cost of electives is also high for students and, where there are bursaries or grants, students are keen to apply for them

A study at the Royal Free Medical School found that most students and teachers believed teaching about disease prevention and health promotion should be integrated into all years of the curriculum and clinical firms. However, teachers were less likely than students to support more learning in these fields or to regard learning about prevention as important as learning about diagnosis and treatment. Megan and Lloyd suggest that, in order to build on their positive findings, aims and objectives should be agreed and that teaching of these disciplines should be integrated both horizontally and vertically throughout the curriculum.[22] There are more examples of integrated health promotion and public health curricula in Part 4.

There is clearly a need for a shared consensus on what constitutes the 'health promotion syllabus' at this level. Developing this shared consensus is an ongoing task within

BOX 5.1 Theoretical framework for integrated teaching of public health and clinical practice

	Epidemiology	Behaviour	Environment	Services
Prevention	Concepts, principles	Individual risk factor identification/modification	Supporting creation of safer, healthier environments	Policies, resources
Diagnosis	Disease frequency Accurate history taking Validity of tests	Risk vs cause Aetiological formulation Role of smoking, alcohol drugs, diet	Housing, climate, pollution, transport, workplace, school Microbes, herd immunity Family, neighbourhood, poverty	Resources, access to NHS
Treatment	Critical appraisal of evidence Clinical guidelines	Compliance Behavioural change	Modification of environmental factors Ameliorating impact of poverty	Rationing, pharmacopoeias Service planning, management
Follow-up	Recurrence rates Prevention of recurrence Adverse effects of treatment Clinical audit	Quality of life Risk of recurrence	Monitoring environmental, familial, social change	Geography, community facilities

the international teaching community. This book endeavours to contribute, in the first instance, by identifying discrete learning outcomes related to health promotion as distince from public health.

No single set of educational objectives will necessarily apply similarly to every medical school, as educational contexts differ. An updated set of public health educational goals (*see* Box 5.2) has recently been proposed by public health teachers in the UK. If applied flexibly, they should contribute to contemporary expectations of medical professionalism.[22]

BOX 5.2 Educational goals that can be used to develop a public health medicine curriculum

Medical students should be able to:
- discuss the nature of health, disease and their population determinants
- take a population perspective on health, disease and medical treatment
- discuss the principles and practice of health promotion and disease prevention
- use epidemiology, data handling and public health skills in the practice of evidence-based clinical medicine
- outline methods of communicable disease control and the scope of the doctor's role and responsibilities in health protection
- describe the principles and practice of population health needs assessment, healthcare planning, resource allocation, and healthcare evaluation
- describe the key features of the National Health Service as a healthcare system subject to organisational change
- discuss the achievements, potential and ethics of public health, and lessons to be learnt from how the public health function has developed.

Several medical schools have framed learning outcomes in term of the competencies they wish students to acquire. Competencies may be less relevant, however, than the attitudes and knowledge needed to fulfill an appropriate future role in the healthcare system. Safe doctors fit for practice at foundation level require the following:
➤ behaviour change skills
➤ an understanding of the clinical governance in its many different aspects
➤ the ability to make cost-effective clinical decisions that are in the patient's and population's best interests.

Undergraduate medical education should emphasise the essential epidemiological and ethical principles that underpin these transferable skills.

Wylie and Thompson have explored many of these concerns, reporting on their experiences of establishing health promotion in core curriculum in a clinically relevant context.[23] Their preferred working definition of health promotion, based on previous research,[3] is 'the study of, and the study of the response to, the modifiable determinants of health'. They argue that how students look after their own health should be an integral aspect of the curriculum, given that junior doctors need to also demonstrate they are fit to practice and able to care for their own well-being.[24] What is sustainable and what impact health promotion teaching may have on students, teachers and faculty is part of a longitudinal research programme with Monash School of Medicine in Melbourne.

Resources for teaching and learning

Medical faculties are responsible for ensuring that the GMC recommendations on health promotion and public health education are fulfilled. The medical school's 'department of public health' should share in the responsibility, leadership, and coordination of such efforts. The delivery of public health education should involve a range of departments including primary healthcare, occupational health, child health, medicine, or equivalents. However the curriculum committee is organised, which is probably unique to each medical school, public health and health promotion should be represented.

The last major review of UK undergraduate public health teaching, in 2005, found great variability in the amount of public health teaching, content and methods used as well as the resources available to deliver it.[13] There is no single design and management structure for the curriculum that will ensure effective public health education. The local circumstances and context will determine the approaches to be taken. Nevertheless, departments of public health can and should provide access to trained staff with varied experience in education, health services and clinical research (and evaluation) and clinical, social and health promotion services. Traditionally in the UK, there has been no 'service increment for teaching' allocated to support public health staff, which will have affected how local public health involvement in the curriculum has developed. Local arrangements vary, but both KCL and Monash Medical School have introduced a system of rewarding their community-based health promotion facilitators. This has been helpful in gaining and sustaining commitment, both with regard to the facilitators' own training and briefing as well as supporting the students' learning.

Staff development should promote aspects outlined in *Tomorrow's Doctors* such as:

➤ modern educational theory and evidence
➤ role modelling
➤ skills in tutoring
➤ small-group work
➤ assessment
➤ programme evaluation
➤ facilitating active learning, where appropriate
➤ participating in student selection.

Web-based resources are an increasingly critical source of educational material. Effective information and communication technology support is therefore vital for effective curriculum implementation. Some of the resources developed at KCL are already available to a wider audience through the International Virtual Medical School (IVIMEDS). An innovative repository website, hosted by Monash Medical School in association with KCL is described in Part 4, Chapter 17, while assessment is the focus of Part 5.

It is inevitable that students attach most significance and devote most learning time to aspects of the course that are formally assessed and therefore 'count'. But public health and health promotion fare poorly in this regard: public health related disciplines feature in 'finals examinations' in less than half of all UK medical schools.[13] Public health related disciplines should, given the directives from regulatory bodies, feature in summative assessments, that is, those that ultimately count towards academic progress and the achievement of an award.

The assessment methods used should relate appropriately to what is being tested, for example:

➤ multiple choice or extended-matching items should explore applied epidemiological knowledge and understanding
➤ written answer questions and written project work should explore critical analysis for clinical practice and related attitudes
➤ objectively structured, directly observed exercises should explore specific practical health-promoting skills.

The development and dissemination of suitable resources for assessment in this field should yield more opportunities for medical schools to include public health related fields in 'high stakes' examinations – but the process requires material support.

Developing the teaching faculty

Successive structural reforms within the NHS have further strained teaching resources. There has been a major expansion in medical student numbers in an attempt to meet the national shortfall in doctor numbers. More than half the medical schools were having difficulty finding teachers and staffing levels had deteriorated.[13] Other studies have highlighted teaching capacity and skills shortages, with students reporting poor role modelling from faculty.[11] Those involved in health professionals' education should be equipped with teaching skills and subject knowledge. For PBL, facilitation skills, with good briefing notes, are essential.[20] As well as possessing teaching and facilitation skills, faculty need to be clear about the content and learning outcomes for public health and health promotion sessions.

A KCL teaching pack, consisting of a CD with PowerPoint presentation and DVD of simulated clinical scenarios, was prepared, piloted, revised and evaluated for use by seminar leaders. The rationale was:

➤ that students could be taught in smaller groups with an opportunity for role play and discussion
➤ there would be consistency for the learners who would be assessed
➤ motivated teachers less familiar with the field of health promotion and public health could gain confidence about content.

The multi-media pack was made available to students online, although they were encouraged to attend the related seminars.

In short, we need to increase the supply of well-trained and motivated teachers and combine the best traditional teaching methods with more innovative, problem-based approaches. Faculties need to share 'learning about what works' and their teaching resources across medical schools, as well as addressing a culture of neglect of teaching in some departments. Many teachers feel that their contributions were undervalued and few are aware of the level of funding received to support teaching.[15]

FUTURE CHALLENGES

Public health and health promotion continue to gain recognition as an important subject within undergraduate curricula. In the UK, recent national policy developments have reinforced the importance of developing the healthcare workforce in these areas.[7,25] This chapter has highlighted several ways in which undergraduate teaching of public health and health promotion could be strengthened.

➤ Consensus on what constitutes the 'public health syllabus' at this level needs to be strengthened.

➤ Further evaluation of problem-based public health learning is required and attempts to integrate clinical teaching need to be evaluated.

➤ The advent of new medical schools offers opportunities to extend the evidence base in support of PBL.

➤ There is scope for much more sharing of teaching materials and experience about 'what works'.

➤ Knowledge and skills in health promotion should be formally assessed and this needs to be reflected in the content of final qualifying examinations.

➤ With a shortage of faculty to deliver in these areas, workforce development is a major priority.

➤ Beyond basic training and induction, teachers need continuing developmental support.

➤ There needs to be appropriate career-long recognition and incentivisation of teaching activities within the relevant academic departments.

International influences on public health provision and priorities will affect different countries in different ways. Nevertheless within core curricula for medical education there can be consistent public health and health promotion content. A recurrent theme of this book is the need to improve learning across international boundaries, providing medical graduates with the skills to apply the core principles of health promotion and public health within the context of their professional practice. This is not the parochial concern of a diminishing cadre of medical educationalists. If health systems are to play their part in addressing global health inequities, this is of paramount importance.[26]

REFERENCES

1 Harden RM, Davis MH, Crosby JR. The new Dundee medical curriculum: a whole that is greater than the sum of the parts. *Med Educ.* 1997; **31**(4): 264–71.

2 Phillips S. Models of medical education in Australia, Europe and Canada. *Med Teach.* 2008; **30**(7): 705–9.

3 Wylie A. *Health Promotion and Medical Education: an exploration of the epistemology and the challenge* [dissertation]. London: King's College; 2003.

4 Flexner A. *Medical Education in the United States and Canada: a report to the Carnegie Foundation for the Advancement of Teaching.* New York: Carnegie Foundation; 1910.

5 General Medical Council. *Tomorrow's Doctors.* London: General Medical Council; 1993.

6 General Medical Council. *Tomorrow's Doctors.* 2nd ed. London: General Medical Council; 2003.

7 Department of Health. *Choosing Health: making healthier choices easier.* [Public Health White Paper]. London: The Stationery Office; 2004.

8 Department of Health. *The Report of the Chief Medical Officer's Project to Strengthen the Public Health Function.* London: The Stationery Office; 2001.

9 Hill A, Griffiths S, Gillam S. *Public Health and Primary Care.* Oxford: Oxford University Press; 2007.

10 Sim F, Locke K, McKee M. *Maximizing the Contribution of the Public Health Workforce: the English experience.* Geneva: World Health Organization; 2007.

11 Rego PM, Dick M-L. Teaching and learning population health: challenges for modern medical curricula. *Med Educ.* 2005; **39**(2): 202–13.

12 Soethout MBM, ten Cate OJ, van der Wal G. Development of an interest in a career in public health during medical school. *Public Health.* 2008; **122**(4): 361–6.

13 Gillam S, Bagade A. Undergraduate public health education in UK medical schools: struggling to deliver. *Med Educ.* 2006; **40**(5): 430–6.

14 Bellas PA, Asch SM, Wilkes M. What students bring to medical school: attitudes toward health promotion and prevention. *Am J Prev Med.* 2000 (April); **18**(3): 242–8.

15 Stone DH. Public health in the undergraduate curriculum: can we achieve integration? *J Eval Clin Pract.* 2000; **6**(1): 9–14.

16 Stone DH. The Beer Sheva experiment and its lessons for community medicine. *Community Med.* 1988; **10**(3): 228–34.

17 Roddy E, Rubin P, Britton J. A study of smoking and smoking cessation on the curricula of UK medical schools. *Tob Control.* 2004 (March); **13**(1): 74–7.

18 Kerr S, Watson H, Tolson D, *et al.* An exploration of the knowledge, attitudes and practice of members of the primary care team in relation to smoking and smoking cessation in later life. *Prim Health Care Res Dev.* 2007; **8**(1): 68–79.

19 Vogt F, Hall S, Marteau T. General practitioners' beliefs about effectiveness and intentions to recommend smoking cessation services: qualitative and quantitative studies. *BMC Fam Pract.* 2007; **8**(1): 39.

20 Wood D. ABC of learning and teaching in medicine: problem-based learning. *BMJ.* 2003; **326**: 328–30.

21 Wylie A, Furmedge D, Appleton A, *et al.* Medical curricula and preventing childhood obesity: pooling the resources of medical students and primary care to inform curricula. *Educ Prim Care.* 2009; **20**(2): 87–92.

22 Gillam S, Maudsley G, editors. *Public Health Education for Medical Students: a guide for medical schools.* Rev. ed. Cambridge: Department of Public Health and Primary Care, University of Cambridge; 2008.

23 Wylie A, Thompson S. Establishing health promotion in the modern medical curriculum: a case study. *Med Teach.* 2007; **29**(8): 766–71 .

24 General Medical Council. *The New Doctor.* Available at: www.gmc-uk.org/education/postgraduate/new_doctor.asp (accessed 30 October 2009).

25 Lord Darzi. *A High Quality Workforce: NHS next stage review.* London: Department of Health; 2008.

26 Commission on Social Determinants of Health. *Closing the Gap in a Generation: health equality through action on the social determinants of health. The final report of the WHO Commission on Social Determinants of Health.* Geneva: World Health Organization; 2008.

PART TWO

Curriculum structures and practical options for health promotion integration

INTRODUCTION
Ann Wylie

Medical education has undergone widespread change, with limited empirical evidence but informed by sound argument and pragmatic responses to call for change, especially in 1993.[1-3]

Change has been influenced by medical educators having an increased engagement with the wider discipline of education and its theories and philosophies.

The approaches to contemporary curriculum design in medical and health professional vocational courses have provided opportunity to consider how health promotion could be integrated. The moves to outcome-based curricula have been advocated and implemented in many universities, with a spiral curriculum[4] similar to that of the constructivist approach described by Hirsch[5] being favoured, in part because this allows the student to build on knowledge and experience. Curriculum development and design is complex, needs to be responsive to context, student need, teacher skill and availability as well as resources, and cognisant of public expectation with regard to healthcare. Whether a problem-based approach or a vertical and integrated approach within health courses, the curriculum should reflect values associated with healthcare provision and the communities in which the health practitioners, when qualified to practice, will work.[6] We also need to consider in the curriculum design that assessment is an integral part of this process, and as such, it must be linked to the measurable, defined outcomes and the requirements of the regulatory and awarding bodies and must, of course, demonstrate reliability. Few medical schools can start with a blank drawing board when planning curricula and there are a number of stakeholders and factors that influence how curriculum evolves.

Part 2 explores curriculum structures and considers the place of health promotion in these structures. Some examples of how health promotion sits within existing curricula are given. Finally, Chapter 9 discusses the importance of assessment within curriculum design, although assessment issues are more fully explored in Part 5.

REFERENCES

1 Morrison JM, Sullivan F, Murray E, *et al.* Evidence-based education: development of an instrument to critically appraise reports of educational intervention. *Med Educ.* 1999; 33(12): 890–3.
2 Wylie A. *Health Promotion and Medical Education: an exploration of the epistemology and the challenge.* London: King's College; 2003.
3 General Medical Council. *Tomorrow's Doctors.* London: General Medical Council; 1993.
4 Harden R, Crosby JR, Davis MH, *et al.* AMEE Guide 14: Outcome-based education: Part 5 – From competency to meta-competency; a model for the specification of learning outcomes. *Med Teach.* 1999; 21(6): 546–52.
5 Hirsch ED. The core knowledge curriculum: what's behind its success? *Educ Leader.* 1993; May: 23–5.
6 Prideaux D. ABC of learning and teaching in medicine: curriculum design. *BMJ.* 2003; 326(7383): 268–70.

CHAPTER 6

Vocational curricula: structures and demands

Ann Wylie

CHANGING THE STRUCTURE: WHY?

Pedagogy within medical education came under scrutiny by a number of agencies and academics in the 1980s and 1990s, leading to major curriculum reform in many institutions. Scrutiny continues as part of academic enquiry, scholarship and account-ability to regulatory bodies. Those involved in early reform offered ideas for change and some early evaluation evidence, notably by Harden and Davis[1] and the Dundee model. Questions being explored included:

➤ What constitutes evidence-based teaching?
➤ How could traditional curricula be radically transformed without harm to learners and patients?
➤ What are the costs involved?
➤ How will change be evaluated?

Evidence and argument, essentially from educational paradigms that draw on eclectic research approaches and occasional quasi-experimental design but rarely randomised controlled trials, were guiding enquiry. This contrasts with the highly valued randomised control trials of scientific medicine. The pragmatists however, saw change as inevitable, particularly because of the community context of healthcare and the reduced access to patients in the teaching hospitals. Patients were spending less time in hospital, mainly because of health reform, with increased community-based care and changing patterns in morbidity such as increased prevalence of chronic disease. Questions about assessment, its validity and reliability, the processes and fairness, were being more openly researched within education generally, as well as within medical education. Debate and evidence were emerging about the limitations of traditional methods of assessment and arguing for improvements.

Educationalists have had minimal involvement with medical education and its curriculum design until reform seemed inevitable. Educationalists had much to offer including the psychology of learning, pedagogy and instructional design, andragogy, self-directed learning and problem-solving principles, evaluation of input, process, outcome and assessment methodologies. That teaching was not the same as learning, that assessment reliability could be examined, that context was a contributory barrier or help to the learner were the fodder of the debates in medical education literature and at conferences.

Curriculum structures could be changed, and with that change could come a revision of content, content being linked to what is considered relevant, and with a focus on outcome-based education.

Additional aspects influencing the need for change were the cost of medical education, the need to expand student intake and to have a more diverse student body and health professional workforce, likely to be more representative of the communities they served. The place for the 'newer themes', such as health promotion, ethics and communications, also had to be worked in and Harden, *et al.* provided an example by integrating these newer themes as vertical threads within a spiral curriculum when they described the New Dundee Curriculum.[2] Educational technology would also play a part in the modernising of curricula and the delivery of curricula, enabling, for example, students in rural and remote areas to have access to their campus via Internet and Intranet links, to have web links and online tutorials and do online assessments. All the elements of curriculum design are linked[3] and therefore planning for change, reviewing and reforming curricula require the basic structure to be fit for purpose.

CHANGING THE STRUCTURE: PLANNING

The curriculum, argues Harden, is:

> . . . a sophisticated blend of educational strategies, course content, learning outcomes, educational experiences, assessment, the educational environment and the individual student's learning style, personal timetable and programme of work.[4]

Integrated curricula require teachers to move away from the focus of their own discipline and content, so as to enable students to have meaningful learning experiences, relevant to future practice and being patient-centred. Harden identified four key areas – learning outcomes, assessment, content and learning opportunities – and then provided additional domains as follows: curriculum organisation; staff; learning resources; timetable; learning location. From each of these, further subdivisions were explained. The curriculum map, although not an easy task to undertake, provides a method of implementing outcome-based education. Whilst Harden located health promotion within an example of curriculum mapping, hyperthyroidism, it is doubtful whether other medical curricula would have included health promotion in a similar manner.

By 1995, Harden and Davis had published the Association of Medical Education in Europe (AMEE) Medical Education Guide for a core curriculum with options or special study modules.[5] Their evidence to support change was well articulated, relating to factual overload, the need to pay attention to newer topics, including health promotion, and the economic issues facing medical undergraduate education as a result of the length of the course. Some thought was given to rationalising the content with a view to developing four-year instead of five-year courses, as has already happened in some countries.

Harden and Davis also used the GMCs *Tomorrow's Doctors* document to support the argument for change. Moving to the evidence to support the planned changes, they drew on Levy's ideas with regard to effectiveness of teamwork in problem solving.[6] The arguments for core curriculum content ideas are informed by Hirsch with regard to students' ability to learn higher-level objectives and enhance critical thinking skills.[7] The paper then describes the New Dundee Curriculum, which has a constructivist core, informed by educational argument and supplemented by study options which involved students making choices. They note that this notion of core curriculum with options is attractive to educationalists, medical teachers, students and the public.

This paper was the prototype for many medical schools, enabling them to modify and, for many, radically change curricula in the next five years. Plans for change were well under way before evidence of effectiveness would be available, but the critical mass for change gave momentum to the transfer from traditional approaches to integrated curricula using adult learning methods.

By 1997 Harden, *et al.* reported on the success of the New Dundee Curriculum, which related to input and process, to the development and implementation of the new curriculum that was theoretically informed, but as yet there was no evidence related to outcome from the student perspective.[2] Evidence began to emerge relating to a variety of aspects associated with curriculum change, including evaluation studies and teacher competence. Increasingly evidence about these educational innovations became available, with questions about access and quality being asked. Concern about the evidence-based education and how to critically appraise reports of educational research was seen as increasingly important. Morrison, *et al.* argued that medical education would impact on patient care and therefore should be thoroughly evaluated. Still they noted that medical education had undergone widespread change with limited evidence to inform the changes or evaluation evidence to support change.[8]

The principles of integrated and spiral curricula were theoretically plausible and as research papers emerged reporting on evaluation and impact of change, the reflexivity process could further enhance contextual education research.[9]

In many medical faculties traditional curricula were based on subjects such as anatomy, basic sciences and physiology, and these were taught in lecture theatres and laboratories during a preclinical phase with the following clinical years providing opportunities for clinical skills.

Other healthcare professional vocational courses, although usually of three to four years' duration rather than four to six years' duration, had similar approaches, some providing a degree and other diplomas, or professional qualification. Educational theory played a limited role in both medical education and health professional vocational courses and course providers were in close association with healthcare providers.

This situation, which had seemed pragmatic for so long, was not underpinned by educational principles and was becoming 'overcrowded' as new findings were added in without other topics being modified. Nursing education was first to be revised in the UK and go to a degree programme. The rationale for this was that it would better prepare nurses to be lifelong learners and critically review their practice, relate it to evidence and be in line with many other countries.

However medical education was guided by the GMC's recommendations,[10,11] which set out curricula in regard to learning outcomes and made recommendations to consider the learner. In the meantime, the call for education theory to be applied to proposed change had been heeded, and exemplars such as the New Dundee Curriculum[2] were being described in the literature.

Whilst simultaneously structure and content were to be revised, the diverse needs of the student population also became significant. Student admission procedures were reviewed with the requirement to accept students coming from underrepresented groups such as those on lower incomes, those with poor education experiences but deemed able to meet the needs of university education, and those from minority ethnic groups. In England the scheme is called Widening Participation and is managed by the Higher Education Funding Council for England (HEFCE).[12]

Other factors also changed, including an increased number of students with first degrees and work experiences applying for places, the development of 'fast track' graduate four-year courses similar to the USA, with the majority of other admissions, especially in the UK, coming from school. Admissions policies changed and modernised. So many changes were happening concurrently, and as the momentum gathered, many medical schools were seeing out the old and bringing in the new curriculum. How would health promotion find its place?

CHANGING THE STRUCTURE: THE OPTIONS AND HEALTH PROMOTION

Conventional or traditional medical curricula had covered individual subjects (e.g. anatomy, biochemistry, microbiology, pathology, pharmacology, sociology) and students would then apply this knowledge to clinical problems. One of the drawbacks is that it is not clear just how much of each individual subject is relevant and necessary for a student in a vocational course such as medicine. The tendency has always been to include more and more and consequently conventional curricula tend to get very crowded. These traditional curricula started with a disease or system, building the science content to enable students to comprehend.

Problem-based learning (PBL) was the most innovative option for most schools to consider and this related to Socrates' and Plato's philosophy of posing questions to explore beliefs, values, prior knowledge and what line of enquiry is needed to reach wider deeper understanding. Unique to PBL, in contrast with traditional curricula, is the starting point for students, this being the patient or case, as opposed to the disease.[13]

PBL additionally aligns well to modern theories of higher education and adult education, but designing PBL curricula for medical schools was more complex than the ideology. Maastricht in the Netherlands and McMasters in Canada pioneered PBL medical courses and described the guiding principles, which also allowed for vertical integration and a spiral concept. In the UK both Liverpool and Manchester medical schools have opted for PBL curricula. PBL, according to the University of Manchester's website:

> . . . is an educational approach that is particularly designed for active self-directed learners, which doctors must be throughout their professional lives.

Short clinical case scenarios (cases) are used to start and guide the process of learning. The emphasis is on the gaps that students discover in their knowledge and skills, and how to remedy them. PBL aims to enable students to discover and learn for themselves, with experienced tutors to facilitate the process, but not to subject them to formal tuition under a different name.

> Each semester consists of a series of clinically related problems, which students use to define their specific study objectives in the biological, pathological and psycho-social sciences week-by-week. Students work together in developing a sound understanding of the science fundamental to clinical practice.[14]

In a problem-based curriculum, students begin with relevant clinical problems and with the help of a facilitator or tutor work out how much they know and understand of the underpinning biomedical sciences from the knowledge they already have (and what they do not know). They then define what they need to learn in order to gain a fuller insight and understanding of the problem(s). These cases have to be skillfully written and according to Manchester's website relate to 'key issues of health and illness as well as key concepts in the sciences fundamental to medicine.'[14]

PBL involves students, in small groups, having a 'case' to consider and in a week or two doing a presentation on their findings. Over the course of each year a set number of cases will have been given to the same small group of students. These cases become increasingly complex as the students progress, with more confounding aspects to be considered. Overarching the PBL process are usually four or five themes and the students will relate their presentation to these. At Liverpool Medical School for example there are four themes as follows:

➤ structure and function
➤ individuals, groups and societies
➤ population perspective
➤ professional and personal development.

Each one could have some health promotion related aspect but in reality students put most of their effort into structure and function in a clinical and scientific way. What health promotion is explored is likely to be within the population perspective and dominated by public health aspects.

A PBL facilitator helps the student group negotiate their tasks, has access to briefing notes but is not there as an expert or clinician, rather as a facilitator for learning. Students can, during the intervening time, access lectures, seminars, textbooks and journals as well as other reliable sources, and the amount of guidance will vary. The students learn to work in groups in a collaborative way as will be needed when they are qualified. They will experience uncertainty of what is required, become familiar with self-directed learning and critiquing evidence, which are essential experiences to prepare them for professional practice. Their learning is considered to be deeper than surface learning, which is where rote learning can be discredited, but inevitably critics of PBL concern themselves with the limited factual knowledge that students have. Critics also question the concept of the facilitator role, the variability of student experience and the difficulty of establishing evidence of effectiveness of PBL in the short- and mid-term. Epstein's review of the PBL literature[15] explores the debate, the opportunities and limitations of PBL *per se*.

PBL offers opportunities for health promotion learning but this is dependent on how the case is focused, the overall learning outcomes, what the briefing notes indicate to the facilitator about health promotion aspects and how skilled or favourably disposed the facilitator is with regard to health promotion. For example, a case with a patient who has poorly managed asthma and is a smoker may focus on treatment review, the patient's inhaler technique, the patient's exposure to workplace allergies, and thus pay little attention to smoking and smoking cessation other than to advise the patient to stop. If the facilitator is aware of smoking cessation interventions and the evidence base, either through the briefing notes or their own experience, students may be 'guided' towards this.

Whilst there are health promotion opportunities in PBL curricula, they could be fragmented, marginalised, limited to lifestyle advice, omitted or ineffectively explored. There may be limited opportunity for deeper understanding of principles and intervention evidence, and indeed disagreement as to whether students need this at a particular stage. This is possible for other topics as well as health promotion and needs to be considered by curriculum planners. To ensure students are able to identify and learn about health promotion aspects relevant to the case it will be necessary to have appropriate facilitator training, briefing notes and signposting to key resources.

PBL hybrids have however become more usual in new curricula and at new medical schools such as The University of East Anglia and Peninsula Medical School. For example, Monash Medical School in Melbourne uses a PBL approach with cases and small group tutor groups. But in addition there are core taught components, with explicitly defined objectives and linked to assessment. An example of a typical PBL week in senior years at Monash Medical School is given in Table 6.1.

TABLE 6.1 An example of a PBL week in senior years at Monash Medical School

Monday	Tuesday	Wednesday	Thursday	Friday
Ward Theatre (2 hours)	Identify patient for PBL Practice case presentation (2 hours)	Ward Theatre (2 hours)	Ward Theatre (2 hours)	Clinico-pathologic correlation (CPC) or other dedicated pathology teaching (2 hours)
Clinical bedside teaching (1.5 hours)	Study (1.5 hours)	Clinical bedside teaching (1.5 hours)	Study (1.5 hours)	Study (1.5 hours)
Paper PBL 1 & 2 (2 hours)	Patient PBL 1 & 2 (3 hours)	Theme teaching (2 hours)	Ward Theatre (1.5 hours)	Ward Theatre (2 hours)
Study (1.5 hours)	Ward Theatre (0.5 hours)	Study (1.5 hours)	Study (2 hours)	Week in review (1 hour)
				Study (0.5 hours)

Many medical and health professional schools have incorporated elements of the PBL approach with small-group teaching where possible and the use of case scenarios. The small-group teaching in PBL hybrid curricula maybe more didactic than the PBL model and may highlight specific areas of learning, be they factual knowledge or complex concepts and skills. Although there is a reduction overall in lecture-based approaches to teaching, the PBL hybrid curriculum retains didactic and large-group teaching, symposia and individual project work.

Health promotion could be presented in a more explicit and direct way, indicating to students the specific learning outcomes and how they are relevant to their wider learning. There could be a level of compulsion to cover specific topics, including health promotion, especially if they are to be assessed. However where and how these topics are presented may influence their long-term value to the student. The integrated spiral

PBL hybrid curriculum provides opportunity for students to learn about the field of health promotion in some depth, critique evidence and evaluate interventions during clinical placements. In the junior years at Monash Medical School, students spend significant curriculum time involved in health promotion (*see also* Chapters 7, 13 and 14) but less so in the clinical years, whereas at King's College London School of Medicine (KCL), also using a PBL hybrid model, more emphasis is placed in the senior years and related to clinical context.[16] The dilemmas, rather similar to basic sciences and other topics, remain; dilemmas such as how much curriculum time, what depth, how will students recall and apply their learnings in the clinical context and what type of assessment is reasonable in the coverage of health promotion.

In summary, both PBL and PBL hybrid curricula are now widespread in medical education, especially in North America, Europe and Australia, and offer many health promotion opportunities. The debates about cost-effectiveness continue but the benefits of such approaches, as indicated by Phillips,[13] are that the starting point for the contextual learning is the patient and the presenting symptoms rather than the speciality of the teacher involved. Such approaches should, in theory, be conducive to exploring health promotion issues for the patients. Table 6.2 summarises the key elements of each. However with PBL hybrids, there is more opportunity to ensure health promotion aspects will be presented and will be explicit.

TABLE 6.2 Key elements of PBL and PBL hybrid approaches to medical education

PBL	PBL hybrid
Paper or patient case	Paper or patient case
Facilitator-managed sessions	Tutor-managed sessions
Resources available	Support for learning explicit
Self-directed	Seminars and lectures integral

Modular curricula are much in evidence in higher education, where a coherent whole is made up of defined modules that are both self-contained and cumulative. Medical courses have rarely adopted this curricular structure but there are similarities where for example system-based curricula and topic-specific rotations inform the structure. In traditional courses, subjects in basic sciences and behavioural sciences are taught in the preclinical phase, with students moving to clinical firms in the clinical phase to learn about specific illnesses. Clearly defined basic science topics are rarely taught but instead have been integrated into systems-based curricula in the early years of the course. Students in the clinical phase then have rotations with defined outcomes and where possible are taught in small groups within firms. Justifying and locating health promotion can be difficult and may become marginalised. But as health promotion crosses many specialities within medicine, relevant aspects can be integrated to the clinical rotations. Family health however is the most likely rotation to accommodate applied health promotion.

In the UK, regardless of the curricular structure, special study components or modules (SSMs) occupying about 20–30% of curriculum time are available for students. Provided the schools have the enthusiasm and staff, health promotion could be a visible choice and even some element of requirement.[17] At KCL a range of health promotion

SSMs are offered but in the penultimate year students must do an elective portfolio, including within that about 1000 words regards their own health and well-being. *See* Chapter 14 for more details.

It is therefore the *structure* that will inform how and where health promotion fits, how explicit or implicit, how well integrated yet visible, and what the assessment possibilities are. It is unlikely that those who champion health promotion will be central to curriculum design unless, that is, they are also educationalists, possibly with another clinical speciality, able to see health promotion in relation to the other essential learning outcomes and how best these can be achieved within the restraints and opportunities of the specific school.

MEETING THE DEMANDS FOR HEALTH PROMOTION IN CURRICULA: HIGHER EDUCATION

A number of external factors influence and impact upon health promotion in higher education *per se* but also in health-related courses. Adult education principles, such as those based on Schon's reflective practice,[18] Dewey's scientific enquiry[19] and experiential learning and Kolb's cycle[20] are significant in what is seen as quality in education.

The work of Schon is placed within the tradition of 'adult learning', while John Dewey emphasised the creative, human, self-corrective aspects of scientific enquiry. The notion of reflection as a contributor to the improvement of practice has its roots in the work of John Dewey. Reflective practice involves examining strongly held beliefs, and through this, discovering how actions are the results of beliefs, some that are examined and some that are not. Kolb's experiential learning cycle compliments the ideas of Dewey and Schon, as represented in Figure 6.1.

This cyclical process impacts on the design of curriculum, the pedagogy, the assessment of learning, evaluation of the learning process and modification of the curriculum based on feedback. When regulatory bodies inspect medical and health-related vocational courses, the educational process and the 'quality' will be reviewed as well as content and other factors.

Is the medical curriculum student-centred and does it consider students' own health and welfare needs? When curricula are reviewed, one key question will be linked to how modern approaches to adult learning are incorporated. The curriculum should not hinder students' learning but indeed should ensure that students are coping and, where there are difficulties, that students are able to access adequate and relevant support. Attention is given to these aspects within the General Medical Council's (GMC) *Tomorrow's Doctors*.[11] Medical schools are usually part of a university or higher education institute, where much of the supportive infrastructure is shared across faculties. However medical students, especially in their senior years, may find their workload and financial situation increasingly difficult, while simultaneously being in a clinical learning environment rather than at their campus base. The way the curriculum is designed and delivered in the clinical context still needs to promote the well-being of students and offer appropriate support for their learning. This becomes an opportunity to integrate health promotion principles within the learning context as well as within the curriculum. In the UK for example, GMC inspections will include off-campus site visits to clinical and community settings, discussing such matters with the students.

As well as student well-being, there are the learning outcomes to consider. Prideaux posits that there are three levels of curriculum: the planned curriculum, the delivered

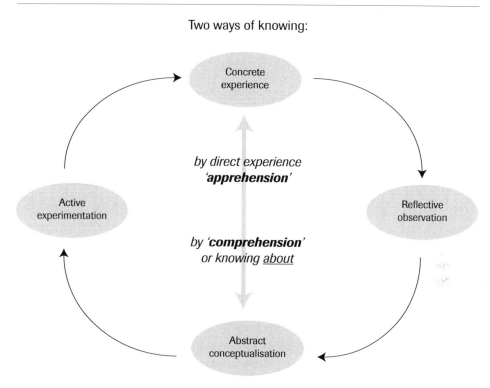

FIGURE 6.1 The cyclic processes of learning

curriculum and the experienced curriculum – what is learnt by the students.[3] It is probable that health promotion is difficult to isolate and map out, especially in PBL programmes. What the students learn may be well linked to the planned and delivered curriculum if they themselves are involved in the process of curriculum review and feedback. Students need to be involved in curriculum, as argued in European and international directives. The Bologna Declaration[21] and various national governments require health promotion to be a component of modern health vocational courses. Medical students should have an active role in new curricula and the Bologna proposals show how they see the students' role in curriculum content. They suggest nine domains with 76 defined outcomes, the nine domains being:

➤ clinical skills
➤ communication
➤ critical thinking
➤ health in society
➤ lifelong learning
➤ professionalism – attitudes, responsibilities and self development
➤ teaching
➤ teamwork
➤ theoretical knowledge.

The curriculum they advocate should maintain and improve the quality of education, healthcare and mobility. It is mainly within the domain of health in society that health promotion can be visible. The opening statement to this domain, health in society, is:

> As future doctors in a rapidly changing environment we are obliged to adjust our attitudes to the expectations of society. We consider knowledge of the basic principles of public health issues as essential for our work as future physicians at a local, national and international level. Therefore we stress the importance of including environmental, cultural and international health-related issues in our medical curriculum.[22]

Specific outcomes are given and include that medical graduates should be able to identify vulnerable populations and respond appropriately and they should be able to promote health in individual patients, and in society, by active education of patients. The proposal also argues that medical graduates should be equipped to formulate their own opinions on these matters and participate actively in shaping health policies.

MEETING THE DEMANDS FOR HEALTH PROMOTION IN CURRICULA: THE MEDICAL PROFESSION

Although smoking cessation is only a small part of health promotion, the basic skills associated with approaches to patients who smoke and wider smoking reduction policies are seen as highly relevant for taught curricula. Yet they are receiving little attention in UK medical schools, according to Roddy, *et al.*[23] Kerr, *et al.* found inconsistencies with regards to smoking cessation referrals in older people and this was associated with lack of confidence and awareness of the potential effectiveness of smoking cessation programmes.[24] Similar findings by Vogt, *et al.*[25] argue for interventions to improve the situation, given that helping people to stop smoking is one of the most effective ways of reducing health inequalities. Likewise the concerns about GPs' responses to obesity have highlighted limited confidence and awareness of how to intervene.[26,27] More recently, a study on sexual activity and older people suggested that doctors are uncomfortable asking about patients' sexual health and well-being, even though sex is important in the well-being of older people.[28] Kleinplatz suggests that every doctor should be trained to ask patients if they have any sexual concerns, thereby normalising and affirming the importance of sexual well-being for health.[29]

The above papers relate to already qualified doctors and topics that would be part of their applied health promotion practice; the question is then at what point should doctors acquire health promotion skills – undergraduate or postgraduate? Key questions also arise such as:

➤ Are doctors adequately prepared to address these issues?
➤ Are they competent and who decides?
➤ If they are prepared and competent then why are they uncomfortable?

For current practitioners these issues have to be part of postgraduate training and continuing professional development, given the evidence is relatively recent to support interventions and the situation is evolving. Both the Royal College of Physicians (RCP) and the Royal College of General Practitioners (RCGP) specifically make reference to the rationale for health promotion in their programmes. The RCP campaigns on key public health issues in the UK and in the European Union. It founded 'ASH', the anti-smoking body, and has produced guidelines and teaching materials. Its current public health issues are concerned with the health damage resulting from excessive alcohol consumption and the impacts of climate change.[30] The RCGP gives details of its curriculum, with its Domain 5 being Healthy Lives.

> General practitioners have a crucial role to play in promoting health and preventing disease. More important than the general practitioner's role is that of the patient through self-care. During the consultation there are excellent opportunities to discuss healthy living with the patients and for the early detection of illness. To put patients at the centre of their care, general practitioners need to possess appropriate skills to support people to self-care, taking them through a range of approaches, in partnership, recognising that the individual should make the choices, decisions and take the actions themselves. The general practitioner's defined practice list offers a framework to provide appropriate diagnostic, therapeutic and preventative services to individuals, and to the registered population. Gaining a better understanding about inequalities in health and strategies to address inequalities in health are important aspects of training to be a general practitioner.[31]

If the medical profession are to respond and adapt to changing public health and health promotion priorities, as well as to government and other directives, then it would seem to be imperative that medical graduates leave medical school with the basic health promotion outcomes described earlier.

In part, we have to return to the definition of health promotion, the parameters and the challenge of shifting priorities. We also have to distinguish the needs of those health professionals who will specialise in various aspects of health promotion and public health from those who will be integrating health promotion into their clinical and professional practice.

There are a number of topics, mainly associated with health-related behaviour and risk factors, that all have special skills, but for the most part there are overarching principles. That said, smoking behaviour and policy offers a very useful framework for exploring health promotion at undergraduate level. It is relevant to many branches and specialist fields of medicine and clinical care. Smoking behaviour is linked to health inequalities and is a major economic burden to healthcare service providers. Yet without a specifically defined curriculum outcome and location it could be 'lost' during undergraduate years. If, for example, smoking cessation and policies are within the respiratory/chest rotation, without learning objectives detailed or briefing notes provided, it may fall outside a nominated teacher or facilitator's perceived responsibility, it may be considered 'common sense' and covered as part of patient-centred communications, the task being simply to provide information and advice. Equally, social determinants of health may sit within behavioural sciences and public health where students are aware of the determinants, the epidemiology and demographic studies associated with smoking, but are not aware of how to apply intervention knowledge and skills within the clinical context and may lack role modelling of such skills.

MEETING THE DEMANDS FOR HEALTH PROMOTION IN CURRICULA: THE EMPLOYERS

Within the UK since the New Labour Government came to power in 1997, a number of health targets, policy directives and health-related documents have emphasised the need to improve public health, and the NHS is expected to be a major stakeholder improving the nation's health. In the recent report about the needs of a high-quality workforce, Lord Darzi recommends that health professionals should be engaged in keeping people healthy and should have expertise in prevention and health promotion within the context of their professional practice. Whilst some health professionals will be part of continuing professional development, there is an expectation that new graduates will have the basic skills related to health promotion for their occupation.[32] There are similar aspirations across Europe where there is a need promote health for such benefits as a reduction in health inequalities. The main focuses here are on children and young people, workforce health and strategy papers on mental health and sexual health.[33] Although many stakeholders are involved in health promotion, there is an expectation that health professionals will have a defined role; higher education, preparing this workforce, therefore has responsibilities in this regard.

Junior doctors in their first year of paid work in the UK enter the Foundation Year 1 category. This is regulated by the GMC and in order to be eligible for registration and progression to Foundation Year 2 they must demonstrate a number of outcomes. In particular they should be able to 'demonstrate that they can recognise and use opportunities to promote health and prevent disease and show they are aware of the wider worldwide health priorities and concerns and health inequalities'. With regard to their own health they must be able to demonstrate 'a knowledge of their responsibilities to maintain their health including a suitable balance between work and personal life and know how to deal with personal illness. They must take appropriate action to maintain their own health.'[34]

The collective demands of higher education, the medical profession and employers for substantive and visible health promotion content in curricula makes it imperative that there is demonstrable progress in medical education endeavours. Integrating curricula is complex, whatever approach is taken and whilst there is clear opportunity for the social and behavioural sciences, which include health promotion, there is much to be gained by sharing and disseminating experiences, as Muller, *et al.*[35] have done.

The following two chapters provide examples of how health promotion has been integrated, with reference to issues of responsibility as well as accountability to the faculty.

REFERENCES

1 Harden R, Crosby JR, Davis MH, *et al.* AMEE Guide 14: Outcome-based education: Part 5 – From competency to meta-competency; a model for the specification of learning outcomes. *Med Teach.* 1999; **21**(6): 546–52.

2 Harden RM, Davis MH, Crosby JR. The new Dundee medical curriculum: a whole that is greater than the sum of the parts. *Med Educ.* 1997; **31**(4): 264–71.

3 Prideaux D. ABC of learning and teaching in medicine: curriculum design. *BMJ.* 2003; **326**(7383): 268–70.

4 Harden RM. Curriculum mapping and outcome-based education. Paper presented at 10th International Ottawa Conference on Medical Education. Ottawa, ON; 2 A.D. 13–16 Jul 2002: p. 212.

5 Harden RM, Davis MH. AMEE Medical Education Guide No. 5. The core curriculum with options or special study modules. *Med Teach.* 1995; **17**(2): 125–48.

6 Levy P. *Transferable Personal Skills and the Higher Education Curriculum: an annotated bibliography.* Sheffield: Personal Skills Unit, University of Sheffield; 1992.

7 Hirsch ED. The core knowledge curriculum: what's behind its success? *Educ Leader*. 1993; May: 23–5.

8 Morrison JM, Sullivan F, Murray E, Jolly B. Evidence-based education: development of an instrument to critically appraise reports of educational intervention. *Med Educ*. 1999; **33**(12): 890–3.

9 Usher R. Textuality and reflexivity in educational research. In: Scott D, Usher R, editors. *Understanding Educational Research*. London: Routledge; 1998. pp. 33–51.

10 General Medical Council. *Tomorrow's Doctors*. London: General Medical Council; 1993.

11 General Medical Council. *Tomorrow's Doctors*. 2nd ed. London: General Medical Council; 2003.

12 Higher Education Funding Council for England. *Widening Participation*. Available at: www. hefce.ac.uk/widen/ (accessed 19 August 2008).

13 Phillips S. Models of medical education in Australia, Europe and Canada. *Med Teach*. 2008; **30**(7): 705–9.

14 School of Medicine, University of Manchester. *Problem-based learning*. Available at: www. medicine.manchester.ac.uk/undergraduate/medicine/pbl/ (accessed 31 October 2009).

15 Epstein RJ. Learning from the problems of problem-based learning. *BMC Med Educ*. 2004; **4**: 1. Available at: www.biomedcentral.com/1472–6920/4/1 (accessed 16 November 2009).

16 Wylie A, Thompson S. Establishing health promotion in the modern medical curriculum: a case study. *Med Teach*. 2007; **29**(8): 766–71.

17 Wylie A. Health Promotion Special Study Module – whose agenda? Paper presented at the 1999 AMEE Conference. Sweden; September 1999.

18 Schon D. *Educating the Reflective Practitioner*. San Francisco, CA: Jossey-Bass; 1987.

19 Dewey J. *How We Think: a restatement of reflective thinking to the educative process*. 2nd ed. Lexington, MA: Heath; 1933.

20 Kolb DA. *Experiential Learning: experience as a source of learning and development*. Englewood Cliffs, NJ: Prentice Hall; 1984.

21 Hilgers J, DeRoos P, Rigby E. European core curriculum: the students' perspective. *Med Teach*. 2007; **29**(2–3): 270–5.

22 Ibid.

23 Roddy E, Rubin P, Britton J. A study of smoking and smoking cessation on the curricula of UK medical schools. *Tobacco Control*. 2004 (March); **13**(1): 74–7.

24 Kerr S, Watson H, Tolson D, *et al.* An exploration of the knowledge, attitudes and practice of members of the primary care team in relation to smoking and smoking cessation in later life. *Prim Health Care Res Dev*. 2007; **8**(1): 68–79.

25 Vogt F, Hall S, Marteau T. General practitioners' beliefs about effectiveness and intentions to recommend smoking cessation services: qualitative and quantitative studies. *BMC Fam Pract*. 2007; **8**(1): 39.

26 Walker O, Strong M, Atchinson R, *et al.* A qualitative study of primary care clinicians' views of treating childhood obesity. *BMC Fam Pract*. 2007; **8**(1): 50.

27 King LA, Loss JHM, Wilkenfeld RL, *et al.* Australian GPs' perceptions about child and adolescent overweight and obesity: the Weight of Opinion study. *Br J Gen Pract*. 2007 (February); **57**: 124–9.

28 Beckman N, Waern M, Gustafson D, *et al.* Secular trends in self reported sexual activity and satisfaction in Swedish 70 year olds: cross sectional survey of four populations, 1971–2001. *BMJ*. 2008; **337**: a279.

29 Kleinplatz PJ. Sexuality and older people. *BMJ*. 2008; **337**: a239.

30 Royal College of Physicians. *Professional Issues and Policy*. Available at www.rcplondon.ac.uk/ Professional-Issues/Pages/professional-issues-policy.aspx (accessed 31 October 2009).

31 Royal College of General Practitioners. *Healthy People: promoting health and preventing disease*. Available at: www.rcgp-curriculum.org.uk/pdf/curr_5_Healthy_people.pdf (accessed 31 October 2009).

32 Lord Darzi. *A High Quality Workforce: NHS next stage review.* London: Department of Health; 2008.

33 European Alliance for Public Health. *European Commission Priorities for Public Health in 2008.* Available at: www.epha.org/a/2842 (accessed 31 October 2009).

34 General Medical Council. *The New Doctor.* Available at: www.gmc-uk.org/education/postgraduate/new_doctor.asp (accessed 30 October 2009).

35 Muller JH, Jain S, Loeser H, *et al.* Lessons learned about integrating a medical school curriculum: perceptions of students, faculty and curriculum leaders. *Med Educ.* 2008; 42(8): 778–85.

Health promotion in curricula: examples of integration

Tangerine Holt and Craig Hassed

with additional contributions from Karen Sokal-Gutierrez, John Edward Swartzberg, Amin Azzam, Elizabeth Garland, Erica Friedman and Richard Bordowitz

INTRODUCTION

Chapter 7 presents a number of educational models of health promotion within existing medical education structures. It highlights the importance of the role of medical education structures in addressing community health issues by transforming the educational process of medical students. This adoption of innovative, systematic approaches in medical education has a number of implications. These implications and challenges will be presented in Chapter 15.

Pomrehn, *et al.*[1] in their discussion on prevention for the twenty-first century raised critical questions about the role of medical education. They are:

➤ How can medical educators best prepare their students to contribute to another century of continued health improvement?
➤ Are students learning about prevention currently?

Three descriptive examples of international models of health promotion across undergraduate (school leaver entry), graduate (those who already have a bachelor's degree) and postgraduate (those who have a graduate degree) levels address these questions. The aim is for the reader to be able to compare and contrast these health promotion education models, the number of students, their context and curriculum structures which promote health through the delivery of preventive services in the community. Both Australian and American examples of community-based practice, the Program in Medical Education for the Urban Underserved (PRIME-US) and the Mount Sinai School of Medicine (MSSM) programmes showcase:

➤ innovative generalist programmes at undergraduate, graduate and postgraduate (residency) levels utilising community-based models
➤ continuity of practice within the community
➤ the training of future medical practitioners utilising a systemic interprofessional approach to care.

Peak educational bodies such as the Australian Medical Council (AMC) and the Association of American Medical Colleges (AAMC) have long recognised that health promotion and preventive medicine are integral components of both medical education and practice. A review of the literature indicates that there are a number of examples of health promotion being taught across medical curricula, some more effectively than others. Garr *et al.*[2] point out that many medical schools indicate the desire to improve their teaching of prevention. A key educational strategy utilised in successful development and implementation of health promotion in medical education is the establishment of community partnerships with higher education. We support Garr, *et al.*'s[3] argument for students to engage in experiential learning opportunities that show them how to apply prevention to patient care in the community.

HEALTH PROMOTION IN CURRICULA AT MONASH UNIVERSITY, AUSTRALIA

Background

Health promotion content has been a major component in the Monash University medical curriculum since the early 1990s. At that time a team-based Health Promotion (HP) project was introduced in order to give a practical and experiential context to the lecture content.[4] Since the introduction of the new Bachelor of Medicine/Bachelor of Surgery (MBBS) problem-based learning (PBL) five-year curriculum in 2002 the HP content and project work has expanded in terms of depth and time commitment. The medical course is structured on four themes.

Theme 1: personal and professional development.
Theme 2: population, society, health and illness.
Theme 3: foundations of medicine.
Theme 4: clinical skills.

Table 7.1 presents the learning objectives and corresponding assessment activities for the community-based practice (CBP) programme, which is an integrated programme of Community Partnerships Placement and Health Promotion components for approximately 300 second-year medical students. Individual theme content in Year 2 is as follows:

> Theme 1: ⎰ community-based practice programme ⎱ CBP
> Theme 2: ⎱ health promotion and knowledge management ⎰
> Theme 3: homeostasis: maintaining the internal environment
> Theme 4: clinical skills.

Educational innovation and learning environment

Health promotion teaching is largely delivered in Year 2 of the five-year programme. It is integrated with knowledge management and, since 2008, has been combined with the community placement programme to form the unit Community-Based Practice (CBP). Prior to this, the HP projects were student-driven research projects implemented in a setting of the student's choosing. The course convenors are authorised by the Monash University's Standing Committee of Ethics Research for Humans (SCERH) to approve the projects provided they address the criteria of low-impact research, meaning that they were not ethically complex; that is, dealing with sensitive issues or vulnerable

TABLE 7.1 Learning objectives and assessment activities for the community-based practice programme for second-year medical students

CBP/HP objectives	Assessment
1 Appreciate the interplay of medical, scientific, social, cultural, political, economic and ethical factors in HP	• 20% for the project proposal • 60% for the final report • 40% for HP fieldwork (3000 words): reporting on the findings and discussion points related to their fieldwork. It is presented in the form of a journal article with introduction, methods, results, discussion and conclusion
2 Define, compare and contrast medical, behavioural and socio-environmental approaches to HP	
3 Understand the application of HP theories of behaviour change used in HP interventions	

4 Understand the basic HP process of programme:
  — Development and planning
  — Implementation
  — Evaluation
	— 10% for hypothetical sections (1000 words): if only one or two of the three phases of the HP cycle are covered in the fieldwork then the other section/s must be covered hypothetically to be sure the students grasp the integrated nature of the HP cycle

5 Identify appropriate strategies for individual (targeted high risk), community and media (population-based) interventions	

6 Knowledge management:
  — Understand the relationships between data, information, evidence, knowledge and informed care
  — Demonstrate skills in information management (literature searching and medical database identification, presentation skills)
  — Apply critical appraisal skills to clinical and research questions
  — Application of a range of knowledge-based systems in clinical practice (bibliographic software, decision support systems)
	— 10% for personal and professional development reflective essay (1250 words): this covers their personal reflections on their placement experience and teamwork
	— 20% for the poster presentation: at the end of the year students present a poster – much as they would at a conference – outlining their fieldwork. This is a major event on campus which showcases all of the group's project work. After presenting the poster students field questions from their assessor

participants. Evaluation suggested that this was challenging but was nevertheless a powerful way of achieving learning objectives with regard to health promotion, research methods, knowledge management, ethics and teamwork.

Learning activities

Table 7.2 provides an overview of key lectures (one hour) and tutorial content (two hours) across two semesters in second-year medicine as part of the CBP programme. The HP content of the course is delivered via three methods:

➤ health promotion projects through the completion of a community placement

➤ lecture content
➤ tutorials.

In 2008 the team-based projects were embedded for the first time in the Community Partnership Program settings. These community placements have been running since 2002 and are an opportunity for students to gain community experience as well as reinforce learning objectives related to the social sciences, social justice, equity, ethics and multidisciplinary teamwork. As such, the emphasis of the HP projects has shifted from research to community engagement and contribution. In 2008, if a group of students wanted their health promotion project to be a formal research project so they could publish their work outside of their placement and project report, or if they were dealing with ethically sensitive issues, then they were required to submit their proposal to SCERH, Monash University. If any project proposal was deemed in a grey area as to whether it constituted research then it was considered by HP convenors and if it was deemed to be research then it was either modified so as not to be considered a research project any longer or refined and submitted to ethics branch on appropriate forms for review.

The students are placed in their community placement for one day a week during the second half of semester 1 and the first half of semester 2 (14 placement days in all). It is also hoped that students learn about themselves and how to work in teams at the same time as they are making a valuable contribution to the community placements by assisting them in fulfilling HP goals that they may not have had the time or resources to previously fulfill. The community placements are varied and include experiences such as working with the homeless and mentally ill, centres working with injecting drug users, schools, social support programmes for chronic conditions, people who have a disability and aged care.

While HP project work is challenging for students, academic advisors and the community, it is also a powerful medium for attaining learning objectives. Guidance is given to ensure that the project is manageable in terms of time and resources. Students work in groups of two to five at their placement. The project work can involve any or all three phases of the HP cycle. They include:
➤ **development** – identify a problem and a strategy to address it in light of existing knowledge
➤ **implementation** (intervention) – carry out the planned programme being careful to use an ethically sound and evidence-based approach
➤ **evaluation** – to what extent was the programme implemented as planned? To what extent was the programme effective in achieving its objectives?

While these steps have been described in a linear fashion, in reality, it is more like an iterative cycle (*see* Figure 7.1), wherein the experience of going through the cycle once is applied to doing it better the next time. In that way, evaluation work in one cycle becomes the 'development' work for the next iteration. This might be done by the same health promotion group over a short period of time, and also can be thought of on an historical scale, where various groups build on each other's work over time (e.g. consider how many different times various health promotion groups have gone through this cycle with smoking cessation over the last 25 years).

All projects must involve fieldwork. For example, student teams may elect to do the following:

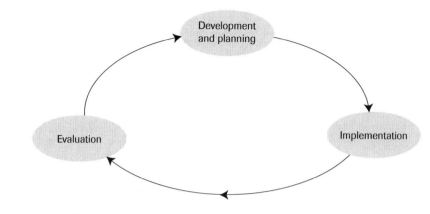

FIGURE 7.1 Health promotion cycle

➤ conduct a survey or needs analysis
➤ develop and deliver an intervention such as a healthy lifestyle or harm minimisation programme for substance abusers, or
➤ evaluate an existing programme being implemented by the community placement.

Some general examples of projects and their corresponding focus include:
➤ identify a problem and develop a novel strategy to address it ('development' focus)
➤ identify an ongoing intervention and evaluate it ('evaluation' focus)
➤ identify a problem and a previous intervention that did not work, and sort out why ('evaluation' focus)
➤ identify an intervention that worked in addressing a particular problem, adapt it to a new context and pilot test it ('development' and 'implementation' focus)
➤ assist a community group or organisation with the planning, implementation or evaluation of a programme. Examples of programmes include pamphlets, wall posters, displays, public outreach/advertising campaigns, and educational sessions
➤ work with staff within an organisation to develop an approach to the promotion of health in an identified problem area (e.g. needle-stick injury among hospital workers)
➤ retrospectively evaluate a health promotion programme that succeeded or failed in achieving its aims in order to better understand why this happened
➤ work with health professionals or others to develop educational programmes to modify clinician knowledge or behaviour.

Students are provided electronic access to the CBP handbook with all the required guidelines and forms. A CBP Reference Guide brochure is provided to students outlining key learning objectives, responsibilities, processes, support, placement dates and assessment deadlines. They also have a faculty-based academic advisor (tutor) who guides the project throughout the year and a placement-based field educator who assists and supervises. HP projects are decided upon by the students themselves according to their interest in cooperation with the placement's needs and resources.

Given that our medical students are working with the community and health professionals to contribute to the development and delivery of healthcare which meet the needs of the community, SCERH, on meeting with the academic convenors of the Community Partnerships and Health Promotion programmes, recommended that all HP projects in 2009 be considered formal research projects. Students are expected to meet high standards of methodological and ethical rigour as these are important learning objectives required for the successful implementation of their project work. Even more important is the need for students and academic advisors to consider the ethical implications of their health promotion project and fieldwork, especially in dealing with vulnerable populations. As in 2008, this ensures the emphasis of the HP projects is still central to community engagement and contribution, which is encompassed with ethical rigour, sound methodology and publishable outcomes for both students and community partners.

Before the students commence their placement days they conceptualise and prepare their projects. The HP project proposal is submitted electronically on a modified ethics form for marking at the end of semester 1 and must be approved by the tutor and course convenors before proceeding to fieldwork in semester 2. After their final placement day in mid-semester 2, students are engaged in analysing data and preparing their final project report and posters. The mandatory components of the health promotion proposal are:

➤ literature review
➤ hypotheses, rationale and aims
➤ methodology
➤ outcomes
➤ discussion
➤ ethics.

Lecture series

The project work is underpinned and informed by a lecture series throughout the year (*see* Table 7.2). The lectures deliver background principles and information to provide students with a generic understanding of HP principles so that they are able to apply them to particular projects. The knowledge management content serves to provide knowledge and skills which are reinforced through application of the HP project work. International health promotion is also covered in the lecture series.

Tutorials

Five two-hour tutorials are provided each semester to help reinforce generic health promotion principles as well as provide support and feedback for the HP projects. Each tutor (academic advisor) has five to eight project groups within their tutorial group.

Assessment

The mark for the CBP project accounts for 19% of the total mark for Year 2 medical students. This is a significant assessment load that students do not take lightly. Added to this, HP content appears in written exams and an objective structured clinical examination (OSCE) station at the end-of-year OSCE, resulting in an overall of 25% of the assessment.

Feedback and formative assessment is provided in tutorials and meetings with project supervisors (academic advisors and field educators). Students are also asked to

TABLE 7.2 Lecture and tutorial content (two-hour tutorials throughout each semester are shaded)

Semester 1 topics	Semester 2 topics
CPP selection procedures	Information management for chronic disease
Vic Health 1	HP challenges and future directions
Vic Health 2	International health 1
Detailed project outline	Clinical decision support and analysis 1
Social, cultural and international contexts in HP	Clinical decision support and analysis 2
Psychosocial factors, health and mind-body medicine (MBM) 1	Project update • Progress reports • Fieldwork/questions • Quiz
Health psych/behaviour and lifestyle change 1	International health 2
Health psych/behaviour and lifestyle change 2	Making decisions: evidence-based diagnosis 1
Applied HP research and evaluation 1	Writing a paper
Health promotion principles and practice	Project work • Writing journal articles • Project report writing • Fieldwork • Quiz
Applied HP research and evaluation 2	Clinical practice guidelines
Psychosocial factors, health and MBM 2	CBP debrief
Medical professionalism	Optional: meetings between tutors and groups if needed by mutual arrangement
HP in medical practice	Evidence-based diagnosis 2
International health promotion	• Progress reports and feedback • Project write-up • Hypothetical sections • Poster
KM (Knowledge Management): Data to information to knowledge: Introduction to systematic reviews	Project report and paper briefing
Health promotion projects in community settings	• Finalising reports • Hypothetical sections • Revision and review
KM: Finding knowledge lost in the information	Knowledge management
KM: MEDLINE searching	HPKM revision
KM: Critical appraisal of a therapy article	

(*continued*)

TABLE 7.2 (*cont.*)

Semester 1 topics	Semester 2 topics
KM: Where are data stored? Who has access?	
Research ethics and project proposal submissions	
CPP Integration	
Literature appraisal and evaluation	
KM: Management of medical knowledge & online communities	
International health promotion	
Project proposals	

submit a peer assessment form for their group members at the end of each semester to help tutors monitor how well the project teams are working together.

Conclusion

Our experience has been that the delivery of theoretical HP content is significantly enhanced by an experientially and community-based HP project. A wide number of important learning objectives can be attained through the one project. For such a project to be successfully implemented it needs to be integrated with wide-ranging learning objectives, and assessment that is adequately supported by both academic and community-based faculty.

US CONTEXT OF DEVELOPMENT OF HEALTH PROMOTION AT GRADUATE AND POSTGRADUATE LEVELS

A Cooperative Agreement between the Centers for Disease Control and Prevention (CDC) and the AAMC was established in 2000 to facilitate improved and increased collaborations between public health and academic medicine to include a population health component in graduate medical education (GME) programmes. The reason for the introduction of this content in residency curricula was to help doctors contribute to long-range improvements in the health of the public.[5]

In 1998, the second Medical School Objectives Project Report, *Contemporary Issues in Medicine: medical informatics and population health*[6] recommended that all medical students receive training in epidemiology; biostatistics; disease prevention/health promotion; healthcare organisation, management and financing; and environmental and public health as part of their population health education. Enhancing the education of the medical community about population health, the public health system, prevention, and the role of physicians in public health is a well-recognised need. The Institute of Medicine (IOM) has continued to explore the challenges facing the American health system and has defined public health broadly as 'what we as a society do collectively to assure the conditions in which people can be healthy'.

The Institute of Medicine has played a leadership role in the US in advocating a bridge between clinical medicine's focus on individual health and public health's focus on population health.[7] Furthermore Gebbie *et al.*,[8] in the 2003 IOM report, *Who Will Keep the Public Healthy*, recommended that all physicians learn both the ecological model of the determinants of health and 13 population-health content areas (i.e. epidemiology, biostatistics, environmental health, health services administration, social and behavioural sciences, informatics, genomics, communication, cultural competence, community-based participatory research, global health, policy and law, and public health ethics).

In its 2007 report, *Training Physicians for Public Health Careers*,[9] the IOM reinforced the findings in the 2003 report by recommending that 'each graduate medical education programme identify and include the public health concepts and skills relevant to the practice of that specialty' and also move toward assessing competencies; the IOM also added leadership, clinical and community preventive services, and public health emergency preparedness to its recommended content areas. It supported the inclusion of this content through the continuum of physician education, regardless of specialty.

JOINT MEDICAL PROGRAM AT UCSF AND UC BERKELEY
Historical background of the programme
Karen Sokal-Gutierrez, John Edward Swartzberg and Amin Azzam

The University of California, Berkeley Joint Medical Program (JMP) was developed in 1971 to train doctors for practice as primary care physicians in the community. It was established as a health sciences and medical education programme based on a broader definition of health than medical care alone. It was designed to be responsive to societal and student needs and flexible enough to change as these needs changed. However, the Liaison Committee on Medical Education (LCME) of the Association of American Medical Colleges did not then accredit two-year programmes and so recommended concurrent registration at the University of California, San Francisco (UCSF). The LCME recommendation was adopted in 1973 and that year the LCME approved the shared programme. In 1974, funds for planning were allocated from the State to support the UC Berkeley-UCSF Joint Experimental Program in Medical Education, since renamed the UC Berkeley-UCSF Joint Medical Program. In 1978 the JMP became the five-year Master of Science/MD programme it remains today. Students spend three post-baccalaureate pre-clerkship years at Berkeley in simultaneous pursuit of a health-related Master's thesis and the pre-clerkship medical curriculum, followed by the two clinical years at UCSF. The JMP programme was established to teach 12 medical students each year at the Berkeley campus.

Educational innovation and learning environment
UC Berkeley's unique pedagogy in medical education focuses on training physician-leaders who are knowledgeable in the social, behavioural, ethical and human aspects of medicine, and who can play key roles in a rapidly shifting healthcare system. The course utilises a pure PBL process to deliver content known as contextual, integrated case-based curriculum (CICBC) integrated within a community context. Given the small a number of students, they attend 10.5 hours of PBL seminar per week, introducing principles of basic medical science, health policy, public health and clinical aspects of medicine taught in a contextual, integrated case-based format. The sequence includes curricula in biochemistry, histology, microbiology, immunology, neuro-anatomy,

pathology, physiology, pharmacology and clinical sciences. In a separate course, Clinical Skills, community-based and faculty-based physicians teach clinical skills utilising extensive facilities of the San Francisco Bay Area community hospitals, physician's offices and clinics.

The JMP is academically housed within the UC Berkeley School of Public Health. This affiliation provides leading-edge medical education that meets the needs of a changing healthcare environment. There are specific components of this educational innovation that have an impact on medical education, workforce issues and the community. The whole curriculum is purposefully integrated with the nature of health, illness and community while promoting discovery, self-reflection and lifelong learning.

PRIME-US curriculum: the genesis of the programme

For almost 30 years the enrolment within California medical schools had not increased. A comparison between student demographic data within medical education versus state demographic data showed that there was a mismatch with the growing diverse population in the communities in California and the type of medical practitioner being produced or not being developed to address the domestic healthcare needs of the community. This scenario raised a number of concerns for medical education in particular and higher education in general. It required an intricate response and comprehensive educational strategy to address these concerns at political, social and education levels. Consequently this process raised a number of competing values and questions, relating to ensuring equity while increasing diversity in student admissions. According to Komaromy, et al.,[10] the State of California classifies Medical Service Study Areas (MSSAs) as:

➤ 'Rural MSSA' – population density less than 250 residents per square mile and contains no city with a population of 50 000 residents or greater
➤ 'High minority' MSSA – population of African-American or Latino residents greater than or equal to 85th percentile of all areas of the state
➤ 'High poverty' MSSA – mean household income in the lowest quartile of mean incomes for the state.

As the University of California has a number of campuses, a statewide medical education funded strategy in the state of California resulted in University of California campuses adopting PRIME (Program in Medical Education) into its medical education programme based on the community health needs and the MSSA classifications previously outlined. The PRIME focus across University of California campuses includes:

➤ UC, San Francisco and UC, Berkeley Joint Medical Program focused PRIME on 'Urban Underserved' (known as PRIME-US)
➤ UC, Davis focused PRIME on 'Rural Health'
➤ UC, San Diego focused PRIME on 'Health Equity'
➤ UC, Los Angeles focused on 'Leadership' and 'Health Disparities'
➤ UC, Irvine focused PRIME on 'Latino Community Health'.

PRIME-US program at University of California, Berkeley and San Francisco

Within the JMP and UCSF medical school, an innovative Program in Medical Education for the Urban Underserved (PRIME-US) was developed for those medical students committed to working with the urban underserved. The programme includes

11 students at the UCSF School of Medicine and four additional students from the JMP on the UC Berkeley campus. These students are required to complete normal academic admission processes for entry into medicine plus an additional selection process of an essay and interview with the admissions team which consists of PRIME faculty, staff and students. The establishment of this programme adopted key strategies to alleviate physician shortages across the following categories: applicant pool, medical education and practice environment.[11]

Table 7.3 provides an overview of the details of the PRIME-US curriculum incorporating an MS degree across a five-year curriculum across two campuses. For detailed information on the clerkship years, please visit www.medschool.ucsf.edu/curriculum/clinical/.

MOUNT SINAI SCHOOL OF MEDICINE (MSSM)
Elizabeth Garland, Erica Friedman and Richard Bordowitz

Mount Sinai School of Medicine (MSSM) has a four-year graduate curriculum. The underlying pedagogy is a combination of lectures, labs, small-group discussion, case-based learning, longitudinal patient experiences and self-directed learning. It actively engages students through various teaching and learning opportunities between the preclinical and clinical years with the surrounding community, its affiliate community hospitals, its tertiary hospital and its research departments and institutes. The primary aim of the curriculum is to transform the student from layperson to doctor through the acquisition of knowledge, skills and attitudes that are patient-centred.

The first year of medical school, although taught by scientists and clinicians, is focused on the fundamental principles of science and its application of this knowledge to the *care of the patient*. During this year, Epidemiology and Preventive Medicine is introduced through small-group exercises and case studies in preventive medicine and critical appraisal of published research. The course emphasises the logic of inquiry and concepts relevant to the decision-making process in clinical medicine and these concepts are aligned with the two-year longitudinal doctoring course called 'The Art and Science of Medicine', where health policy and ethical decision making are taught.

The focus of the second-year MSSM programme is on exploring the basic pathophysiology of organs, the body's major systems and continued clinical skills development, including clinical reasoning. At the end of the second year, through the longitudinal patient experiences, The Art and Science of Medicine and the Epidemiology courses, key issues of critical importance to the practice of medicine are addressed, which are expanded upon in Years 3 and 4 of the programme. At this point, students should be successful reporters and progressing towards being successful interpreters of the issues impacting on the care of patients.

Year 3 marks the beginning of the transformation into a caregiver. The third-year curriculum is designed to assist students with applying the principles learned in the first two years to the diagnosis and treatment of patients in both inpatient and outpatient settings. Equally important is the honing of the attributes of an exemplary professional, applying ethical principles to patient management, providing patient-centred, culturally competent care, respecting the value of team interactions and developing and refining communication skills. The third year is made up of four 12-week clinical clerkship modules covering paediatrics, internal medicine and geriatrics, obstetrics and

TABLE 7.3 PRIME-US curriculum, goals, activities and outcomes

PRIME-US goals	PRIME-US curriculum	PRIME-US activities	Outcomes
Attract medical students from diverse backgrounds who have a strong interest in caring for the urban underserved in the United States	*Summer Introduction* Students participate in a 1–2 week stipend-supported immersion experience in the Bay Area	In addition to and coordinated with the JMP medical curriculum, the PRIME-US curriculum includes: • biweekly seminars on community-based experiences by experts on homelessness, immigrant health, the prison system and healthcare disparities	Students have contributed to scholarship in their area of interest through studies that explored questions through diverse lenses, including: • epidemiological • ethical • policy
Provide a medical education experience for these students to equip and support them to become leaders in the care of urban underserved communities	*Core Seminar Series* Regularly scheduled afternoon seminars provide students with a solid foundation in the principles, practices and populations of urban underserved care	• an immersion clinical experience across three years at a community site focused on providing care for underserved populations	• economic • historical • anthropological • artistic • clinical, and • scientific aspects of human health and disease
Enable these students to serve as a catalyst for others at UCSF and the JMP to appreciate the rewards and challenges of caring for the urban underserved	*Clinical Immersion* Students are placed in community-based clinics to learn about direct patient care in community settings	• clinical clerkships with UCSF PRIME-US, with rotations in underserved communities including San Francisco General Hospital and the Fresno campus of UCSF	
Increase the number of UCSF medical school graduates who choose to pursue careers devoted to improving the health and healthcare of the urban underserved through leadership roles as community-engaged	*Community Engagement Program* Students learn a framework for building community partnerships and participate in service learning and community-based projects *Masters Degree* A fifth year of study is included in PRIME-US	• master's thesis work related to healthcare and social advocacy for the urban	

PRIME-US goals	PRIME-US curriculum	PRIME-US activities	Outcomes
clinicians, educators, researchers and social policy advocates	*Mentorship* A formal mentorship programme ensures personal, professional and academic success	underserved in the community supported by a coherent scholarly programme approved by the Master's Faculty • strong academic and social support provided by dedicated staff and faculty to ensure personal, professional and academic success	

gynaecology, anaesthesiology, neurology, ambulatory medicine, psychiatry, surgery and clinical skills, and one-week periods in which the entire class comes together to explore the interdisciplinary nature of patient care and revisit health policy issues. For example, the focus of the paediatrics clerkship is on principles of health promotion, disease prevention and the recognition of common health problems that are unique to the newborn period, childhood and adolescence. By focusing on growth and development, medical students begin to understand the impact of family, community and society on child health and well-being. During the ambulatory medicine four-week rotation, students learn to provide comprehensive healthcare for individuals and families by focusing on disease prevention and health/wellness promotion. They also work in teams to complete a service learning project after they have identified a systems issue impeding patient care (e.g. health literacy, insurance coverage restrictions, etc.).

The focus in the fourth year at MSSM is on facilitating professional practice with required rotations in critical care, emergency medicine, anatomic radiology and a four-week sub-internship in either medicine or paediatrics. Throughout the year students meet with course directors, chairs and specialty advisors to tailor a fourth-year curriculum that permits exploration of each individual's interests.

Mount Sinai School of Medicine residency training programme in general preventive medicine

Background

In 2004, the Healthy People Curriculum Task Force provided more detailed recommendations regarding the content of health professionals' education in clinical prevention and population health in four domains: evidence base for practice; clinical preventive services; health systems and health policy; and community aspects of practice.[12] It recommended that models be developed for integrating public health principles and practice into physician education at both undergraduate and graduate levels and that each graduate medical education programme identify and include public health concepts and skills that are relevant to the practice of that specialty.

Because limited opportunities had existed for the medical and public health practice communities to work together on educational agendas for medical students and residents, a pilot programme was implemented in 2003 through the AAMC-CDC Cooperative Agreement to establish Regional Medicine–Public Health Education Centers (RMPHECs) in seven medical schools. The RMPHECs were required to partner with a local and/or state health agency to improve the public health/population health education for their medical students. In 2006, funding became available to build on the pilot programme across 11 medical schools to pursue the 'full integration' of population health into their curricula through collaborations with their public health colleagues. The MSSM residency training programme is an example of such 'full integration'. Table 7.4 provides an overview of the Medicine–Public Health course requirements for residents participating in this integrated programme.

Purpose

The purpose of the MSSM residency training programme is to educate and train physicians in the application of the population aspects of medicine for problem solving in the planning, administration, organisation and evaluation of healthcare systems to improve health, while focusing on the promotion of wellness and the prevention of disease.

TABLE 7.4: Mapping of ACPM and MSSM goals and objectives

American College of Preventive Medicine's published competencies for its programme goals and objectives	Goals and objectives for the MPH Degree
I Generic preventive medicine competencies	*Goals for instruction*
• Communicate to target groups and to the media in a clear and effective manner, both orally and in writing, the levels of risk from potential hazards and the rationale for selected intervention	*To educate our students to enhance the health of populations*
• Communicate to health professionals in a clear and effective manner, both orally and in writing, the findings and the rationale for selected interventions	• Provide instruction in how to assess the health status of populations, design appropriate interventions and evaluate the success of such interventions
• Prepare and critique a proposal for programme resources	• Evaluate students' mastery of these skills within the curriculum by examination and through their participation in small-group discussions
• Order priorities for major projects and/or programmes according to definable criteria	*To educate our students to consider the health of individuals within the context of community and environmental influences*
• Use computers for specific applications relevant to preventive medicine	• Provide training in community health, preventive medicine and environmental health that allows our students to identify and recognise a variety of avenues and mechanisms through which community, cultural and environmental factors can influence health
• Interpret legal and regulatory authority relating to protection and promotion of the public's health	
• Identify ethical, social, and cultural issues relating to policies, risks, research and interventions in public health and preventive medicine contexts	• Evaluate students' understanding of these issues by examination and through their participation in small-group discussions
• Identify the processes by which decisions are made within an organisation or agency and their points of influence	*To educate our students to work in an interdisciplinary milieu*
• Identify and coordinate the integrated use of necessary and sufficient resources to improve the community's health	• Provide small-group participatory activities with our courses that involve interaction among students and faculty from multiple disciplines
• Disease or injury and to promote wellness	• Include faculty and guest lecturers throughout the curriculum from a variety of disciplines
II Epidemiology and biostatistics competencies	
• Design and conduct an epidemiologic study	

(continued)

TABLE 7.4 (cont.)

American College of Preventive Medicine's published competencies for its programme goals and objectives	Goals and objectives for the MPH Degree
• Select and describe limitations of appropriate statistical analysis as applied to a particular data set. Translate epidemiologic findings into a recommendation for a specific intervention to control a public health problem • Design and operate a surveillance system *III Management and administration planning* • Formulate policy for a given health issue • Develop goals and objectives for a given health issue • Design an implementation plan to address goals and objectives • Conduct an evaluation and/or quality assessment based on measurable criteria (process and outcome) • Manage the operation of a programme or project, including human and fiscal resources *IV Clinical preventive medicine competencies* • Develop, implement and refine screening programmes for groups to identify risks for disease or injury and opportunities to promote wellness • Design and implement clinical preventive services for groups and individuals • Implement individual and community-based interventions to modify or eliminate identified risks for of significance within general preventive medicine and public health	*To educate our students to critically evaluate published research* • Evaluate students' abilities to critically evaluate published literature within the epidemiology curriculum through written examinations and student participation in small-group discussions. Provide students with opportunities to practise critical evaluation of research through regularly convened journal clubs and grand rounds • Evaluate students' abilities to critically appraise the literature related to their thesis topic through critical, mentored assessment of the introductory sections of the thesis *Goal for research* *To equip students with the appropriate tools to conduct community-based research that will provide a scientific basis for health promotion and disease prevention* • Evaluate students' mastery of the principles of epidemiology and biostatistics within those courses in the curriculum, by examination and through their participation in small-group discussions • Provide each student with an academic advisor who will assist in identifying one or more thesis advisors to provide strong mentorship throughout the student's research activities. These advisors will mentor, advise and support each student through their time in the MPH Program and especially in the process of developing the student's thesis

American College of Preventive Medicine's published competencies for its programme goals and objectives	Goals and objectives for the MPH Degree
V Occupational and environmental health competencies • Assess individual risk for occupational/environmental disorders using an environmental and occupational history • Identify potential occupational and environmental hazards in defined populations, and assess and respond to identifiable risks	*Goals for service* *To collaborate with communities in initiatives to improve health and prevent disease* Conduct an annual faculty survey and maintain a database that documents the service activities of our programme faculty and students in community-based activities. This database will serve as a resource for students seeking mentors and advisors on particular topics *To provide students with opportunities to apply their public health knowledge in the public and private sectors* • Create partnerships with the public health community in New York and nationally to develop and maintain a set of field practicum offerings for students • Create stated, written learning objectives for each field practicum experience to ensure that each student has guidelines that they can follow in the practicum • Evaluate each student's fulfilment of the stated learning objectives for each practicum experience through formal written evaluation by the practicum preceptors

Program goals

➤ To maintain a high-quality, accredited residency program that enables the resident to apply for board certification by the American Board of Preventive Medicine.
➤ To create qualified physicians for the practice of general preventive medicine for academic medical centres, Departments of Health and other health agencies.
➤ To provide a broad and flexible preventive medicine training program, able to meet the needs of a diverse group of residents.

The residency program is fully accredited by the Accreditation Council for Graduate Medical Education and adheres to the American College of Preventive Medicine's published competencies for its programme goals and objectives as mapped in Table 7.4. The two-year residency program includes concurrent academic and practicum phases, each equivalent to one full year leading to a Master of Public Health degree. The full general preventive medicine program requirements can be accessed at www.acgme.org, click on Review Committees then Preventive Medicine or go direct to the site at www.acgme.org/acWebsite/RRC_380/380_prIndex.asp.

General preventive medicine residents MPH course requirements

General preventive medicine residents must complete 41 required credits, with a further credit accrued though electives, seminars and independent study. Residents must meet early on with the Residency Director to plan for completion of a total of 42 credits. The breakdown of credits is outlined below.

Year 1

➤ Clinical Environmental & Occupational Medicine	3 credits
➤ Introduction to Epidemiology	3 credits
➤ Advanced Occ. & Envir. Pulmonary Disease	2 credits
➤ Research Methods	1 credit
➤ Introduction to Biostatistics	3 credits
➤ Strategic & Program Management	3 credits
➤ Epidemiology of Infectious Disease	3 credits
➤ Multivariable Methods	3 credits
➤ Current Topics in Clinical Preventive Medicine	3 credits
➤ Journal Club for Health Professionals (year-long)	1 credit
➤ Seminar in Applied Preventive Medicine (year-long)	1 credit

Year 2

➤ Seminar in Applied Preventive Medicine (year-long)	1 credit
➤ Journal Club for Health Professionals (year-long)	1 credit
➤ Case Studies in Epidemiology: Envir. & Occ.	2 credits
➤ Elective	3 credits
➤ Practicum	0 credits
➤ Master's Thesis	4 credits

One course from below
Socio-Behavioural Health:

➤ Behavioural Medicine	3 credits
➤ Culture, Illness & Community Health	3 credits

One course from below
➤ Underserved Populations   3 credits
➤ Introduction to Medical Anthropology   3 credits
➤ Health Literacy   3 credits
➤ Addiction Medicine   2 credits
➤ Life Cycle of Violence: Implications for Public Health   2 credits
➤ What's Sex Got to Do With It? Teen Pregnancy   2 credits
➤ Prevention & Intervention

One elective from below
➤ Global Health
➤ Outcomes Research
➤ Occupational and Environmental Tracks
➤ Individually arranged independent study

CONCLUSION

Eriksson and Lindström[13] argue that health promotion is a human right that requires a humanistic approach, with coordination of activities between professions and professionals in societies where the individual becomes an active participant. The three examples described above attempt to inculcate a 'culture of prevention' into practice by ensuring that health promotion is a core component that is vertically and horizontally integrated across the medical curriculum. It also highlights a range of teaching approaches in a variety of settings including the development of specific competencies to identify and strengthen health promotion practice.

The MSSM example in particular highlights the importance of such integration within its graduate medical programme. By linking the residency training program with the Masters degree in Public Health and the American College of Preventive Medicine's published competencies, their residents will be equipped to address contemporary health promotion needs within the community. The JMP/PRIME example highlights not only the educational outcomes for the students but the development of health promotion competencies in relation to addressing community health issues, morbidities, cross-cultural issues and innovative approaches to quality care across a number of settings. The community-based practice example highlights the importance of community partnerships where second-year medical students experience first-hand the role of continuity of care across health professional disciplines. They learn about the fundamental skills of the doctor-patient relationship while working with clients from community organisations to:
➤ understand their health needs and the impact of social determinants on health
➤ change unhealthy behaviours through programme development
➤ promote healthy behaviours through implementation of a health promotion project.

Health promotion in medical education also requires students to utilise effective communication, relationship-building, facilitation, negotiation and partnership skills in the provision of preventive services.[14] Koo and Thacker[15] strongly advocate a multipronged approach that includes opportunities for academic and experiential learning, so as to establish population health concepts with physicians at all stages of their education.

The three prototypes of health promotion curriculum show that medical education has an opportunity to foster student learning in preventive medicine at various levels of medical education. Of course our experience has shown that there is a need at an institutional level for uncompromising support from medical educationists across the spectrum of disciplines; this often brings with it its own challenges in shifting attitudes and behaviour throughout medical education.

REFERENCES

1 Pomrehn P, Davis M, Chen DW, Barker W. Prevention for the 21st century. *Acad Med.* 2000; **75**(7): S5–13.
2 Garr D, Lackland D, Wilson D. Prevention education and evaluation in U.S. medical schools: a status report. *Acad Med.* 2000; **75**(7 Suppl.): S14–21.
3 Ibid.
4 Jones KV, Hsu-Hage BH. Health promotion projects: skill and attitude learning for medical students. *Med Educ.* 1999; **33**(8): 585–91.
5 Association of American Medical Colleges. *CDC-AAMC Cooperative Agreement.* Washington, DC: AAMC; 1998. Available at: www.aamc.org/members/cdc/about/start.htm (accessed 20 March 2009).
6 Association of American Medical Colleges. *Contemporary Issues in Medicine: medical informatics and population health.* Washington, DC: AAMC; 1998. Available at: https://services.aamc.org/publications/index.cfm?fuseaction=Product.displayForm&prd_id=199&prv_id=240 (accessed 31 October 2009).
7 Strelnick AH, Swiderski D, Fornari A, *et al.* The residency program in social medicine of Montefiore Medical Center: 37 years of mission-driven, interdisciplinary training in primary care, population health, and social medicine. *Acad Med.* 2008; **83**(4): 378–89.
8 Gebbie K, Rosenstock L, Hernandez LM, editors. *Who Will Keep the Public Healthy? Educating public health professionals for the 21st century.* Washington, DC: The National Academies Press; 2003.
9 Hernandez LM, Munthali AW, editors. *Training Physicians for Public Health Careers.* Washington, DC: The National Academies Press; 2007.
10 Komaromy M, Grumbach K, Drake M, *et al.* The role of black and Hispanic physicians in providing healthcare for underserved populations. *New Engl J Med.* 1996; **334**: 1305–10.
11 Grumbach K, Coffman J, Liu R, *et al. Strategies for Increasing Physician Supply in Medically Underserved Communities in California.* Berkeley, CA: California Program on Access to Care, California Policy Research Center; 1999.
12 Allan J, Barwick T, Cashman S, *et al.* Clinical prevention and population health: curriculum framework for health professions. *Am J Prev Med.* 2004; **27**(5): 417–22. Available at: www.aptrweb.org/resources/publications.html#AJPMArticles (accessed 31 October 2009).
13 Eriksson M, Lindström B. A salutogenic interpretation of the Ottawa Charter. *Health Promot Int.* 2008; **23**(2): 190–9.
14 Dube CE, O'Donnell JF, Novack DH. Communication skills for preventive interventions. *Acad Med.* 2000; **75**(7): S45–54.
15 Koo D, Thacker S. The education of physicians: a CDC perspective. *Acad Med.* 2008; **83**(4): 399–407.

CHAPTER 8

Health promotion in curricula: levels of responsibility and accountability

Tangerine Holt and Ann Wylie

with additional contributions from Markus Herrmann,
Andreas Klement, Craig Hassed, Pat Nolan, Albert Lee and Richard Shircore

The responsibility is old; only the context is new.[1]

THE INTERNATIONAL CONTEXT

The voices of noted academics from around the world have emphasised that standards of excellence in medical education are required to ensure medical graduates have the requisite knowledge, skills, expertise and professional attitudes required to tackle contemporary health problems. There is little doubt that accountability in medical education is a social responsibility which emphasises the importance of framing adequate educational strategies and paradigms for the advancement of medical education. The quality of medical education is dependent on an integrated setting of academic rigour and clinical excellence. A socially responsible medical school has the ability to perceive the needs of society and reacts accordingly, and a socially accountable school also consults society about priorities and provides evidence of impact of its deeds.[2]

Walton[3] in his critical analysis of primary healthcare in Europe highlighted that medical education was scarcely cognisant of the importance of primary healthcare development despite major international developments, statements and approaches to healthcare. These include: the Alma-Ata Declaration (1978); the 'Health for All' movement which has become the official policy of the World Health Organization (1981); and the 'Mobilizing Universities for Health' approach, which was the topic of the technical discussions at the World Health Assembly in May 1984, resulting in the educationally significant resolution WHA.37.31 of 17 May 1984. The focus of the World Conference on Medical Education in 1988 considered how medical schools and other educational bodies should respond to the challenge set out in the Alma-Ata Declaration to achieve the aims of 'health for all' by the year 2000.[4] Amos, *et al.*[5] linked medical education with the fundamental need to reorient health services in order to achieve improvements in health, as expressed in the Ottawa Charter on Health Promotion.[6]

For example, *Australia's Health*[7] is based on the conceptual framework where the levels of health and well-being, including diseases and disability, are influenced by a complex interplay between health determinants, interventions and resources, including systems. In Australia, almost 70% of total health expenditure is funded by government.[8] In 2002, the Australian Health Ministers' Advisory Council (AHMAC) endorsed a set of 10 priorities to guide the development of health information, which included population health, equity and access and the health labour force which was later published.[9] In Britain health promotion has been identified as a major priority for the National Health Service (NHS) in the provision of preventive services and health education through primary care. In the USA, Schroeder[10] raised an important discussion around the role and responsibility of academic medicine with the health of the public. By doing so, leaders of medical schools are required to set an example that health professionals have a responsibility to serve the public. McIntosh, et al.[11] noted that such recommendations have been made by serious entities such as:

➤ the World Health Organization:[12] medical education should emphasise public health and preventive medicine training
➤ the Pew Health Professions Commission:[13,14] health professions schools must ensure that their students are competent in community-based care
➤ the Association of American Medical Colleges, in its 1998 Medical School Objectives Project report:[15] develop educational outcomes which cultivate physicians who are *dutiful* and who 'collaborate and use systematic approaches for promoting, maintaining, and improving the health of individuals and populations'.

EDUCATIONAL DEVELOPMENTS

The assumption that teaching occurs naturally as a result of content expertise is challenged.[16] The paucity of formal education about the subject, 'health promotion', has been one of the most important impediments to teaching about health promotion at both undergraduate and postgraduate levels. Hence, it is not surprising that many doctors have not developed their role in health promotion as they are not fully aware of their potential contribution or feel they lack the knowledge and skills necessary to be effective in this role.[17]

Since the 1990s, medical education has been fundamentally reformed in the developed world in response to societal trends towards increased accountability from the public, profession and government bodies; with quality assurance in the establishment of academic standards for the achievement of graduate outcomes by accreditation bodies. The process of change is continuing, in how medical educators teach and what they teach to educate medical students. The greatest change taking place is in the underlying pedagogy of medical education.[18] These changes include:

➤ application of a variety of teaching and learning approaches in medical education which is more student-centred, using small-group discussions and self-directed learning through exposure to aspects of healthcare that reflect the needs of society
➤ utilisation of experiential learning in community sites so that students understand the context of people's lives and not as patients who present with illness at a hospital
➤ application of technology to discover new information which adds to the evidence base of professional practice

➤ integration of curriculum components both horizontally across discipline-based content and vertically across the medical programme, with assessment closely aligned to the principles being taught.

Such educational developments, together with the increasing complexity of the curriculum whether at undergraduate or postgraduate level of training, have led to the recognition that all those who teach require some form of training in education.[19] As faculty members are central to the successful adoption of any new curriculum paradigm, the active involvement of faculty early in the process of change is necessary.[20]

The following examples are a collection of reports on the pedagogy that underpins the curriculum structure on health promotion in medical education. The authors raise issues about governance structure, curriculum management, teaching activity, learning outcomes, assessment and clinical experience. The content provides the reader with an understanding of curriculum governance and its approach to health promotion curriculum organisation, and the philosophy of teaching and learning as expressed in international models of health promotion in medical education. Each example outlines its schema on how best to educate medical students in health promotion by highlighting the principles of curriculum design, educational encounters and the learning environment, use of education strategies, assessment and evaluation in medical education on health promotion.

FUTURE DIRECTIONS

Koo and Thacker[21] believe that doctors who are fully trained to use population health skills are more likely to improve health using an integrated model of healthcare. These doctors focus on protecting the health of their patients, not just caring for them after they become ill. To achieve this vision of multipronged health promotion, education throughout undergraduate, graduate and postgraduate levels is required. A shortcoming of most medical school curricula is their focus on the 'medical model', which addresses health at an individual level.[22,23] This was illustrated by the Association of American Medical Colleges' GQ Graduation Questionnaire (available at www.aamc.org/data/gq/allschoolsreports/start.htm) by McIntosh, et al.,[24] which highlighted the following problem:

> [Approximately] 32.1% of graduating medical students in 2006 reported that inadequate time during medical school was devoted to the role of community health and social service agencies; 32.1% noted this for public health, 21.4% for community medicine, 19.5% for clinical epidemiology, and 14.3% for health promotion and disease prevention.

Medical schools and other stakeholders can pursue optimal patterns of healthcare most effectively through partnerships with one another.[25] Furthermore, medical educators have a responsibility to address the expectation of the community of producing doctors who serve community needs. They are central to the successful adoption of any new curriculum paradigm.[26]

The examples that follow in this chapter demonstrate the importance of building partnerships between community and higher education. The teaching and learning approaches outlined in the examples emphasise important adult education themes of student autonomy; learning from experience; collaborative learning; and health professional as educator in the teacher–learner relationships. These international examples showcase prevention content, educational opportunities, and a range of learning environments and experiential learning in health promotion in medical education.

> Ultimately, the successful integration of disease prevention and health promotion principles into medical student education does not depend on new curriculum, curriculum coordination and integration, or the use of new educational technology. Ultimately, the academic health sciences centres and schools of medicine must reconnect with the health needs of people, forming alliances with community groups and programs that focus on prevention. This reconnection demands a shift in core institutional values – from the paradigm of healing to the paradigm of health.[27]

To bring about change, a way forward may be for medical education to view health promotion teaching and learning through community collaboration *as analogous to medical student placements in clinical education.*[28]

EXAMPLE 1: INSTITUTE OF GENERAL PRACTICE AT THE MEDICAL FACULTIES OF THE UNIVERSITIES OF HALLE-WITTENBERG AND MAGDEBURG, GERMANY

Markus Herrmann and Andreas Klement

Are curricula fit for purpose?

Prevention and health promotion are of increasing importance in modern health systems due to economic and demographic factors. In response, German legislators have, since 2003, introduced the 'Cross-Sectional Term 10' (Q10), called 'Prevention and Health Promotion', as one of 12 'new' interdisciplinary subjects in the undergraduate medical curriculum. A national catalogue of educational objectives, evaluation requirements and central scientific steering of this extensive reform were waived on political reasons.[29] Thus, teaching evaluation and curriculum development is conducted regionally at both medical faculties in Saxony-Anhalt.

Successful prevention and effective health promotion in medical practice require training in specific abilities, skills and attitudes. Important aspects include: patient-oriented shared decision making, risk communication and focus on key resources. Till now it is unknown whether support of these characteristics at a national level has been achieved through the introduction of Q10. A survey of 5000 physicians who completed their medical undergraduate curriculum in Germany during 1998–2003, however, indicates that little is to be expected: only 15% of medical school graduates felt themselves to be 'very well' or 'well' prepared for professional practice based on their university studies. The relevance of curricula to practice is rated with an average value of 4.2 on a five-point Likert scale (5=insufficient).[30] These results are confirmed by a questionnaire conducted in 2002 on 671 prospective physicians at seven German universities, who evaluated their medical studies retrospectively. Blatant deficits are seen primarily in the imparting of practical medical skills and psychosocial competencies when dealing with their patients.[31]

In 2007 before the start of the cross-sectional term in prevention and health promotion, medical students in Halle were surveyed before starting the term in the effectiveness of their education in 'prevention and health promotion'. A five-point Likert scale (5=insufficient) for the questions was used. Those responding gave a predominantly negative assessment with 3.4 as average degree of agreement (n=93; sd=0.79). It appears that until now at the Medical Faculty in Halle, prevention and health promotion have been inadequately integrated into the whole context of the medical curriculum – whether this can be changed meaningfully by a curriculum segment at the end of the course of study remains open for future analysis.[32]

How are standards for content and skills set?

Regarding conceptualisation of the new Cross-Sectional-Terms the German legislators have left universities a wide range of freedom in performance of content and methods. As products of local expert consensus, different educational concepts were generated at each of 36 medical schools. In Halle, the educational objectives, curriculum design and evaluation were developed based on an initial literature survey and the academic prevention textbook most widely used in Germany. Consensus was reached among the participating institutions through a simplified three-step Delphi procedure.

The variation in curriculum content among universities could be disadvantageous to students, particularly regarding the written part of the second state medical examination, which is administered in a nationally standardised manner. In individual cross-sectional areas, such as the cross-sectional term ('medicine for the elderly'), there are now national recommendations from interdisciplinary author groups concerning educational objectives; the national decisions made by the Institute for Medical and Pharmaceutical Examination Questions (IMPP) concerning exam-relevant knowledge could orient themselves toward these recommendations.[33] For the cross-sectional term, 'prevention and health promotion', this desirable development has yet to occur. Few universities have published detailed educational objectives catalogues with elaboration on operationalised educational objectives, identification of competence levels and requirements regarding teaching formats; relevant development is presently under way at the University of Halle.[34]

A first 'stocktaking' of Q10's implementation at the German medical faculties was presented in 2007. Here, considerable differences in lengths of time allotted for the curriculum, elements of practice with patients, and the format for the graded certificates are visible. While extensive conformity exists among the universities regarding prevention-related topics, there are very different foci set in health promotion.[35]

To reach consensus across universities on educational objectives catalogues and teaching formats, knowledge of area-specific student attitudes, expectations, learning strategies and even preliminary estimations can be helpful.[36] But there is currently no published information on this for the German-speaking countries.

How are links between practitioners and the university used to inform curriculum development and implementation?

For the conduct of a mandatory two-week-long clerkship in general practice during the semester preceding the cross-sectional term, 'prevention and health promotion', the University of Halle supports a network of 80 accredited teaching GPs. Due to very positive experiences – not only in Halle – regarding student and instructor motivation in a decentralised one-on-one learning situation, this model was integrated into the Q10 curriculum.[37] In this context, a predetermined number of students are randomly assigned to their former teaching practice for a case-based graded certificate including patient contact. The instructing physician refers a risk-stratified patient to the student and supervises the student's assessment and suggestions made during consultation. In a seminar of 20 students, five presentations on 'prevention cases' with risk assessments and documented risk communication by 'medical students as health coaches' can be discussed at each meeting.[38] Students with other, more theoretical 'problem-based prevention projects' can profit synergistically from the experiences of their classmates who have patient contact.[39]

The university supports the problem- and case-based graded certificates in Q10 through the reservation of a two-week block free of competing examinations for the students and through the prestige of accreditation as 'university-associated teaching practices' for the instructing physicians. The participating institutions learned interdisciplinary cooperation first-hand with the cross-sectional term, prevention and health promotion. University instruction comes into direct contact with real (preventive) practice with all its possibilities and limitations.[40]

How are these links and partnerships maintained?

Participating faculty holds two or three regular pre- and post-meetings annually for Q10. As post-work, the evaluation data are presented and individual teaching experiences discussed. During the preparatory phase, possible changes to curriculum design or evaluation are addressed. For practitioners giving instruction, four to six 'teacher to teacher' sessions are conducted annually by the Institute of General Practice. An internet-based evaluation system as benchmarking for decentralised instruction is under construction, as is a practice network for research projects.

EXAMPLE 2: MONASH UNIVERSITY, AUSTRALIA

Craig Hassed

The broad overview of the Monash University health promotion program, objectives and delivery were given in Chapter 7. Here we will discuss some of the other issues relating to integration, accountability and links with outside agencies.

Where HP sits within the curriculum

The formal health promotion (HP) content in the curriculum is embedded in the subject Community-Based Practice (CBP) alongside the Community Partnership Program (CPP). It accounts for 15% of curriculum time and is spread over the whole of second year in Monash's five-year undergraduate course. HP belongs in Theme 2 of the curriculum – Population, Society, Health and Illness – and CPP belongs within Theme 1 – Personal and Professional Development.

Who is responsible?

The two convenors of the HP content of CBP are from the Department of General Practice – part of the School of Primary Healthcare (SPHC) – and the Department of Epidemiology and Preventive Medicine – part of the School of Public Health and Preventive Medicine (SPHPM). The knowledge management component of the HP program is convened by the Monash Institute of Health Services Research (MIHSR), which is also part of SPHPM. MIHSR has its background in applied research, education, advocacy and innovation in the areas of clinical management, service delivery and health policy, with the aim of improving health services delivery.

HP content is congruent with the core business of the key departments involved in its delivery. The approach was taken that HP embraces a broad spectrum of HP activities including the biomedical, psychological and socio-environmental perspectives. It is hoped that students will see HP as relevant all the way from its being promoted by clinicians with their patients to the population perspective. It has always been a core aim of the course to help students to see the relevance of HP content to their future work as medical practitioners rather than its merely being seen as an activity carried on by non-medical community-based groups or epidemiologists.

These departments of General Practice and Epidemiology are deemed to have the necessary skills, resources and personnel to be able to deliver what is a resource- and labour-intensive program. The most intensive part of the program is the HP project.

How does HP relate to other parts of curriculum?

At Monash HP is a central part of a vertically and horizontally integrated curriculum (*see* Table 8.1). Thus, skills and knowledge taught in one part of the curriculum are relevant to other parts. For example, the generic skills of literature appraisal, understanding research methodology and ethics, understanding behavioural psychology and being able to work in multidisciplinary teams are skills which the students will hone in the HP course and they are highly likely to need such skills for the rest of their working lives.

Accountability to regulatory bodies and partnership agencies

The HP course is implemented through the Theme 2 committee, which looks after Theme 2 content across the five years of the medical course. HP is also overseen by

TABLE 8.1 An example of vertical and horizontal integration of HP content and themes across the medical curriculum

Year	HP content	Description
Year 1	Health Enhancement Program[41] (HEP)	The HEP is an experientially based lifestyle and mindfulness-based stress management program which is part of the Theme 1 content of first year. In this program students learn to apply various health promoting strategies to themselves so as to be able to benefit their own personal well-being as well as to understand how to apply behaviour change strategies for patients, to learn clinical skills and to better integrate the biomedical, psychological and social sciences. The HEP is described in more detail in Chapter 14
Year 1	Epidemiology	In Year 1, students learn the basics of epidemiology, population health and statistics. This knowledge is applied in the Year 2 project work in particular
Years 1–3	Patient-centred learning/ Problem-based learning (PCL/ PBL)	Throughout the first three years of the course students have weekly cases. In Year 1, PCL presents weekly cases which often have lifestyle and preventive issues, many of which arise from the HEP content. In years 2 and 3 students have PBL via weekly cases which reinforce lifestyle issues and content from the HEP lectures and project work
Year 2	International health	In Year 2, three hours of lecture time and two hours of tutorial time is dedicated to international health promotion covering such topics as the health issues which impact on other countries around the world, understanding the impact of war and natural disasters, the particular challenges faced by developing countries, the impact of HIV/AIDS and the various ways in which a medical student or doctor can pursue an interest in international health
Years 2–3	Evidence-based medicine (EBM)	This is a subtheme which recurs throughout the entire curriculum. Students are required to apply the principles of EBM, literature searching and critical appraisal to their project work and perform literature reviews as part of their project proposals. In Year 3 students have a more extensive series of 10 two-hour tutorials where they go into this topic in far more detail
Year 3	Occupational health	In Year 3 students have a series of eight two-hour tutorials where many of the health promotion principles they learn are applied in the workplace setting
Year 4	General practice	The main GP rotation takes place in Year 4. Students learn clinical and consulting skills, part of which includes applying lifestyle, stress management and behaviour change strategies to a variety of cases. Preventive opportunities need to be considered in every case

(continued)

TABLE 8.1 (*cont.*)

Year	HP content	Description
Years 2 and 4	Psychology	The psychology content in Years 2 and 4 includes content related to health behaviours. Students perform a behaviour change project in Year 2 where they apply one of these strategies to a personal behaviour of their own choosing
Years 1 to 5	Biomedical knowledge	Great effort is made throughout all years to ensure that Theme 3 content – Foundations of Medicine – is integrated with the psychological and social sciences and clinical skills. For example, the HEP and HP lectures are heavily referenced to establish the scientific underpinnings of the program

the Year 1 and 2 Management Committee who are responsible for the implementation and horizontal integration of Years 1 and 2. The entire curriculum is overseen by the Faculty's Five-year Curriculum Committee. Because of the project work being implemented through Theme 1, CPP, input is also received from the Theme 1 Academic Convenor.

The community placements involve nearly 80 community organisations who apply to be community partners. Briefing sessions are provided and then, provided they are still interested and can demonstrate that they meet the criteria, the placements sign up to take anywhere from two to 15 students on placement for the year.

Once students have made their choices for placements early in Year 2 they contact the agency field educator to request an interview. On this visit they will also meet with staff and discuss the requirements of the placement, clarify placement expectations and requirements, formulate learning agreements, start to formulate HP project ideas, and ensure that they are genuinely committed to engage with the agency. Following the interview, if it is decided that the placement is not suitable, then the CBP convenors are informed and an alternative placement is found. Placement is finalised after the interview and an orientation with the community partners is then organised.

Quality issues and links to agencies and partnerships

Students and placements sign agreements regarding their expectations and obligations. If at any time students or placements are not performing according to expectations then contact is made with the CPP convenors and the matter is either resolved or an alternate placement is found.

To monitor this, CPP convenors and academic advisors visit the placements during the year and ensure that the placement is happy with the student's performance, the student is happy with the placement's performance, and that the learning agreements and HP project requirements are being met. The list of potential placements is adjusted every year according to such feedback. Any placements which do not provide a suitable learning experience and adequate support are removed from the placement list.

Standard-setting for content and skills

The standards and skills required of the students and placements are set by the CBP convenors with oversight given by the Themes 1 and 2 curriculum committees.

Assessment activities such as project work and poster presentation are set by the

HP/CBP convenors and marked by the academic advisors according to agreed pre-set criteria. HP-based exam questions and OSCE stations are offered by the HP convenors and then independently assessed by the Year 2 assessment subcommittee before being accepted for exams. Post hoc statistical evaluation of exam questions is undertaken to remove any questions which perform poorly.

The curriculum is revised annually according to feedback from students, community partners, convenors and tutors.

Conclusion

The Monash programme requires the cooperation and hard work of staff within the medical faculty along with community partners. The program provides a rewarding but sometimes challenging experience for the students. Through these combined efforts students are able to make a valuable and significant contribution to the placement agencies at the same time as they are meeting valuable learning objectives.

EXAMPLE 3: HEALTH PROMOTION AT BROWN UNIVERSITY, US

Pat Nolan

The curriculum for the first two years of study at Warren Alpert Medical School (WAMS) is at Brown University, Providence, Rhode Island underwent a major change in the academic year beginning in 2005. The change was intended to provide an integrated basic science curriculum and to prepare students for the clinical curriculum in the final two years of medical school.

The 'Doctoring Course' occupies a central role in instilling medical professional behaviour and skills in preparation for a clinical career. This two-year required course of study is designed to teach the skills, attitudes, knowledge and behaviours essential to competent, ethical and humane medical practice. Coursework combines instruction, practice and assessment in medical interviewing and physical examination with medical ethics, cultural competence and professional development. The course design uses an educational paradigm that models interdisciplinary teaching and collaboration to promote patient-centred care, reflection, teamwork and teacher-learner partnerships. Students observe demonstrations of techniques in the lecture theatre. They discuss and practise skills in small groups (eight students) with a preceptor team consisting of a physician and a behavioural health practitioner. In small groups, the students interview and examine 'standardised patients'. The students also observe physician mentors in practice in the community. They also practise their skills with patients in this setting. A teaching academy conducted by more advanced students provides additional skills practice in informal settings.

First-year medical students have had limited opportunities to go beyond the interviewer-examiner role and practice skills essential to therapeutic interventions. Recognising the importance of learning to educate, motivate and communicate effectively with patients, the course directors incorporated health promotion into the course content. Opportunities to participate in interventions to improve health while developing skills in motivational interviewing and behaviour change counselling are provided to students at this early point in their development. Students are expected to master basic interviewing skills to allow evaluation of dietary intake, physical activity levels, sleep, alcohol intake and tobacco use. They practise assessing readiness for behavioural change and apply concepts of motivational interviewing specifically for reducing or quitting smoking.

In the second year of the doctoring course, emphasis on physical examination skills increases. Students are gaining knowledge of pathologic processes and become more focused on detecting normal and abnormal physical findings. Additional opportunities for learning health promotion skills have been identified for second-year students. This aspect of the course continues to evolve. Women's health screening is a paradigm for health promotion in the second-year course. Students learn health promotion strategies to address osteoporosis prevention in the context of the life cycle. They practise communication of risk and motivational interviewing, to encourage increased screening, physical activity, calcium intake and other interventions.

As students move into clinical settings in their third year of medical studies, they have had exposure to key elements of the physician role in health promotion. They have skills in history taking that allow them to ask about health behaviours and health risks and recognise the extent of a person's risks for adverse health outcomes, advise specific health promotion strategies, assess the person's readiness for change and offer assistance tailored to readiness for change. They have knowledge of the importance of arranging follow-up and continuing to support and promote changes in health behaviours and maintenance of therapeutic interventions.

The next steps in their medical education take place in clinical clerkships. Sustained attention to health promotion is a part of clerkship curricula, particularly in family medicine, internal medicine, paediatrics and community health. By developing students' skills in health promotion early in their medical school courses, the medical school seeks to increase the perception of their importance to practice. As students spend time with their mentors in the community and practise these same skills, the medical school is also sustaining the interest in and attention to health promotion among practising physicians.

EXAMPLE 4: OVERVIEW OF THE TEACHING OF HEALTH PROMOTION AT THE FACULTY OF MEDICINE, CHINESE UNIVERSITY OF HONG KONG

Albert Lee

(This review is based on the contributor's analysis of the curriculum.)

The teaching of health promotion and disease prevention for medical students in the Faculty of Medicine at the Chinese University of Hong Kong spreads from Year 1 to Year 4, since a revision of the medical curriculum in 2001. It is broadly categorised under six key themes.

1 Understanding of the wider determinants of health.
2 Ability to implement strategies for risk reduction for individual patients and population.
3 Understanding of the concepts of multidisciplinary and multisectoral collaborations in health promotion and disease prevention.
4 Planning for health promotion and disease prevention for both individual and population health, with an understanding of the barriers and obstacles.
5 Multidisciplinary and multisectoral approaches in health promotion and disease prevention.
6 The importance of patient health education and the role of doctors as patient health educators.

Medical students begin to learn health promotion and disease prevention during Year 1 under the course 'Health and Society'.[42] This course consists of six units (around 72 contact hours of teaching) during Year 1. It enables students to understand some of the broader concepts of health, disease and disease prevention. Teachers of the health and society course come from various academic departments (Community and Family Medicine, School of Public Health, Psychiatry, Paediatrics, Obstetrics and Gynaecology, Medicine and Therapeutics, Clinical Oncology, Biochemistry, Sociology) and also from the Health Authority, reflecting the medical school's multidisciplinary and multisectoral approach to health promotion.

The specific learning objectives of health and society are described as follows:

A understanding the wider concepts of health and disease prevention, and essential public health principles and practices
B understanding the determinants of health including the ecology of health and the impact of environmental and socioeconomic factors on health
C becoming familiar with various modes of healthcare delivery and financing
D developing a regard for patients in their holistic setting, as members of a family and a community
E establishing caring attitudes
F valuing the importance of medical ethics and the need for clinicians to meet high ethical standards.

Learning objectives A to D, in particular, are intended to demonstrate to students that health promotion is directed towards action on the determinants of health. The course combines diverse but complimentary methods or approaches including education, communication, organisational change, community development, fiscal measures, legislation and local actions.[43] Attention to aspects of public health is demonstrated through the following examples:

➤ *physical environment* covers the important area of urban design, housing and transport as well as traditional areas of public health – clean water, adequate sanitation and unpolluted air
➤ *social environment* includes measurement of community involvement and participation in education at all ages as well as crime and domestic violence
➤ *economic environment* covers poverty and level of employment, which affects people's ability to access good food and decent housing
➤ *political environment* covers legislative measures and guidelines such as smoke-free zones, school lunches, food labelling.

Table 8.2 presents the broad learning objectives and content focus on the social determinants of health component of the course in the years 2001–08.

TABLE 8.2 Learning objectives and content focus for the social determinants of health

Learning objectives	Content focus
• Examine the relationship between socioeconomic condition and health status among the residents of Hong Kong • Explore the effects of cost of healthcare services on the utilisation of healthcare services across different social classes in Hong Kong • Assess social class differences in health belief and health lifestyle among the people of Hong Kong • Review the association between economic development and health status and disease patterns over the last few decades in Hong Kong	• Look at health from a biomedical, social, psychological integrative perspective • Assess some of a person's behavioural health risks and give advice regarding their reduction • Value the 'patient-centred' approach in health behaviour change and health promotion • View measures to promote health and prevent disease through behaviour change as just as important as treating illness through other methods

There are also lectures on health and social care systems in Hong Kong and worldwide, as well as debate on healthcare systems so students can develop some insight about the impact of health and social care systems on the health and well-being of the population. Other lecture topics include addressing work and health, exercise and health, health psychology and environmental health. The teaching of health and society in Year 1 is intended to serve as a building block for learning health promotion in the clinical context.

During Years 2–4, there are no formal lectures by the health and society panel; teaching is provided under the 'Family Follow-Up Project'.[44] From Year 1 to Year 4, students are required to conduct a family follow-up study. Groups of two to three students are each assigned a newborn during Year 1, and they follow the child until the age of three years. The project provides a unique opportunity for students to observe the growth of a child from birth to three years in a normal family environment rather than in a hospital setting. It is intended that at the end of the project, the students have some understanding of the influences of the socioeconomic background of the family, their health beliefs and practices, and the available social support on childcare and family adjustment. The project also provides an opportunity for students to learn about interviewing techniques and the development of long-term relationships with a family. All of these opportunities facilitate students' learning about health promotion and disease prevention from early childhood.

From the first clinical year (Year 3) onward, different clinical specialties integrate health promotion perspectives into their teaching programmes. During Year 3, specific health promotion and disease prevention teaching will be covered for women and elderly groups by the Department of Community and Family Medicine.[45] Within the programme on musculoskeletal aging (*see* Table 8.3), one lecture specifically addresses 'promotion of musculoskeletal health for the elderly', and is delivered by a family physician. Case examples are explored throughout the lectures so that students gain a deeper understanding of the importance of health promotion and prevention, apart from conventional treatment and management of this common disorder among the elderly.

TABLE 8.3 Learning objectives and lecture series on musculoskeletal aging

Learning objectives	Lecture series
• Understand musculoskeletal problems among the elderly in the community and the impact of those problems on daily life • Review the general principles of primary care management of musculoskeletal problems among the elderly • Examine preventive measures at primary, secondary and tertiary levels • Explore the role of lifestyle modification	• Basic science of aging in the musculoskeletal system (by research scientist) • Clinical aspects of musculoskeletal aging and geriatric rehabilitation (by geriatrician) • Geriatric fracture and fall prevention in the elderly (by orthopaedic surgeon) • Promotion of musculoskeletal health in the elderly (by family physician)

The lecture on 'cervical cancer screening', part of the 'sex and human development' unit of study within the Department of Community and Family Medicine, also emphasises screening as preventive strategies to reduce disease incidence.

During Year 4, students rotate through four modules: community and family medicine; obstetrics and gynaecology; paediatrics; and psychiatry. Obstetrics and gynaecology, paediatrics, and psychiatry cover the health promotion perspectives of their own specialties. During the community and family medicine module, students learn more on epidemiology and public health practice, including screening and occupational and environmental medicine.[46] They also learn about prevention of communicable and non-communicable diseases as well as risk reduction for occupational and environmental hazards. The learning objectives for this component of the course include:

➤ define health education, and understand the concept of patient-centred health education

➤ understand the important role of health education in healthcare delivery systems and patient management

➤ understand the different models of health education and ways of changing people's behaviour

➤ understand the different modes of delivery of health education messages, and appreciate the new approach to health education
➤ appreciate the role of doctors as patient educators.

The primary care setting is where the majority of health problems first present to health-care providers. From the discipline of family medicine, the clinical attachment to family physicians enables students to observe and learn the important role of family physicians in health promotion and disease prevention and improving the health of the population.[47,48] There are seminars on (i) disease prevention and health promotion: primary care perspective; (ii) community-based rehabilitation: the role of family physicians; and (iii) chronic disease management. The first of these addresses the importance of health promotion in primary care and how an effective primary care system would improve population health.[49] Basic concepts of motivating people to change health behaviour and adoption of healthy lifestyles are also covered.[50] The second seminar examines the mobilisation of community resources to prevent complications and deterioration in the condition of patients with chronic illness; the empowerment of patients and families in self management; and the provision of psycho-social rehabilitation.[51] All these contribute to tertiary prevention and promotion of quality of life and well-being for patients with chronic illnesses.[52] The Community Rehabilitation Network of the Hong Kong Society for Rehabilitation is also involved in teaching and in the organisation of site visits for medical students.

During their final year, students are attached to the Rehabilitation Medicine unit. This provides them with the opportunity to gain further experience to promote better health for patients with chronic disorders and disabilities. The basic principles and concepts of determinants of health, behaviour change and models of health promotion are designed to assist students to identify the barriers to health promotion and disease prevention for such patients at both personal and societal levels. During the planning process, strategies can be developed to overcome those barriers.

In summary, health promotion teaching within the Faculty of Medicine, Chinese University of Hong Kong is integrated across different subject areas and different clinical specialties. Direct topics are addressed in units covering 'health and society', musculoskeletal studies and 'sex and human development', and in rehabilitation, community and family medicine modules. Students are assessed accordingly within those study areas on relevant topics related to health promotion.

EXAMPLE 5: DEVELOPING INTERPROFESSIONAL SKILLS IN HEALTH PROMOTION AND PUBLIC HEALTH PRACTICE: A UK EXAMPLE OF DEVELOPING PROFESSIONAL CAPACITY AND COMPETENCY

Richard Shircore

Introduction

Health promotion and public health are fascinating fields of work – yet like other areas of professional endeavour the very 'open air' nature of their work creates unique challenges. Not for the health promoter the environmental control of the laboratory, nor the certainty of a sequential positivist approach. Health promotion and public health is more like civil engineering, where the nature of the challenge requires careful assessment and options of response need to be weighed not only in terms of effectiveness but also in terms of cost and sustainability – all the while being aware of the stresses and strains within the very structures in which we are working.

The University of Reading hosts a Level 2 programme of 60 Credit Accumulation Transfer Schemes (CATS),[53] 'Developing Interprofessional Skills in Health Promotion and Public Health Practice', co-written by Dr Ann Wylie and Richard Shircore. The current programme has evolved over many years from a professional development programme originally written for the Health Education Council in the 1980s. It is in its tenth year of existence.

The course has undergone many revisions but its core aims of developing skilled, competent and capable public health and health promotion professionals is an ever-present requirement. Particular attention is paid to grounding students in appropriate methodologies and congruent methods of implementation and application.

The level and syllabus was developed with the intention of producing self-contained practitioners. Many students graduating will be operating in the UK or overseas in environments where professional support and mentoring may be limited. They need enough knowledge and skills to be self-contained. Therefore it is crucial they can think through problems from a 'first principles' perspective. The core syllabus of six modules is presented in Table 8.4. In order to support the teaching and learning that takes place in these modules, professional training events described in Table 8.5 are organised to extend the professional development aspect of the course. An example of a specific training event on 'Working with Aims and Objectives' is presented in Table 8.6 and its associated agenda appears in Figure 8.1.

TABLE 8.4 Core syllabus of six modules

Core modules	Description
Epidemiology	Focuses on use to data and health intelligence to carry out an effective 'needs assessment'. Appreciation of the different types of need is crucial
Communications	This covers 1:1 communication, through to group work and on to the basics of using the mass media. Particular attention is paid to engaging with clients and populations by the use particular forms and methodologies of personal skills[54]
Theories and methods	The authors believe the difference between the professional practitioner and the enthusiastic amateur is in the professional's use and application of relevant theories and methods. Using set texts[55] and specially written course materials, students are introduced to the major contemporary theories and models. Students are also encouraged to be alert about utilising other theories and models from other disciplines if circumstances require it
Designing and implementing	This module further develops the professional competency aspect by requiring students to identify, plan and implement a short program of work which is assessed by the tutors. In this module the challenge of assessing needs and audience/population characteristics is coupled with the professional need to create a sequential body of learning. The importance of session planning is also covered as well as the basics of operational planning
Practitioner-based enquiry (PBE)	The PBE is designed to bring together the previous core syllabus elements. Students are required to carry out a piece of research using data they have obtained themselves and to use the data to either inform a proposal for a health promotion/public health development or to assess the impact/effectiveness of a health promotion/public health development
Dissemination/Review	The final module gives students the opportunity to disseminate the findings of their particular PBE to each other in a safe environment. This allows for further professional experience as successes can be acknowledged, as well as learning from each other as to mistakes and omissions. This process is particularly important to the development of the reflective practitioner

TABLE 8.5 Professional development components

Topic	Description
Working with aims and objectives	A core competency which all professional staffs need to master
Professional communication skills	Focus on understanding the nature of effective communication and the prerequisites for effective engagement with clients
Inequalities in health promotion	Review of how social conditions affect health status and how health promotion can be used in the pursuit of social justice
Planning and implementing	Students are introduced to the fundamentals of strategic and especially operational planning
Problems-solving	Consider how problems present and how they can be analysed to indicate a way forward. Partnership and responsibility issues tend to feature prominently
Introduction to management skills	Professional staff from one discipline will frequently be asked to pioneer organisational change with no grounding in organisational change management theory or practice. Students are briefed on key management skills; e.g. constructing agendas for effective meetings

TABLE 8.6 Session sample: training day on working with aims and objectives

Topic	Description
Rationale	Professional practice requires precision and accuracy. The use of language to describe and explain action is therefore crucial
Focus	The training day 'Working with Aims and Objectives' focuses on how to break down the task (health promotion) and to accurately describe the ultimate aim (outcome desired) and the key steps required for its accomplishment (objectives)
Key concepts	Within this training module students are introduced to other key concepts necessary for programme development: *Content* – the factual element; *Process* – the organisational structure of the programme, e.g. partnership programme with external funding utilising local venues; *Context* – the situational and environmental aspects which may influence delivery; and lastly *Format* – structure of the delivery, e.g. seminar, press release, drop-in clinic etc.
Conclusion	It is frequently observed that students have significant difficulty separating out aims and objectives and the aims and objectives from content, process, context and format. The mastery of understanding these concepts is crucial to future evaluation and assessment and is therefore the foundation of much health promotion and public health work

Agenda: Writing aims and objectives

Tutors – Richard Shircore and Ann Wylie

09.30 Group review and understanding of aims and objectives   RS
- Current methods of planning and organising activity
- Aims and objectives – putting their importance in context
- Why start with aims and objectives?
- Professional standards, technical writing

50.50 The programme aims and objectives – handout   RS
- Aims and objectives in educational practice
- Aims and objectives in health promotion management and organisation

10.10 Introduction to the concept of an aim   AW
- What is an aim?
- Relevance to: success, methods and methodologies, planning, joint working and evaluation

25.25 Introduction to the concept of an objective   RS
- Types of objectives – focus on drafting behavioural objectives
- Relevance to success, methods and methodologies, planning, joint working evaluation
- Recognising an aim – exercise
- Recognising an objective
- The difference between educational and behavioural objectives
- Recap

11.10 *Break*

11.30 Introduction to associated concepts: content, context, format, process   AW
- The importance of congruence – exercise

11.55 Time scheduling with aims and objectives – exercise   AW

30.30 *Lunch*

13.15 Critical appraisal of aims and objectives of a health promotion programme   RS
- Exercise – Community practitioner

13.45 Briefing for practical   AW

14.00 Exercise in groups

14.45 *Break*

15.00 Report back by group   All

16.00 Review and reflection

16.20 Quiz ————————— [Using a quiz format allows review and reflection on key points and enables a check on learning outcomes]

Close

FIGURE 8.1 Agenda for writing aims and objectives for health promotion/public health workshop

REFERENCES

1 Boelen C. Adapting health care institutions and medical schools to societies' needs. *Acad Med*. 1999; **74**(8): S11–20.

2 Ibid.

3 Walton HJ. Primary health care in European medical education: a survey. *Med Educ*. 1985; **19**: 167–88.

4 Warren K. World Conference on Medical Education, Edinburgh. *Lancet*. 1988; 8608: 462.

5 Amos A, Church M, Forsters F, *et al*. A health promotion module for undergraduate medical students. *Med Educ*. 1990; **24**: 328–35.

6 World Health Organization/Health and Welfare Canada/Canadian Public Health Association. *Ottawa Charter for Health Promotion*. World Health Organization: Copenhagen; 1986.

7 AIHW (Australian Institute of Health and Welfare). *Australia's Health 2006*. Canberra: Australian Government Printing Service; 2006.

8 Ibid.

9 NHIMG (National Health Information Management Group). *National Health Information Development Priorities*. Canberra: Australian Institute of Health and Welfare; 2003.

10 Schroeder SA. Understanding health behavior and speaking out on the uninsured: two leadership opportunities. *Acad Med*. 1999; **74**(11): 1163–71.

11 McIntosh S, Block RC, Kapsak G, *et al*. Training medical students in community health: a novel required fourth-year clerkship at the University of Rochester. *Acad Med*. 2008; **83**(4): 357–64.

12 World Health Organization. *Health: a WHO global strategy for changing medical education and medical practice for health for all*. Geneva: World Health Organization; 1996.

13 Pew Health Professions Commission. *Recreating Health Professional Practice for a New Century: the fourth report of the Pew Health Professions Commission*. San Francisco, CA: Pew Health Professions Commission; 2006.

14 Pew Health Professions Commission. *Critical Challenges: revitalizing the health professions for the twenty-first century*. San Francisco, CA: Pew Health Professions Commission; 1995.

15 The Association of Medical Colleges. *Medical School Objectives Project, Report 1. Learning objectives for medical student education: guidelines for medical schools*. Washington, DC: Association of Medical Colleges; 1998.

16 Davis MH, Karunathilake I, Harden R. AMEE Education Guide No. 28: the development and role of departments of medical education. *Med Teach*. 2005; **27**(8): 665–75.

17 Amos *et al*., op cit.

18 Anderson, M. Brownell. A snapshot of medical students' education at the beginning of the 21st century: reports from 130 schools. *Acad Med*. 2000; **75**(9 Suppl.) S10–14.

19 Davis, *et al*., op. cit.

20 Sachdeva A. Faculty development and support needed to integrate the learning of prevention in the curricula of medical schools. *Acad Med*. 2000; **75**(7 Suppl.): S35–42.

21 Koo D, Thacker S. The education of physicians: a CDC perspective. *Acad Med*. 2008; **83**(4): 399–407.

22 Gottlieb LK, Holman HR. What's preventing more prevention? Barriers to development at academic medical centers. *J Gen Intern Med*. 1992; **7**: 630–5.

23 Chamberlain L, Wang NE, Ho ET, *et al*. Integrating collaborative population health projects into a medical student curriculum at Stanford. *Acad Med*. 2008; **83**: 338–44.

24 McIntosh, *et al*., op. cit.

25 Boelen, op. cit.

26 Sachdeva, op. cit.

27 Stine C, Kohrs FP, Little DN, *et al*. Integrating prevention education into the medical school curriculum: the role of departments of family medicine. *Acad Med*. 2000; **75**(7 Suppl.): S55–S59.

28 Chamberlain *et al*., op cit.

29 The Federal Ministry of Health. Medical licensing regulations for physicians; dated 27 June 2002. *Bundesgesetzblatt.* 2002; **I**: 2405–35.

30 Jungbauer J, Kamenik C, Alfermann D, *et al.*, How do young physicians assess their medical studies in retrospect? Results of a medical graduates' survey in Germany. *Gesundheitswesen.* 2004; **66**(1): 51–6.

31 Jungbauer J, Alfermann D, Kamenik C, *et al.*, Psychosocial skills training: unsatisfactory results from interviews with medical school graduates from seven German universities. *Psychosom Med Psychol.* **53**(7): 319–21.

32 Klement A, Lautenschläger C, Bretschneider K, *et al.*, Interdisciplinary teaching of prevention and health promotion at the Medical School of the University Halle-Wittenberg (Part I): Evaluation of students' attitudes and estimates before entering the curriculum. *Gesundheitswesen.* 2010 (in press).

33 Mau W, Gülich M, Gutenbrunner C, *et al.*, Educational objectives in the new interdisciplinary subject 'Rehabilitation, Physical Medicine, Naturopathic Techniques' under the 9th revision of the licensing regulations for doctors: consensus recommendations of the German Society for Rehabilitative Sciences and the German Society for Physical Medicine and Rehabilitation. *Rehabilitation.* (Stuttg.) 2004 (December); **43**(6): 337–47.

34 Studiendekanat der Medizinischen Fakultät der Albrecht-Ludwigs-Universität Freiburg. *Lernzielkatalog für das Fach Prävention und Gesundheitsförderung.* Freiburg: University of Freiburg; 2006. Available at: www.uniklinik-freiburg.de/kinderklinik/live/lehre/schein/Lernzielkatalog.pdf (accessed 2 November 2009).

35 Walter U, Klippel U, Bisson S. Implementation of the 9th revision of medical licensing regulation for physicians in the cross-sectional area 'prevention and health promotion' at the German medical faculties. *Gesundheitswesen.* 2007; **69**(4):2 40–8.

36 Blue AV, Barnette JJ, Ferguson KJ, *et al.*, Evaluation methods for prevention education. *Acad Med.* 2000; **75**(7 Suppl.): S28–34.

37 Litaker D, Cebul RD, Masters S, *et al.*, Disease prevention and health promotion in medical education: reflections from an academic health center. *Acad Med.* 2004; **79**(7): 690–7.

38 Wagner PJ, Jester DM, Moseley GC. Medical students as health coaches. *Acad Med.* 2002; **77**(11): 1164–5.

39 Worley P, Prideaux D, Strasser R, *et al.*, Empirical evidence for symbiotic medical education: a comparative analysis of community and tertiary-based programmes. *Med Educ.* 2006; **40**(2): 109–16.

40 Stine *et al.*, op cit.

41 Hassed C, de Lisle S, Sullivan G, *et al.* Enhancing the health of medical students: outcomes of an integrated mindfulness and lifestyle program. *Adv Health Sci Educ.* 2009; **14**(3): 387–98.

42 Faculty of Medicine, University of Hong Kong. *Professional Undergraduate Programme in Medicine (MB ChB): Student Handbook 2007–08.* Hong Kong: The Chinese University of Hong Kong; 2007.

43 Lee A, Fu J, Ji C. Health promotion activities in China from the Ottawa Charter to the Bangkok Charter: revolution to evolution. *Promot Educ.* 2007; **XIV** (4): 214–23.

44 Faculty of Medicine, op. cit.

45 Ibid.

46 Ibid.

47 Ibid.

48 Lee A, Kiyu A, Milman HM, Jara J. Improving health and building human capital through an effective primary care system. *J Urban Health.* 2007; **84** (Suppl. 1): 75–85.

49 Ibid.

50 Lee A. Effective lifestyle change. In: Wong WCW, Lindsay M, Lee A, editors. *Diagnosis and Management in Primary Care.* Hong Kong: The Chinese University Press; 2008. pp. 45–57.

51 Lee A. Partnership with NGOs in healthcare. In: Wong WCW, Lindsay M, Lee A, editors. *Diagnosis and Management in Primary Care.* Hong Kong: The Chinese University Press; 2008. pp. 105–12.

52 Lee SH, Lee A, To CY, *et al. Consultancy Report to Hong Kong SAR Government on Evaluation of Community-Based Rehabilitation Network.* Hong Kong: Department of Community and Family Medicine, The Chinese University of Hong Kong; 1999.

53 This is an accepted way for students to acquire university-level credits to lead to a degree. CATS was pioneered by the Open University.

54 Davis *et al.,* op cit.

55 Ewles L, Simnett I. *Promoting Health: a practical guide.* 5th ed. London: Bailliere Tindall; 2003.

CHAPTER 9

Assessment drives learning: the case for and against formal health promotion in curricula

Ann Wylie and Kathy Boursicot

Although Part 5 focuses on assessment, this short chapter presents argument about the concepts of assessing and linking core content to assessment, the benefits and the burdens.

AN ASSESSMENT CULTURE

Assessment, regardless of the format, has a central role in health professional education given that the ultimate role of a vocational course is to enable candidates to become safe practitioners on graduation. Graduates will have or should have been assessed by demonstrable valid and reliable processes against a set of expected outcomes.[1] Such high-stakes assessments may result in some students failing to reach the demonstrable required standard. When this happens there are varied individual reasons. If the assessment is reliable, valid and fair, the student's ability will have been judged correctly to be suboptimal. However, there may be other reasons, which could include:

➤ flaws in the assessment processes
➤ assessor ability or shortcomings
➤ student's lack of preparedness or other student-related factors
➤ course structure poorly matching assessment
➤ deficiencies in course content and resources
➤ issues surrounding how the course was taught and by whom.

For students investing in many years of learning at high cost, failure has serious implications for all protagonists. Far from being a separate but necessary aspect of curricula, assessment is an integral aspect of the whole, linked to defined learning outcomes and pedagogical approaches.

As assessment has an emphasis on concerns of measurable reliability, medical schools and regulatory bodies have nevertheless had to develop approaches to assessment of the 'less easy' – such as professionalism and ethics – to define learning outcomes.[2,3]

111

These are some of the more challenging components of curricula for assessment, but if taught as part of core curricula it follows that assessment should be designed appropriately to demonstrate competence, skills and/or knowledge. There is much ongoing work on developing reliable assessments of professionalism.[4]

Students themselves are judicious about their learning strategies, with concerted effort for aspects of the course they know will be assessed and perhaps less emphasis on those areas of the course they judge to be 'optional' or carry minimal weighting in the assessment stakes.

Students who find the so-called 'optional' aspects of their course very interesting may do well but without requiring any stressful additional input to their learning. For those who find some aspects of their course stressful, they may decide to put minimal effort into these and more effort into other aspects of core curriculum topics that will be assessed.

Assessment takes many formats and in the interests of all protagonists, curricula should clearly state learning outcomes and the assessment processes and how these are linked. For example, the in-course assessments for a cohort may include presentations, log book sign-ups and attendance and participation in group sessions. These may be 'hurdle' assessments in that regardless of their weighting, students must achieve a satisfactory pass mark. Such an arrangement could in theory prevent a student progressing if one small component was not satisfactory.

The end-of-course assessment may include written examinations with a mix of short answer questions and multiple-choice questions. In addition there may be a test of clinical and communication skills, most commonly in the format of an objective structured clinical examination (OSCE)[5] or a variation of this original model.[6] The details about these summative assessments will include the weighting for each of the components, but as with the 'hurdle' assessments in in-course assessment, the students may be required to reach a pass mark in all components of the examinations. The non-compensatory model is based on the premise that a student should not be reliant on small foci of knowledge or skills, but should have sufficient knowledge and skills across a broad range, and be able to integrate and safely apply their learning in clinical context.

For those who lead on specialist aspects of core teaching, there is an imperative to be part of the overall assessment process, so that students and others value these specialists sessions. But is that the best way to present health promotion in contemporary curricula? Is health promotion a special case, will it be marginalised without robust assessment and is it possible to have reliable and valid assessment for this discipline?

ASSESSMENT DRIVES LEARNING

The notion that assessment drives learning is rarely contested, although for students, how to approach assessment and concerns about what has to be learnt and to what depth cause considerable anxiety. How to prepare for assessments, and how much guidance and signposting should be part of the curriculum or the function of medical teachers is debatable. There are also cost implications for both assessment approaches and the support given to preparation for assessment. Given that health professionals need to qualify with the ability to be lifelong learners, the questions of balance between guidance for assessment and how much the student should manage their own learning, as well as these costs, are all part of the debate.

More recently however studies have indicated that an approach to learning that includes testing can be beneficial. In other words where the curriculum design integrates 'testing' as part of the approach to teaching, assessment outcomes improve.[7]

In contrast, the ad hoc arrangements of medical electives are challenged by Jolly, where he posits 'how do we know what skills and capacities our students are developing'? He argues for a much stronger approach to assessment even though there is a culture that advocates self-directed learning.[8] Could it be that the 'learning' during electives is different and not necessarily without merit but neither is it easily measured?

For students the value of assessment is essentially twofold. It enables them to progress, start their career and access an income, but successful assessment also provides students with the confidence and self-esteem they need to develop their professional and practice skills, identify their ongoing learning needs and take steps to address them.

What must be evident for students is why they need to learn, what they need to learn and how this is weighted overall. The apparently more abstract aspects of core curricula may require practice and feedback from peers and teachers but Wood also warns of the potential for erroneous learning.[7]

Study skills are sometimes lacking in those students who had previously done well, are good at time management yet learn inappropriately – their efforts being without reward.

Contemporary curriculum anticipates that if the student needs support they should have it and that no health, social or physical impairments should be a factor in failure. And for students who have no specific learning needs they too should have access to opportunities and resources for assessment preparation.

The increasing access to skills laboratories, to OSCE practice, to computerised mannequins and practice examination questions all reinforce the value put on assessment so even if this is not seen as an integral part of the curriculum, students will find time to access these resources. Many medical teachers experience reduced numbers of students attending their sessions as examinations approach. This is not just because of revision time but optional 'practice sessions' may have been arranged at this same time for the students, be they arranged by the faculty or other agents such as student support groups or commercial revision providers. Students, it seems, will prioritise time for revision opportunities to enable them to perform well in assessment.

THE SCIENCE AND RESEARCH AGENDA FOR ASSESSMENT

International medical education conferences frequently feature a major theme in and around assessment, with keynote speakers who are experts in educational assessment research such as Professor Dylan Wiliam.[9] He argues that student do not learn what we teach and hence assessment must be central to the teaching process to allow us to identify the impact of teaching on student learning. His research has also included the margin of error and the impact of this as suboptimal conditions ensue.[10] A number of medical education researchers concern themselves with the science of assessment and regularly sections of conference proceedings are associated with assessment. Attention is given to the research findings and the recommendations for faculties by faculties themselves as well as by regulatory bodies.

There is a debate relating to the major differences between the UK and other countries such as the US and Canada. In the UK, each school manages its own assessment procedures under statutes within the context of the awarding university body but meeting the requirements of the regulatory bodies; for medicine this being the General Medical Council (GMC). The situation in the US and Canada is that there is one national qualifying assessment process – this is run by national bodies, the National Board of Medical Examiners in the US and the Medical Council of Canada in Canada. The US and Canadian schools with have their own curricula and assessments during the course, which vary from school to school, but all with the ultimate goal of satisfactorily preparing the students for the national qualifying examinations.

Other research themes include the reliability of examinations, the validity of test instruments, the best formats for testing knowledge and application of knowledge, the best formats for testing clinical and communication skills, how to assess professionalism, the value of portfolios and the impact of assessment on learning. Research findings and conclusions yield recommendations not only for the assessment processes but for curricula and how well matched both are, as well as how practical and cost-effective assessment is. Some key questions are how many written items or OSCE stations are needed for a test to be reliable, how many elements of the course should be selected for testing, and what proportion of the tests should be devoted to different parts of the curriculum.

For example, if smoking cessation has been taught and students have had in-course formative assessment, will it need to be included as a separate station in OSCEs or be included in written papers? Could students be expected to demonstrate they can effectively manage a patient with behavioural change issues in a cardiovascular station? Consider a student for whom smoking cessation has been poorly taught, been optional or has been seen as marginal by his or her medical teachers, and the student performs poorly on this aspect, but well on history taking, clinical examination and pharmacological aspects. How would this student be marked and could such weaknesses be a cause for failure? Much depends on what aspects are prioritised by the faculty setting the examination.[11] Statistical models can identify and differentiate the student who is good and safe, good enough, borderline or failure, with the caveats that few students will excel in all aspects, especially under examination conditions. The challenge for researchers has been around the borderline students and how to reliably distinguish between those who are safe to pass and those who are not yet ready.[12,13]

ASSESSMENT METHODS – LINKED TO CONTENT AND PROCESS?

Although the examinations at the end of a course are frequently seen as all encompassing, requiring many hours of preparation, modern educational theory has embraced in-course assessment, formative assessment and ongoing assessment which enable students to gain expertise or at least competence in favourable and perhaps realistic contexts.

The problem-based learning (PBL) approach for example requires the students to work as a small group on a 'case' and then present their findings. Students are less likely to involve themselves in rote learning but in deep learning. Such 'cases' can integrate health promotion, ethics and communication skills as well as search skills and working with groups.

Major assignments linked to modules are also valued by both students and educationalists. The portfolio, the dissertations, reflective reports on placements as well as log book sign-ups all offer opportunities for assessment to be integrated into the process of learning, and much of what is broadly defined as health promotion can be incorporated into such work. Examples of health promotion content and assessment include the use of applied communication and behaviour modification skills, the critiquing of evidence from non-scientific sources such as sociology, public policy and health economics, and the recognition that research and inquiry into many social determinants is complex and needs ethical committee approval. What changes can be attributable to health-promoting interventions are complex to measure as some students will have discovered if they were required as part of their module to address risk factors such as alcohol consumption, diet and diabetes.

There are many difficulties in large medical and health professional faculties with such demanding processes. For example:

➤ How many portfolios can one assessor cope with?
➤ How many assessors can mark assignments with the same level of consistency?
➤ What are the acceptable margins of error when dealing with work that is variable?
➤ Does the assessment account for each student doing highly individual work?
➤ How many assignments need second marking and moderation to be fair to all?
➤ Are assessors adequately trained and monitored?

It is the students who may hold the answers as they now have established a culture of questioning, of expecting constructive feedback and having the confidence to challenge the marks they are awarded if they have feel these are unjust. These student evaluation processes as well as the student representative bodies have become an integral part of the quality process expected in higher education. They will challenge curriculum content, teaching and assessment if there are inconsistencies, a lack of coherence or unjust assessment practices.

The challenge may be to ensure that health promotion is valued enough that assessments count, that there should be consistency, and that students feel confident when applying health promotion in clinical context and able to critique evidence.

LEARNING OUTCOMES: ACHIEVABLE, MEASURABLE AND DEMONSTRABLE

Students have been keen to concern themselves with curricula, and regulatory bodies also indicate what learning outcomes are essential.[2] These essential learning outcomes have to be more than rhetoric, but they need to be achievable, measurable and demonstrable.

For example the GMC in *Tomorrow's Doctors* refers to outcomes in good clinical care and state that students on graduation should:

> Know about, understand and be able to apply and integrate clinical, basic behavioural and social sciences on which medical practice is based . . . They must also know about and understand the role that lifestyle, including diet and nutrition, can play in promoting health and preventing disease.[14]

These statements may seem self-evident but equally nebulous. What basic behavioural sciences are being referred to and how will the student demonstrate knowledge and applied skills? With regard to diet and nutrition, what exactly do they need to know about and understand?

In the first instance, outcomes may be related to epidemiology knowledge – for example, prevalence and trends, demographic variables – but when it comes to integrating into clinical practice then one assumes intervention skills and the evidence base associated with these interventions is required. Such fields are relatively new to medical education and there is fragmentation of teaching between and within faculties in this area as well as variation in clinical practice.

With regard to diet and nutrition, the knowledge base may be about the science, the factors associated with poor nutrition, healthy balanced nutrition and excessive consumption. The learning outcomes may relate to risk factors for poor nutrition such as physical problems, social circumstances, skills and income. Outcomes could however be focused on successful interventions, best evidence-based approaches, debating the pros and cons for mandatory supplements to staples, such as folic acid.

It will therefore be necessary for individual faculties to redefine their learning outcomes around these and identify for students and tutors alike the specific learning outcomes that can be implemented, taught with some consistency, are relevant to wider learning and can be assessed, as well as the format(s) for the assessment.

IS HEALTH PROMOTION A PROBLEM FOR ASSESSORS?

There are two factors that could be challenging for assessors with regard to health promotion.

First, the emerging epistemology and the contested nature of this discipline present curriculum developers with uncertainty. What are the parameters for this field of research and practice and are the various terms interchangeable – terms such as health improvement, public health and lifestyle behaviour modifications? The second factor is the limited teacher experience of the discipline and therefore how it can be successfully taught with consistency and equitable student experiences. Without clarity and consensus, assessment will be of limited value and reliability.

On one side of this debate is the growing argument that health promotion should be taught and assessed, enabling students to demonstrate two broad attributes. First is that they are able to respond within the clinical context to patients' needs such as weight reduction or smoking cessation in a context-appropriate way. This will usually mean motivational interviewing and brief intervention, with referral to appropriate services, agencies that have best evidence. Second, students should be able to demonstrate an ability to access and critique intervention evidence, be it focused at the individual or community level.[15]

A move towards common agreement and goals, hence this book, is evident within the international medical education community. These issues are also now more readily appearing in high-impact medical journals, enabling practitioners and academics to become more aware of the need for knowledge and skills associated with health promotion to improve healthcare overall. The striking example of this is the November 2008 issue of *The Lancet* (Volume 372, Issue 9650) being almost entirely dedicated to the search for health equality, health improvement and health promotion.

SUMMARY

Regardless of the format for curricula, assessment is a substantial and integral part of curriculum development that needs to be linked to education processes and external requirements and be answerable to a number of protagonists including students themselves. The requirement for modern assessments to demonstrate validity and reliability has become a driver for medical education research, and the challenges associated with teaching and assessing health promotion are to be embraced rather than ignored. Faculties have to be pragmatic, they have consider cost-effective assessment methods, the quality of teaching and assessing and the quality assurance process for their assessors, and they need to be accountable to students, regulatory bodies and the public. Assessment is therefore more than a series of disconnected tests but as much a part of the curriculum as the content and the approaches. *See also* Chapter 18 in Part 5.

REFERENCES

1 Carraccio C, Wofsthal SD, Englander R, *et al.* Shifting paradigms: from Flexner to competencies. *Acad Med.* 2002; **77**(5): 361–7.
2 General Medical Council. *Undergraduate Education.* Available at: www.gmc-uk.org/education/undergraduate.asp (accessed 3 November 2009).
3 General Medical Council. *Good Medical Practice.* London: GMC; 2001.
4 Arnold L. Assessing professional behavior: yesterday, today, and tomorrow. *Acad Med.* 2002; **77**(6): 502–15.
5 Harden RM, Gleeson FA. Assessment of clinical competence using an objective structured clinical examination (OSCE). *Med Educ.* 1979; **13**(1): 41–54.
6 Boursicot KAM, Roberts TE, Burdick WP. *OSCEs and other Assessments of Clinical Competence.* Edinburgh: ASME; 2007.
7 Wood T. Assessment not only drives learning, it may also help learning. *Med Educ.* 2009; **43**(1): 5–6.
8 Jolly B. A missed opportunity. *Med Educ.* 2009; **43**(2): 104–5.
9 AMEE Association of medical education in Europe. *Conference program, AMEE 2009.* Conference held 29 August–2 September 2009, Málaga, Spain. Available at: www.amee.org/index.asp?lm=108 (accessed 3 November 2009).
10 Wiliam D. Keeping learning on track: classroom assessment and the regulation of learning. In: Lester FK Jr, editor. *Second Handbook of Mathematics Teaching and Learning.* Greenwich, CT: Information Age Publishing; 2007.
11 Norcini JJ. Setting standards on educational tests. *Med Educ.* 2003; **37**(5): 464–9.
12 Boulet JR, De Champlain AF, McKinley DW. Setting defensible performance standards on OSCEs and standardized patient examinations. *Med Teach.* 2003; **25**(3): 245–9.
13 Norcini JJ, Guille RA. Combining tests and setting standards. In: Norman GR, van der Vleuten CPM, Newble DI, editors. *International Handbook of Research in Medical Education.* Dordrecht: Kluwer; 2002. pp. 811–34.
14 General Medical Council. *Tomorrow's Doctors.* 2nd ed. London: General Medical Council; 2003.
15 Kane P. Sure Start Local Programmes in England. *Lancet.* 2008; **372**(9650): 1610–12.

PART THREE

Learning outcomes regarding the knowledge base, skills and needs of facilitators

INTRODUCTION
Ann Wylie

There are many ways of considering and defining learning outcomes for education in general and for medical and health professional education in particular. These outcomes are predetermined not usually by the learner but by those with responsibilities within a faculty and with regard to the subject and discipline area. Outcomes may also be determined by agencies that regulate the professional practice related to the vocational course in question and by those with academic and professional expertise within a subject. Harden, for example, links outcomes to professionalism, intellectual and emotional decision making and technical intelligence.[1,2] Whilst the public may have limited direct involvement in defining outcomes, their needs and expectations will need to be given due consideration for two essential reasons: first, they will be the recipients of healthcare and have anticipations of what skills and quality are acceptable; and second, for many countries health profession education is funded out of public funds and given that medical education in particular is at very high cost to the taxpayer, even though some students self-fund, the public are indirectly stakeholders in these endeavours. This is not controversial of course until we start to reflect on the field of health promotion, an eclectic and contested field,[3] and on the parameters of professional practice.

In Chapter 10, Duncan looks some of the values, ethics and philosophies that contribute to the debate about the nature of health promotion, about professionalism and what might differentiate outcomes from a first-degree student course to a master's student course, and whether the master's course is focused on health promotion or health promotion is a modular or component part of that course.

In Chapter 11, we deviate somewhat from the academic script and have a narrative about health promotion in practice in a small community, demonstrating practical

119

outcomes. This narrative provides the opportunity to identify and highlight specific learning outcomes that could otherwise seem vague and elusive to curriculum designers.

In Chapter 12 Wills also brings together some pragmatic studies illustrating where and how health promotion learning outcomes could be useful in primary healthcare.

Finally, in Chapter 13 Soethout and Wylie look at defined outcomes and consider how resources and materials, written by those with public health and health promotion expertise, enable facilitators and their learners to meet these outcomes.

REFERENCES

1 Harden R, Crosby JR, Davis MH, *et al.* AMEE Guide No. 14: Outcome-based education: Part 5 – From competency to meta-competency; a model for the specification of learning outcomes. *Med Teach* 1999; **21**(6): 546–52.

2 Harden RM. Curriculum mapping and outcome-based education. Paper presented at the 10th Ottawa Conference on Medical Education. Ontario, Canada; 2 A.D. 13–16 Jul 2002: p. 212.

3 Wylie A, Thompson S. Establishing health promotion in the modern medical curriculum: a case study. *Med Teach.* 2007; **29**(8): 766–71.

CHAPTER 10

Values, contest and the health promotion curriculum in medical education

Peter Duncan

INTRODUCTION

The promotion of health is an ideological enterprise, laden with competing and contested values. If this is so, then design and delivery of the health promotion curriculum in medical education must necessarily involve ideological and values-related choices. My aim in this chapter is to justify and discuss both of these premises. I want to demonstrate how and why health promotion is charged with values and contest. And I also want to present and analyse some of the implications of this state of affairs for those involved in planning health promotion curricula in medical education.

The idea of health promotion as an ideological enterprise is not a new one.[1] Equally, analysis of education itself as a project of ideology is long-standing (see, for example, Peters[2] and Carr[3]). What remains relatively unexplored, though, is the connection between ideological health promotion, on the one hand, and ideological education on the other. In this context, two factors take on an importance. The first is the generalised belief that health promotion, by virtue of its apparent desire to improve the lives of individuals and populations, is *de facto* a 'good thing'.[4] The second is the comparatively embryonic state of work on understanding the source and nature of the ideologies and values present in processes of medical education.[5]

Taken together, these factors suggest the importance of exploring the ideologies and values that might underpin health promotion in medical education. They perhaps indicate a requirement to shift attention towards the nature of the 'fit' between health promotion and medical education. To what extent do the ideologies and values of health promotion (often unreflectively considered a 'good thing') align with those of medical education and the ideologies and values that might be shaping it? Is there reason to be concerned about any tensions that might emerge between the two? Are there ways of dealing with tensions for the benefit of educational process? These are the kinds of questions that I seek to explore in this chapter, approaching them from the perspective of a health promotion academic with a strong interest in values, health and education.

HEALTH: IDEOLOGIES AND VALUES

In a social and political world that is consistently shifting and subject to alteration, subscribing to a particular ideological position provides us with a degree of certainty. Ideologies offer us sets of principles that help us make sense of the elusive, changing world and form moral perspectives and values in relation to it.[6] Of course, ideologies are also instrumental in shaping the world. The ideology of Marxism, for example, not only allows its adherents to understand the world through its construction of the nature of labour and the importance of capital, it also provides a framework for challenge and change to the world from its present state.

This is equally so when we consider ideologies connected to health and healthcare. The most fundamental of these is our ideological understanding of 'health' itself. Debate on the nature of health has been well rehearsed and is very often characterised as being between those adhering to the so-called medical model of health on the one hand, and adherents to the so-called social model on the other.[7] I do not want to offer a further airing of this debate here. My intention instead is to mark and emphasise this debate as essentially an ideological one. This is in contrast to its frequent presentation as one that is mainly to do with differences of approach, background or interpretation.

It requires attention to recognise alternative understandings as representative of *ideological* difference rather than simply differences of approach and so on. In a well-known paper, the physician JG Scadding, for example, claims and argues that those believing 'health' to be anything other than the absence of disease are making a simple *conceptual* mistake.[8] They are failing to recognise, he claims, that there just cannot be a sense in which 'health' is more than disease absence, given our understanding of 'disease' as abnormality of human structure and function. If this isn't present, then how can I possibly regard somebody as anything other than 'healthy'? Thus a 'medical model' view of health (as disease absence) must necessarily satisfy our understanding. There are good reasons to challenge Scadding's argument. However, my point here is not to contest, but rather to observe two points.

➤ In this, and many other arguments to do with the nature of health, the assumption is that difference is a question of (mistaken) interpretation. Those who don't adhere to the medical model are subscribing to, or offering, *too broad* an interpretation of the nature of health. (We could equally point to the argument of somebody adhering to the social model of health and their claim – explicit or implicit – that the medical modeller's interpretation was just *too narrow*.)

➤ However, given the understanding of ideology that I proposed above, Scadding's medical model position is ideological (as is that of the putative social modeller). It is ideological because making the claim that health is no more or less than the absence of disease is the first in a set of principles that help us form our view of the world. If health is disease absence, then we can measure it, research it using quantitative methods, build hospitals to house the technology and the people concerned with improving health through treating and curing disease. We could think of a similar set of principles flowing from the social modeller's belief that health is a product of social circumstance, or a social construction.[7] In both cases, the explanatory power of the founding and subsequent principles frame the medical model on the one hand, and the social model on the other, as ideologies.

What's more, the separate ideological positions are difficult, if not impossible, to reconcile. This is because each of them carries an associated set of *values*. At the simplest level, we can understand values as those things that we find valuable.[6] If I believe in a medical model of health, my values will centre on the requirement to treat individual disease (and possibly also to prevent it at the individual level). I will value professional expertise, patient compliance, resources spent on new technologies and treatments, and so on. Equally, because disease (and health) are located and caused in bodies, I will value individual responsibility for the prevention of ill health. If on the other hand I adhere to a social model, my values will orient much more towards the use of resources and skills (not necessarily professional) for improving health through social change. I will value communitarian (rather than individual) responsibility for ill-health.

It might be argued that we can embrace both the set of values related to the medical model, and the set connected to the social model at one and the same time. My inclination would be to suggest that this might just be possible in a rhetorical sense (although even here we would be in the grip of considerable confusion about exactly what values were important to us). But an important part of the purpose of values is to *enact* them – we want to see more of what we believe to be valuable existing in the world. Now, holding the set of values entailed by the ideology of the medical model and the social model interchangeably becomes very problematic.[9] Do we value professionally controlled technology and treatments above skills within communities? Do we value individual or collective responsibility for health? It might be claimed that we could value all of these things, but at some point we will have to choose between values that are sharply contradictory. (At the very least, when we have to decide how we prioritise work or where to devote resources; employing another practice nurse, say, against allowing the money for the post going to fund a community worker in a voluntary organisation.)

HEALTH PROMOTION: CONTEST AND DISPUTE

The potential partisanship that plays out in healthcare as a result of differing health-related values and ideologies is especially prominent in health promotion.[1] Here we are presented with a further set of models, each of which claims to represent authentic practice. Broadly, these are:

➤ the medical model (health promotion as expert-led, disease prevention – focused and based on individual responsibility)
➤ the educational model (health promotion through informed decision-making)
➤ the empowerment model (promoting health through support to enable individuals and communities to act for themselves and make the choices that they wish in relation to health)
➤ the social change model (health promotion through altering wider social structures).

There is a need, however, to be cautious and point to the limitations of this kind of description of health promotion. Models are, after all, just that: attempts in some way to *represent* reality. They are not reality itself. This, as we know from experience, is much messier and more complex than model-making can allow. So we might be presented with a situation in which social change health promotion is being enacted with just as much expert-led vigour as individual, medical model health promotion. Indeed, social change health promotion can be (and often is) conducted with a set of what we might call 'medical model values' dominating. Take, for example, the introduction of the ban on smoking in enclosed public places instituted in the UK in July 2007. If this involved consultation at all, it was consultation dominated by professional and expert interests. The evidence supplied to support the legislation that provided for the ban was evidence that, generally speaking, had been constructed and disseminated by experts via the House of Commons Health Committee Report.[10] The overall belief was that it was possible to solve a public health problem by putting strong pressure on individuals to behave in certain ways. There is no need necessarily to disagree with what is happening here. It is important, however, to recognise that banning smoking in public places, for example, is more than a technical act. It fundamentally involves an ideology and set of values that we might share, or we might not.

It has been argued that contest and competition over the purpose, scope and limits of health promotion is especially fierce.[11] We might generally be able to agree on the purpose of at least some aspects of acute healthcare. (The purpose of cardiac services, say, is treatment for and rehabilitation of individuals with heart problems.) We might also be prepared to define the scope and limits of, say, cardiology provision. I want to argue that it is difficult for us to do the same with health promotion. Are we preventing disease? Are we promoting health in a more holistic way? If so, what exactly does or should this entail?

The cause of the especially fierce contest that exists over the purpose and scope of health promotion lies in part, of course, in the fact that we find it hard to agree what exactly the 'health' is that we are supposed to be promoting. But this is only part of the answer to the ferocity of differences in relation to the field. Dispute is also fierce because health promotion, in the eyes of some, has been deliberately constituted as a 'reform movement', a counterpoint to the all-pervasive and (it is often argued) limiting power of medicine.[12] This idea is particularly potent when the historical context for the emergence of health promotion is considered. The beginnings of health promotion can be aligned with mid-twentieth-century moves away from accepted and imposed authority, towards individual rights (for example, the women's and disability rights movements).[13] Health and healthcare were not necessarily seen any longer as the preserve of the expert. Part of this tendency stemmed from powerful critiques of medicine and its methods (see, for example, Illich[14]). Yet at the same time, medicine quite naturally sought to maintain its power, if not through explicit attack on those who wished to reform it then at least through attempts to absorb the 'new' creation.[15] The result is the potential for, and often the reality of, deep conflict between the medical traditionalists and the reformers. Even those from medicine with sympathies towards reform might baulk at the consequences of the enterprise (or at least some versions of it). For example, can health promotion *truly* be about empowerment in the sense that peoples' actual health choices don't matter so long as they have been enabled to make the choices that they want? Does this mean that we shouldn't care whether people carry on smoking or not, say, so long as they are empowered? A more reasonable view might be that those working in medicine, and healthcare more generally, operate with the belief that there are indeed better and worse ways to live one's life.[16]

HEALTH PROMOTION: PROFESSIONAL PERSPECTIVES

Within what I have just said lie the seeds of a further reason why health promotion purpose, scope and limits are so heavily contested. We come to believe what we do about the nature of health and the purpose of healthcare through our professional persona.

And this persona might well find it hard to accommodate the kind of liberal health promotion reformist view that I have just outlined.

The idea of the 'hidden curriculum' will be a familiar one to those involved in medical education. This is the notion that running parallel to the formal curriculum through which the values, beliefs and practices of the profession of medicine are officially conveyed is a further process that reinforces and embeds these things in the persona of those who are professionals-in-training. Indeed, it has been argued that this 'hidden curriculum' is immensely powerful in the socialisation effects it has on those striving to become members of the profession concerned.[5] It would be impossible to deny that doctors become doctors partly through their formal training. But they also learn to become and be doctors through processes of vicarious observation, modelling and informal participation that present themselves in the daily (and nightly) lives of wards, clinics, surgeries, student accommodation, staff messes and so on. The importance of the 'hidden curriculum' is not confined to medical education alone, but can also be traced within other professions.[6]

Despite attempts at shifting orientation through policy and other means (see, for example, the General Medical Council),[17] it can reasonably be argued that medical training and practice is by and large wedded to the so-called medical model of health. Belief in the power of the expert to deal with difficulties, and for this to occur largely in the context of individual patient-professional consultations remains central to medical ideology. Part of the reason for this lies in the pervasiveness of the 'hidden curriculum'. Formal policy may dictate one thing, but prejudices and practice encountered every day suggest something quite different.

HEALTH PROMOTION: THE 'DRIVEN CURRICULUM'

Against the generalised background of competing understandings about the nature of health, we are therefore presented with very real conflict about the nature and purpose of health promotion. Liberal reformists ('health promotion is a social movement challenging in some way the status quo in healthcare') lock horns – at least potentially – with conservative traditionalists ('health promotion is a useful adjunct to medicine but its function is to supplement the kind of practice that has always been engaged in'). We can move from thinking about the 'hidden curriculum' within medical education in general to thinking of health promotion as a particularly 'driven curriculum' within the overall project of medical education.

By 'driven curriculum' I mean one that is fundamentally based on values, and that depends on those values to shape, direct and move it forward. In this sense, much of the medical education curriculum is 'driven'. However, my conception of health promotion as a 'driven curriculum' involves one further, fundamental aspect: *the curriculum is 'driven' (and thus derives at least part of its energy) from the fact that there is a diametrically different and competing version of the curriculum that drives the one chosen and followed forward*. In this sense, I would argue that the 'driven-ness' of the health promotion curriculum is unique within medical education. Let me explain what I mean.

Imagine for a moment another curricular aspect of medical education – gross anatomy. We can conceive of this as a traditional basic science course, focusing on the human structure. Or we can understand it as providing an opportunity to extend beyond this and engage with students on issues such as respect, responsibility, self-policing and so on.[18] Such issues extend beyond, but can be integrated with, the basic science. Although it is possible to imagine some level of disagreement about this kind of extension and integration, many would probably see the sense in it. Importantly, we could see the 'revised' gross anatomy curriculum as driven by values, but these would be values that it would be hard not to subscribe to. Exactly how can we argue against the incorporation of teaching and learning about respect, say, in a basic science course that is a foundation for a profession where concern for humanity is so fundamental? In other words, while the gross anatomy course is driven by values, they are values that most would share.

Consider now a possible health promotion curriculum, based on the so-called medical model of health promotion, in the process of development by Dr A. He thinks that this might include material around strategies and practices to change individual 'risky' behaviour, the mechanics of screening for particular diseases and so on. He is beginning his development from the premises that health is the absence of disease and the achievement of good health requires the intervention of the expert (the medical practitioner). However, it is easy to imagine his colleague in another institution, Dr B, framing a quite different health promotion curriculum, one that focuses on the so-called empowerment model. Here, material Dr B might include would be the assessment of health need as identified by lay people and communities, strategies and practices for enabling people to become more skilled at recognising and getting what they feel they need from health and other services, and so on. The premises for this version of a health promotion curriculum would be that 'health' is subject to individual or community interpretation and that what matters is that people feel enabled to do what they themselves think is best, regardless of professional expectations.

The two separate proposed curricula of Dr A and Dr B are quite different because radically alternative premises are driving them. And these premises are not in any sense wholly factual; they are based primarily in values. What makes these health promotion curricula different from the gross anatomy curriculum – what causes them to be especially 'driven' – is that there is every likelihood that many will disagree with one or other set of values. Dr A will find it hard to comprehend the value of empowerment ('how can we justifiably let people do whatever they want?'); while Dr B will quite possibly recoil from the idea of professional judgement trumping all ('how can we force people to do things they have no interest in doing?'). More than this, it is the conception of the other's values-related position that is a principal driver of his or her own. Dr A's belief in the benefit of professional expertise will take strength from a further belief that there are limits to individual or community capacity to create 'health' and deal with 'health problems'. Notions that the unfettered power of the medical expert can be highly damaging will feed Dr B's commitment to the central importance of empowerment. So it is possible to see that dramatically different versions of health promotion curricula, and their completely separate underpinning values, have their power reinforced because, in the different view of each, the alternative is so problematic, even damaging. This is what makes the idea of the health promotion curriculum such a 'driven' one, in the way that I started out arguing it to be.

TOWARDS THE RECONCILIATION OF VALUES

At this point, somebody might reasonably ask whether this kind of 'competitive drivenness' is inevitable for health promotion and for how it might be conceived by those involved in the medical education curriculum. Why can't it be possible for some kind of middle ground to be reached? Why can't we occupy a territory where due regard is given to both the expertise of the professional and the intuition of the lay person, where health is seen as both an individual matter as well as socially mediated and influenced? This may well be the pragmatic conclusion of health promotion curriculum planners. After all, we cannot continue forever with possibly irresolvable arguments to do with ideology and values – at some point we have to stand up and engage in teaching and learning!

While I certainly agree with this pragmatism, there is also a need to balance the suggestion of it with caution. In a field so filled with contest between competing ideologies and values, we cannot simply proceed to the pragmatic without reference to these. That is why the kind of discussion I have tried to engage with in this chapter is such an important one. If we miss out on it, we run the very real risk of teaching and learning in an environment where much is unspoken and where conflict between those with different values, if it surfaces, is either misunderstood or becomes very hard to deal with. Learning and teaching about health promotion in this sort of climate will be deeply difficult, if not impossible.

This seems to draw attention towards ideas about how we might begin to go about dealing with values contest in the health promotion curriculum, and even possibly achieving some degree of reconciliation. I want to suggest that if we are serious about the place of health promotion in the wider curriculum of medical education, we need to engage in four processes.

➤ To begin with, we need to acknowledge that in teaching and learning about health promotion, we are not engaged with a morally neutral activity. It needs to be understood as a field that extends well beyond the factual and into the realm of ideologies, beliefs and values. This recognition needs to involve not only thought of how we might go about promoting health (medical *versus* empowerment model, for example) but also of how we conceive of *effectiveness* in health promotion work, and *evidence of effectiveness*. Views on these things that we might encounter in our preparation for teaching and learning about health promotion are not in any sense simply descriptive. They are laden with values.

➤ This acknowledgement needs to extend beyond an analysis of what is going on in the field, its theories and practices, and embrace our own attitudes towards the promotion of health. It is unlikely that we will have no view whatsoever about health promotion and its purpose. If we have not already done so, we need to engage in a rigorous self-assessment of our own attitudes towards the territory. To what extent are we wedded to the idea of the importance of professional expertise? Are we *really* happy with the idea of conceding control to others? Are there limits to individual responsibility for health, and if so where and how are they drawn? These kinds of questions might form the beginning of a kind of 'self-audit' of our own health promotion-related beliefs and values. And as I have discussed in this chapter, delving into our own professional backgrounds and histories might play an important part in undertaking this exercise.

➤ We need to engage in similar work with the students whom we teach. However, this cannot be a one-sided process. Teaching and learning about values needs the active involvement of the teacher as well as the learner in the process of uncovering exactly what these might be and how they could play out in the practice of health promotion. The separate values positions of teacher and learner can only be discussed if all are involved in the process. If not, there is the risk of one group or another feeling vulnerable and exposed.[19]

➤ Values are deeply personal. As I have discussed, this is a major reason why such strong contest often exists in relation to them. There is a need, then, to be careful about the process of unpacking values. Additionally, many medical education students are at highly formative stages of their lives and for this reason may find it hard to engage in dialogue on values.[20] Helpful approaches to the discussion of values in health promotion might therefore include the use of resources that allow vicarious commentary and discussion on values. For example, students could be asked to examine and discuss the issue of legislation to ban smoking in public places. To what extent do they think values are present in this kind of intervention? What sort of values? Do they agree with those values? These sorts of 'trigger' questions would centre the debate about the intervention clearly on the values and motivations underlying it, but would also allow people to position themselves in relation to it in a non-threatening way.

CONCLUSION

None of this is meant to imply, of course, that the health promotion curriculum in medical education becomes solely concerned with discussions on values. It is, after all, a *health promotion* curriculum, and this is what needs to be taught and learnt about! What I have been arguing in this chapter is that the central place of values in health promotion activity, and consequently teaching and learning about the field, needs to be explicitly acknowledged. In turn, discussion on values needs to be one of the threads running through the health promotion syllabus.

Understanding of the curriculum and construction of the syllabus in these terms is likely to have at least two effects. The first is that students will have more confidence about their attitudes towards health promotion and its place in their future practice. The second is that by 'bringing values out into the open', we are enabling ourselves to discuss the broad range of activities and interventions that might promote health. It is quite right for us to believe that there are better and worse ways to lead lives; and therefore better and worse ways to engage in health promotion. But this belief can only be justified when we have carefully considered the range of possibilities that are contained in our own and others' views of what is better and what is worse.

REFERENCES

1 Tones K, Green J. *Health Promotion: planning and strategies.* London: Sage; 2004.
2 Peters RS. *Authority, Responsibility and Education.* 3rd ed. London: George Allen and Unwin; 1973.
3 Carr D. *Making Sense of Education.* Abingdon: Routledge; 2003.
4 Gillon R. Health education: the ambiguity of the medical role. In: Doxiadis S, editor. *Ethics in Health Education.* London: John Wiley and Sons Ltd; 1990.
5 Cribb A, Bignold S. Towards the reflexive medical school: the hidden curriculum and medical education research. *Stud High Educ.* 1999; **24**(2): 195–209.
6 Duncan P. *Critical Perspectives on Health.* Basingstoke: Palgrave Macmillan; 2007.
7 Earle S. Exploring health. In: Earle S, Lloyd CE, Sidell M, *et al.*, editors. *Theory and Research in Promoting Public Health.* London: Sage/Open University; 2007. pp. 37–65.

8 Scalding JG. Health and disease: what can medicine do for philosophy? *J Med Ethics*. 1988; 14: 118–24.

9 Dougherty CJ. Bad faith and victim-blaming: the limits of health promotion. *Health Care Anal*. 1993; 1(2): 111–19.

10 House of Commons Health Committee. *Smoking in Public Places: first report of session 2005–06*. London: The Stationery Office; 2006.

11 Lucas K, Lloyd B, Hitchin D. Why some children smoke: could measuring personality improve intervention success? *Health Educ Res*. 1999; 14(1): 121–30.

12 Nutbeam D. Health promotion glossary. *Health Promot Int*. 1998; 13(4): 349–64.

13 Duncan P. Dispute, dissent and the place of health promotion in a 'disrupted tradition'. *Publ Understand Sci*. 2004; 13(2): 177–90.

14 Illich I. *Limits to Medicine*. London: Marion Boyers; 1976.

15 Armstrong D. From clinical gaze to regime of total health. In: Beattie A, editor. *Health and Well-Being: a reader*. Basingstoke: Macmillan; 1993.

16 Downie RS, Tannahil C, Tannahill A. *Health Promotion: models and values*. 2nd ed. Oxford: Oxford University Press; 1996.

17 General Medical Council. *Tomorrow's Doctors*. London: General Medical Council; 1993.

18 Pawlina W. *Transformed Gross Anatomy in a Revised Medical Curriculum*. Available at: www. amee.org/video.asp?id 2007 (accessed October 2008).

19 Halstead JM, Reiss MJ. *Values in Sex Education: from principles to practice*. London: Routledge Falmer; 2003.

20 Halper E. Ethics in film. *APA Newsletter*. 2003; 3(1): 191–5.

CHAPTER 11

Defining learning outcomes within a spiral curriculum: from sessions to curriculum

Ann Wylie and Bev Daily

FROM SESSION OUTCOMES TO COMMUNITY OUTCOMES

The content of a typical health promotion session in Year 1 of any health promotion programme would be likely to involve students exploring definitions of health, health as a value, a concept and who the various stakeholders are that define health such as actuaries, politicians and lay public as well as health professionals.

Students would have explicit learning outcomes such as to be aware of complex social factors being determinants of peoples' health, that no single definition exists and that the World Health Organization (WHO) have attempted defining health.[1,2] Students may also be expected to relate health and health belief models to themselves and consider how these may change with time and circumstance.

In addition to this, sooner or later students would be introduced to demographic, epidemiological and public health data. The learning outcomes would be variable depending on the course but would essentially be indicating that measuring health is often limited and subjective whereas measures such as morbidity, mortality rates, infant mortality rates, income, education attainment and housing can provide more substantial and meaningful data for needs assessment and intervention planning. These data may also be resources for learning how to critique studies and be aware of strengths and limitations.

The trajectory of programmes will differ depending on the course, level and context but the following areas, with associated learning outcomes, would be likely to be presented:

➤ the Ottawa Charter and its implications; the main approaches to applied health promotion
➤ the theories, models and concepts; the feeder disciplines and their research paradigms
➤ intervention evidence and evaluation methodology
➤ needs assessment, design, planning and implementing health promotion interventions and strategies.

Students would be looking at these with regard to working with individuals, in partnerships with local agencies, with communities and with national and international policies.

What is especially useful in the narrative below is that we can see how some otherwise vague terms have practical application. The context of the narrative may, however, seem unchallenging, provincial, suburban, well funded, with access to the National Health Service (NHS) and a functioning local democracy. For some the efforts of community-based health promotion are concerned with the underserved, urban deprivation or rural and remote situations, with little or no funding, with poor democratic systems and with civil unrest, violence and crime, drug dependency, oppression and sexual exploitation. Yet the narrative provides the fundamental elements applicable to health promotion community-based outcomes, be they part of a non-government organisation (NGO), a local project in South Africa or an urban strategy for improving physical activity. Whilst Daily has given us a linear and descriptive narrative, Wylie has indicated where these experiences could be linked to specific learning outcomes and concepts.[3] The narrative should also be read with reference to the principles set out in the Ottawa Charter.

The Ottawa Charter set out three principal approaches for health promotion: advocate, enable and mediate, within five domains as follows:

➤ build health public policy
➤ create supportive environments
➤ strengthen community action
➤ develop personal skills
➤ reorient health services.[2]

Further details about the concepts, terms and health promotion practice can be found in the textbooks listed below, which would be familiar to the reading lists on many health promotion courses:

➤ *Health Promotion: foundations for practice* by Naidoo and Wills[4]
➤ *Promoting Health: a practical guide* by Ewles and Simnett[1]
➤ *Health Promotion: professional perspectives* by Scriven and Orme[5]
➤ *Health Promotion: effectiveness, efficiency and equity* by Tones and Tilford[6]
➤ *Hands-on Health Promotion* by Moodie and Hulme[7]
➤ *Health Studies: an introduction* by Naidoo and Wills[8]
➤ 'Health promotion in general practice'[9] (by Wylie), Chapter 11 in *A Textbook of General Practice.*

Information about funding and European programmes that promote and support community action can be found at the European Commission Public Health website (http://ec.europa.eu/health/ph_programme/documents/prog_booklet_en.pdf).

HEALTH PROMOTION OUTCOMES: THE COMMUNITY EXPERIENCE

**HEALTH PROMOTION AT COMMUNITY LEVEL:
THE STORY OF THE BURNHAM HEALTH PROMOTION TRUST**

Background

A cold, wet Friday morning in February 2005. Two individuals sit outside the only public toilets in their village. One a retired GP, the other a community worker, they are counting the number of people entering and leaving. On their clipboards they have collected the information that will help to overthrow a decision that would have had dire consequences, particularly for the elderly and disabled, in the community of Burnham in South Buckinghamshire. Armed with the facts, Burnham Health Promotion Trust (BHPT) mobilised virtually all local organisations to successfully oppose the closure of these toilets by the local authority.

This rather unusual exercise has been one of the many activities carried out by the BHPT, an organisation now at the heart of the life of the village.

Burnham, in spite of its population of 12 000 is, indeed, a village. It is said by some to be the largest village in England. Unique! Possibly unique as well is the local, charity-run health promotion trust, attached as it is to the large, NHS health centre training practice in the middle of the village.

The following Ottawa Charter principles apply to this community initiative
- Create supportive environments
- Strengthen community action
- Reorient health services[2]

The world generally is a place where instructions and advice on how we should live our lives comes down from the top. By contrast, the BHPT is designed to work from the bottom up, to fulfil the need, as is its mandate from the local community.

Among its many activities, BHPT conducted a survey assessing the secondary school students' attitudes to, and requirements from, sex education as delivered at school. There were almost 1000 respondents, aged 12 to 15, across two local secondary schools. At one school, with a 40% Asian-descent intake, the needs of these students as far as sex education was concerned, were substantially different from those at the other school. Thus, it was concluded, from the survey, that sex education must be contextualised for individual schools. And changes were made in Sex and Relationship Education (SRE) at both schools, some almost immediately.

The impact of local health promotion can be immediate in its effect. The need for action can be detected early and easily. The problem can be targeted and assistance given in a very short time.

But how do we define the objectives of health promotion? Getting people to give up smoking? Getting them to stop drinking too much alcohol or eating too much of the wrong kind of food? Getting them to take more exercise? Or do we try and produce an environment where people find it easier to do the things that are generally regarded as 'good for them', indeed, enjoy and feel the benefit of doing the things that are good for them?

At BHPT we aim to do things that help, doing things that are possible and have an effect at a community level. We work with the following health promotion definition, which is 'a study of, and the study of the response to, the modifiable determinants of health'.[9]

Strategy: Explore Ewles & Simnett's Approaches to Health Promotion,[1] Beattie's model[3] and Stages Of Change model[10] to have a coherent, rationale and pragmatic approach to define health promotion objectives.

WHO Principle: Strengthen community action

Outcome: Strengthening community action, advocacy, local democracy and needs assessment

Although this narrative is not scientific it may however be helpful to other small, interested groups, at the sharp end of health promotion, who have thought of setting up a similar type of organisation themselves.

The approach of the Burnham Health Promotion Trust has always been 'Do this, and you'll enjoy your life more . . . and, quite likely, for longer!'

Setting up the Burnham Health promotion trust

In 1997, local philanthropists Louis and Valerie Freedman of Cliveden Stud, Taplow made a gift of £1 million to the adjoining village of Burnham to set up a charitable trust to improve the health and well-being of the residents of the community. A local GP at the Burnham Health Centre who was particularly interested in health promotion, Dr Nigel Lewis, himself a fine sportsman and a particular friend of the Freedmans, was instrumental in setting up this Trust.

The community of Burnham

Burnham is semi-rural, with countryside – including the Burnham Beeches – to the north and west. It is very mixed socially, having both the wealthy and pockets of the very poor. It feels like a village and has a strong sense of community. It sits roughly equidistant from the town centres of Maidenhead, Windsor and Slough.

The usual health-related indices are good: there is low unemployment, low levels of violent crime and virtually no gun crime. However there are relatively high levels of burglary, vandalism, drunkenness, stealing from cars and general antisocial behaviour. There does not appear to be an overwhelming drug problem. There is a small ethnic minority population but little in the way of racial conflict.

The educational system is based on selection at age 11. There are two State secondary schools, Burnham Grammar School, a selective school, and

Burnham Upper School, a secondary modern school. Both schools have specialist school status. Burnham Grammar has a large number of Asian-descent students coming to the school from Slough and West Middlesex. Burnham Upper is a neighbourhood school with a relatively small Asian-descent element, reflecting the ethnic mix of Burnham itself.

The largest unit providing medical care in Burnham is the Burnham Health Centre NHS practice in the middle of the village. This is a training practice with up to three registrars at a time. It also provides training for medical students. The majority of the 18 000 patients come from within the parish. About a quarter come from the adjoining areas of the Slough part of the Burnham Community; indeed, Burnham railway station itself is in Slough.

There are variations in services as there are boundary overlaps with local authority and NHS provisions which can cause problems in the area. So, many people in Burnham, Buckinghamshire live within a few metres of residents of Slough, Berkshire. The BHPT is constantly trying to redress these differences, particularly where Burnham residents do not have access to services freely available to their Slough neighbours living, perhaps, just across the road. Such services as free bus passes for the elderly, Home Start and Age Concern's free toenail clipping services are amongst those that have been financed by the Trust and made available to Burnham residents.

There are many elderly people in Burnham. It is, generally speaking, a pleasant place to live with amenities such as its own high street and shops, and most people do not move away when they reach retirement age.

Consider the following
- Travel, cultural, socioeconomic status of the community
- Generating local demographic data to inform needs assessment, intervention planning

Community profile report

A community profile survey was commissioned to study the health and social needs of the Burnham community. The Community Profile Report published in February 1999 identified nine areas to be addressed and made a number of recommendations for action. The areas identified were:

- Older people
- Young people
- Physical activity
- Communication
- Mental health
- Deprivation
- Lone parents
- Transport
- Alcohol and drug abuse.

As a result of this report, BHPT strategically focused on the following actions:

- Target areas within Church ward and Lent Rise ward where there are some of the highest levels of deprivation in southern Buckinghamshire
- Address the needs of older people
- Focus on facilities for young people
- Increase opportunities for all to improve levels of physical activity.

Strategies utilised

- Recruitment of two health professionals
- Liaison with executive in charge of health promotion at East Berkshire Health Authority who was also a lecturer in health promotion at University of Reading
- Successful management within the Trust
- Allocation of grants and monies for purposeful community development
- Advocacy on behalf of the community to local authorities to prioritise local services.

- Outcomes associated with lessons learned
- Increased clarity as regards the objectives which are indicators of defining success for evaluation
- Community empowerment is evident
- Utilisation of evidence-based interventions

Select examples of activities undertaken by BHPT

Older people

- In partnership with the local health authority, BHPT formed a powerful, popular group for Burnham's elderly – BOPAG, Burnham Older People's Action Group, a very substantial and influential voice. Its activities also include a weekly exercise group.
- Supported the 'Save Burnham Library Campaign' which resulted in partial library closure being averted – indeed the library is now to be extended with a Lottery Fund grant of £300 000!
- In association with Age Concern's 'Happy Feet', free toenail clipping service for elderly and disabled (not eligible for NHS podiatry) brought to Burnham Health Centre, financed by BHPT.

Young people

- A series of after-school discussions was held with groups, mainly girls in Year 10 at local secondary schools, with a health professional, with the aim to build self-esteem, empower, improve self-worth and, manage pressure within peer groups. In follow-up discussions, the effect of the Alpha female and changes to anticipated age for first pregnancy were explored.
- A BHPT survey of 400 primary school and secondary school pupils was carried out on 'Recreational Facilities and Safety in the Community'.
- BHPT researched the condition and suitability of local play areas. With leaders of the Parish Council, it presented its findings to the Trustees of the Louis and Valerie Freedman Charitable Settlement and a large grant

was made to completely refurbish and modernise Burnham's largest play area.

- The Trust carried out its largest survey on all students at Burnham's two secondary schools on lifestyle – eating habits, self-perception, use of computers, exercise, membership of sports clubs, smoking, use of alcohol, use of drugs, and bullying.

Issue to consider include:
- Community empowerment, priorities, and partnerships
- Local politics and the interface with national issues
- Interpretation of directives and use of public funds/resources

This supports the importance of partnerships and working with not-for-profit organisations, often known as the third sector or non-government organisations (NGOs). In North America the term is usually working with the underserved community and in Melbourne the specific scheme for students is the community partnership programme.

Communications
- BHPT financed the first Burnham Access Directory, a comprehensive publication giving details of all Burnham shops, businesses, services, facilities etc. with particular information for the disabled – accessibility etc.
- Development of a website – www.burnhambucks.co.uk for Burnham.

Health and mental health
- 'Round and About', the community newspaper distributed an article to every household on recognising and managing depression.
- BHPT has also been involved in individual, group support and organisational support to families and carers through grants, referrals, education and service delivery on health and mental health issues.

- Questions about the philosophy of equality, empowerment and targeting need to be considered
- Advocate, enable and mediate sustainable outcomes which link with social determinants and medical approaches

Conclusion
A description of the Burnham Health Promotion Trust, how it was started and how it has continued over the last 10 years offers suggestions that might be useful to others thinking of starting a similar venture.

Burnham was very lucky to be in receipt of a most generous gift to start things off and will ever be grateful to Louis and Valerie Freedman, their family and the appointed Trustees of the Louis and Valerie Freedman Charitable Settlement. It has allowed BHPT to put all its energy into health promotion rather than fundraising. Indeed the Trust has been well managed and is a best practice example of community engagement and prudent performance. Volunteerism and staff commitment is strong, with the Trustees being actively involved in a number of roles and sharing their experience and expertise. BHPT's professional working relationships with health professionals, heads of schools, parish and district councillors, police and many local charities, notably the two Rotary Clubs of Burnham and the Lions have enabled participatory action to be taken at a community level.

But most of all, it has the best of relations with the people of Burnham who are very aware of the Trust, the Trustees and what the Trust is able to offer. This has therefore made 'health promotion' in the village of Burnham a very acceptable and helpful concept, with a positive health outcome for the community.

Dr Bev Daily, Trustee, Burnham Health Promotion Trust

SHARED OUTCOMES FOR PROMOTING HEALTH

The context in which students learn will vary and so will any community-based experience for learning about applied health promotion practice.[9] What is possible in terms of local projects, what priority is given in curriculum as well as time, will determine what students can actually do and learn. Doctors and other community-based health professionals will have various levels of involvement with the wider health-promoting community organisations. For doctors and other community-based health professionals, how far beyond the 'clinical remit' should be part of their professional role is constant fodder for debate.

However, whether working in and with affluent, well-educated communities or within poorer, underserved communities, an awareness of local determinants of health is vital.

Studies have demonstrated that students have a good appreciation of local social determinants of health when they have the opportunity to experience involvement with community-based programmes such as these.[11] Effectiveness of advice, for example, to take more exercise, will be enhanced if the advice-giver can enable the patient to access and use local facilities. A good knowledge of the patient's likely income, what resources are available to him and his family, what opportunities there are for physical activity and what barriers exist, all add to the potential for quality of healthcare provision. We are aware that poorer communities suffer poorer health outcomes, so much is to be gained if health professionals, before and after qualification, can work with the community and be proactive partners in community healthcare.[12]

A basic education in community health promotion at undergraduate level would enable health professionals to engage with the principles of the Ottawa Charter, to critique evidence and evaluation data linked to social determinants of health and to consider their role in this context. This would also prepare students for overseas work during electives, whether they are linked with NGOs, small community projects or one of the many charities providing students with popular elective placements.

Health, as the WHO has argued, is not the objective of living but a resource for living, and there are many ways in which health can be enhanced at community level.[2]

REFERENCES

1 Ewles L, Simnett I. *Promoting Health: a practical guide.* 5th ed. London: Bailliere Tindall; 2003.
2 World Health Organization. *Ottawa Charter for Health Promotion.* Geneva: World Health Organization; 1986.
3 Beattie A, Gott M, Jones L, *et al. Health and Wellbeing: a reader.* Basingstoke: Macmillan; 1993.
4 Naidoo J, Wills J. *Health Promotion; foundations for practice.* 2nd ed. London: Bailliere Tindall; 2000.
5 Scriven A, Orme J. *Health Promotion: professional perspectives.* 2nd ed. Basingstoke: Palgrave; 2001.
6 Tones K, Tilford S. *Health Promotion: effectiveness, efficiency and equity.* 2nd ed. London: Chapman and Hall; 1994.
7 Moodie R, Hulme A, editors. *Hands-on Health Promotion.* East Hawthorn, Victoria: IP Communications; 2004.
8 Naidoo J, Wills J, editors. *Health Studies: an introduction.* Basingstoke: Palgrave; 2001.
9 Wylie A. Health promotion in general practice. In: Stephenson A, editor. *A Textbook of General Practice.* 2nd ed. London: Arnold; 2004. pp. 187–210.
10 Prochaska JO, DiClemente CO. Towards a comprehensive model of change. In: Miller WR, Heather N, editors. *Treating Addictive Behaviors: processes of change.* New York: Plenum Press; 1986. pp. 3–27.
11 Holt T, Goodall J, Jones KV, *et al.* Community-based medical professionalism: learning by doing. In: *Proceedings of the 13th International Ottawa Conference on Clinical Competence.* Melbourne, Australia; 2008 5–8 Mar; pp. 469–72.
12 Department of Health. *Tackling Health Inequalities: a programme for action.* London: Department of Health; 2003.

CHAPTER 12

Public health and general practice education

Jane Wills, Jo Reynolds and Tim Swanwick

General practitioners (GPs) have a crucial role to play in promoting health and preventing disease, in consultation with the individual patient, through planned activities such as vaccinations, cervical smears, blood pressure monitoring and through their role in the wider primary healthcare team. At the practice level, health promotion includes the use of education literature in practice waiting rooms, the use of health summaries in medical records, and the use of systematic patient reminders for preventive activity. For many people, general practice is the first point of contact with healthcare provision, and the General Household Survey reveals that since 1972 the average number of GP consultations per person in Great Britain has remained relatively stable at around four consultations per year, with 78% of people consulting their GP at least once during each year.[1]

There have also been calls for primary care in the UK, including general practice, to acknowledge responsibility for the health needs of communities and practice populations, beyond the individual patient in a clinical setting. The Darzi report on healthcare for London emphasised the need for primary care to provide services tailored to the specific needs of their local population and to identify localities or groups with poor health.[2] This reflects the increasing demand for GPs to be able to assess the health needs of the community in which they work, to be involved in practice-based commissioning of services and to contribute towards public health goals.[3] This argument is centred on the idea that GPs, at the forefront of primary care and people's access to healthcare, are well placed to address the wider determinants of health and health inequalities across populations but must do so within a context of limited resources.

Despite a favourable policy context and a recognition of the importance of prevention and health promotion, it plays a minor role in the care by GPs, with low levels of lifestyle advice given and often only when related to the presenting condition.[4] Earlier studies reported that GPs had positive attitudes towards health promotion in principle but reservations about it in practice.[5–8] Barriers cited include lack of training, ambivalence about the effectiveness of interventions, perceived lack of self-efficacy and confidence regarding health promotion, time constraints and a lack of remuneration incentives.[9–11]

Public health can be said to encompass three domains of practice: improving services, health protection and the investigation and control of outbreaks and health improvement, which includes the promotion of good health.[12] Although public health has long been recognised as having a central place in the training of doctors[13] it has struggled to have a place in undergraduate medical training, continuing medical education and even in postgraduate specialty training for GPs. Medical schools have been reluctant to accord public health a central presence in the curriculum and some regard it as an entirely postgraduate discipline.[14] Specialty teachers are in short supply and those from public health tend to regard their subject as exclusively population-based. 'New' medical schools have curricula designed extensively around problem-based learning (PBL), notwithstanding contested evidence as to its benefits.[15,16] Whilst such curricula may exhibit less of the traditional divide between clinical and non-clinical areas, there is no guarantee that epidemiological and preventive principles will be applied in the chosen cases and unless this is specifically assessed, students are unlikely to perceive its importance. A national survey of public health teaching in UK medical schools in 2005[17] highlighted the variable nature of public health teaching and a lack of consensus about what might constitute a public health syllabus, a central concern of many of the regional Teaching Public Health networks funded by the Department of Health. For those who go on to choose general practice as a specialty, the importance of a public health and health promotion perspective is unlikely to have been suggested let alone imbued at this level.

Continuing medical education (CME) can be broadly defined as formal educational events designed to maintain, update or improve professional practice. CME is widely used across healthcare professions, is often compulsory and in general practice is considered to be a means to ensure GPs continue to update and apply their clinical knowledge and skills. There is a body of evidence about effective forms of CME including interactive learning interventions compared to traditional, didactic approaches such as lectures.[18] There is some evidence that CME can improve GP communication skills[19] and this may improve confidence in delivering lifestyle advice and address any concerns over the effect on the doctor-patient relationship by giving this advice.[20,21] Programmes of CME aimed at GPs however rarely address the public health skills, competencies and knowledge to be found in the training curriculum of the Royal College of General Practitioners.[22]

Specialty training for general practice is currently based on a three-year programme which typically involves a series of placements lasting 18–24 months in a hospital or secondary care setting and 12–18 months in general practice. Although it should be noted that following the recent Tooke Report[23] and NHS Next Stage Review[24] there are moves to increase the duration of training programmes to four or even five years. Training programmes are structured by postgraduate deaneries which are organised geographically across the UK. The suitability of current postgraduate medical training schemes for a rapidly changing social, scientific and healthcare environment has come under recent scrutiny.[25–28] In 2007 the Royal College of General Practitioners (RCGP) published a curriculum for GP specialty training. This RCGP curriculum is based on the European Definition of Family Practice[29] which places 'community orientation' as a core domain of competence for the family practitioner. Furthermore, the curriculum's constituent statements highlight the need for GPs to:

➤ move beyond an individual clinical focus to consider patients in a wider social context and address the needs of whole populations and population groups

➤ understand the necessity for, and how to determine, service priorities within available resources, in light of the new practice-based commissioning environment

➤ see general practice as part of wider sector and cross-sector movement for health promotion and improvement.[22]

As an illustration, Statement 5 of the RCGP curriculum 'Healthy People – promoting health, preventing disease' emphasises the need for trainees to discuss healthy living with patients, understand inequalities in health and strategies to address such inequalities, and be aware of the wider health agenda.

To date, there have been very few opportunities created in the UK for training in public health for GPs.[30] A recent survey of GP training in the UK did not include public health in the list of either 'major' or 'minor' specialities covered in standard GP training attachments, and made no mention even of its connection to training programmes or general practice.[31] There are a few examples of evaluations of programmes offering public health-focused training to GP trainees.[30,32,33] However, these programmes, which offered public health training to only a very small proportion of trainees, were evaluated prior to the changes to the RCGP curriculum in 2007 and did not appear to explore trainees' perceptions of how public health training may impact on their future practice.

In 2007 the London Deanery, responsible for the postgraduate education of over 10 000 doctors, developed a number of training attachments based in public health departments and supervised by the Director of Public Health (or a nominated public health trainer).[34] These were offered as part of the three-year GP specialty training programme, alongside traditional clinical attachments, including general practice, accident and emergency medicine, obstetrics and gynaecology, paediatrics and psychiatry. The attachments were located in 10 Primary Care Trusts (PCTs) across London; eight of which provided six-month training posts, and two provided four-month training posts. A competency framework was drawn up for the attachments by mapping key competency areas from the Faculty of Public Health[12] across to five relevant statements from the RCGP curriculum, as shown below with the statement number displayed in brackets:

➤ Evidence-based practice (3.5)
➤ Research and academic activity (3.6)
➤ Teaching, mentoring and clinical supervision (3.7)
➤ Management in primary care (4.1)
➤ Healthy people: promoting health and preventing disease (5).

Additionally, trainees were offered a series of monthly central teaching sessions organised by the London Deanery, and covering the basic principles of public health. Trainees were also required to continue attending their GP specialty training programme teaching sessions.

These attachments enabled GP trainees to address certain areas of the RCGP training curriculum that relate to the changing nature of general practice and the skills required by future GPs in commissioning and assessing health needs and health impact. However, it appears that fulfilling competencies and increasing knowledge of public health may not be sufficient to influence future GPs' perceptions of the importance of the public health, when compared with other specialties in clinical areas of medicine such as paediatrics or obstetrics and gynaecology, or to impact on their future practice. GP trainees had difficulty recognising the role of the GP outside the one-to-one clinical consultation, and how public health skills and knowledge can serve this. Whilst the vast majority of trainees reported a considerable increase in knowledge of public health and understanding of its links with primary care as a result of the attachment, most acknowledged that they had had very little knowledge about it to begin with: 'It's opened my eyes to [the fact] that there's much more to [public health] than chasing salmonella . . . and vaccines!'

The future role of GPs is likely to involve a far greater relationship with public health priorities and initiatives than has been seen before, particularly in relation to practice-based commissioning and health improvement. The aspirations of Lord Darzi's report[2] see GPs at the centre of a new polyclinic organisation, where staying healthy and prioritising the services to facilitate this for population groups will be a core part of primary care. The application of world-class commissioning will affect the relationship of the GP with both the Primary Care Trust and patients: their contribution to tackling or sustaining health inequalities will need to be made clearer as will evidence of successful healthcare interventions as seen by patients. Whilst technical proficiency and partnership-working with patients has traditionally been highly valued by GPs, the changing landscape of healthcare will privilege other skills including those of public health. Public health training can, as one trainer put it, help GPs to gain a population perspective of healthcare provision:

> [The attachment's] . . . preparing them for . . . thinking in terms of . . . the needs of their practice population at population level rather than just at the individual walking through the door, and the relevance of that.

The motivations for becoming a GP may well, for many doctors, relate to the potential to engage in close personal relationships with individual patients as a clinician in addition to the possibility of flexible working.[35] However the reality of the future of general practice requires GPs to understand the managerial, organisational aspects of the role and to recognise that the related skills are as core and essential to being a good general practitioner as traditional clinical and communicative competencies. Within the domains of public health, improving services and the management of communicable diseases are more likely to be recognised as important aspects of the GP role than health improvement. Tackling health inequalities amongst practice populations and promoting healthy behaviours are clearly identified in the RCGP curriculum but are more difficult to provide in experiential education.

REFERENCES

1 Office for National Statistics (ONS). *General Household Survey 2008*. London: Office for National Statistics; The Stationery Office. Available at: www.statistics.gov.uk/StatBase/Product.asp?vlnk=5756 (accessed 4 November 2009).

2 Lord Darzi. *High Quality Care for All: NHS next stage review: final report*. London: Department of Health; 2008.

3 Griffiths S. Editorial: Putting public health practice into primary care practice: practical implications of implementing the changes in *Shifting the Balance of Power* in England. *J Publ Health Med*. 2002; 24(4): 243–5.

4 Lawlor DA, Keen S, Neal RD. Can GPs influence the nation's health through a population approach to provision of lifestyle interventions? *Br J Gen Pract.* 2000; **50**: 455–9.

5 Bruce N, Burnett S. Prevention of lifestyle-related disease: general practitioners' views about their role, effectiveness and resources. *Fam Prac.* 1991; **8**(4): 373–7.

6 Williams SJ, Calnan M. Perspectives on prevention: the views of general practitioners. *Socio Health Illness.* 1994; **16**: 372–93.

7 McAvoy BR, Kaner EFS, Lock CA, *et al.* Our Healthier Nation: are GPs willing and able to deliver? A survey of attitudes to and involvement in health promotion and lifestyle counselling. *Br J Gen Pract.* 1999; **49**: 187–90.

8 Steptoe A, Doherty S, Kendrick T, *et al.* Attitudes to cardiovascular health promotion among GPs and practice nurses. *Fam Prac.* 1999; **16**(2): 158–63.

9 Raupach J, Rogers W, Magaray A, *et al.* Advancing health promotion in Australian general practice. *Health Educ Behav.* 2001; **28**: 352.

10 Brotons C, Björkelund C, Bulc M, *et al.* Prevention and health promotion in clinical practice: the views of general practitioners in Europe. *Prev Med.* 2005; **40**(5): 595–601.

11 Laws R, Kirby S, Powell-Davies GP, *et al.* 'Should I and can I?' A mixed-methods study of clinician beliefs and attitudes in the management of lifestyle risk factors in primary health care. *BMC Health Serv Res.* 2008; **8**(44). Available at: www.biomedcentral.com/1472-6963/8/44 (accessed 4 November 2009).

12 Faculty of Public Health. *Key Competency Areas: 2009.* Available at: www.fphm.org.uk/training/curriculum/learning_outcomes_framework/default.asp#key_areas (accessed 4 November 2009).

13 General Medical Council. *Tomorrow's Doctors.* London: General Medical Council; 1993.

14 Woodward A. Public health has no place in undergraduate medical education. *J Publ Health Med.* 1994; **16**(4): 389–92.

15 Albanese M. Problem-based learning: why curricula are likely to show little effect on knowledge and clinical skills. *Med Educ.* 2000; **34**(11): 729–38.

16 Colliver J. Effectiveness of PBL curricula. *Med Educ.* 2000; **34**(11): 959–60.

17 Gillam S, Bagade A. Undergraduate public health education in UK medical schools: struggling to deliver. *Med Educ.* 2006; **40**(5): 430–6.

18 O'Brien MA, Freemantle L, Oxman AD, *et al.* Continuing education meetings and workshops: effects on professional practice and health care outcomes (review). *Cochrane Database Syst Rev.* 2001; 1: CD003030.

19 Hobma S, Ram P, Muijtjens A, *et al.* Effective improvement of a doctor-patient communication: a randomised trial. *Brit J Gen Pract.* 2006; **56**: 580–6.

20 Tomlin Z, Humphrey C, Rogers S. General practitioners' perceptions of effective health care. *Br Med J.* 1999; **318**: 1532–5.

21 Summerskill WSM, Pope C. 'I saw the panic rise in her eyes and evidence-based medicine went out of the door.' An exploratory qualitative study of the barriers to secondary prevention in the management of coronary heart disease. *Fam Prac.* 2002; **19**(6): 605–10.

22 Royal College of General Practitioners. *The RCGP – GP Curriculum.* London: Royal College of General Practitioners; 2007. Available at: www.rcgp-curriculum.org.uk/rcgp_-_gp_curriculum_documents.aspx (accessed 4 November 2009).

23 Tooke J. *Aspiring to Excellence: final report of the Independent Inquiry into Modernising Medical Careers.* London; NHSME; 2008.

24 Lord Darzi. *A High Quality Workforce: NHS next stage review.* London: Department of Health; 2008.

25 Lyon-Maris J, Scallan S. Do integrated training programmes provide a different model of training for general practice compared to traditional vocational training schemes? *Educ Prim Care.* 2007; **18**: 685–96.

26 McNaughton E, Marsden W, Dousie A. Innovative specialist training programme for general practice in Angus, Scotland. *Educ Prim Care.* 2007; **18**: 35–44.

27 Department of Health. *Modernising Medical Careers: the next steps.* London: Department of Health; 2004. Available at: www.dh.gov.uk/en/Publicationsandstatistics/Publications/PublicationsPolicyAndGuidance/DH_4079530 (accessed 4 November 2009).

28 Postgraduate Medical Education and Training Board (PMETB). *Shaping the Future of Postgraduate Medical Education and Training in the UK: the trainee perspective.* London: Postgraduate Medical Education and Training Board; 2008. Available at: www.pmetb.org.uk/fileadmin/user/Communications/Events/Trainee_Roadshow_Seminar/Trainee_roadshow_report.pdf (accessed 4 November 2009).

29 World Organisation of Family Doctors (WONCA). *The European Definition of General Practice/Family Medicine.* London: WONCA Europe; 2005.

30 Plugge E, Banergee S, Pickard D, *et al.* What can GP registrars gain from training in a health authority public health department? *Publ Health Med.* 2002; 4(1): 17–19.

31 Fraser A, Thomas H, Deighan M, *et al.* Directions for change: a national survey of general practice training in the United Kingdom. *Educ Prim Care.* 2007; 18: 22–34.

32 Morris Z, Bullock A, Cooper R, *et al.* The role of the basic specialist training in public health medicine in promoting understanding of public health for future GPs: evaluation of a pilot programme. *Educ Prim Care.* 2001; 12(4): 430–6.

33 Fisher JA. Medical training in community medicine: a comprehensive, academic and service-based curriculum. *J Community Health.* 2003; 28(6): 407–20.

34 Wills J, Reynolds J, Swanwick T. 'Just a lovely luxury?' What can public health attachments add to postgraduate general practice training? *Educ Prim Care.* 2009; 20(4): 278–84.

35 Lucas H, Hagelskamp C, Scammell A. Doctors becoming GPs: GP registrars' experience of medical training and motivations for going into general practice. *Educ Prim Care.* 2004; 15(1): 76–82.

CHAPTER 13

Facilitators and teachers: are health promotion learning outcomes pragmatic?

Ann Wylie, Marc Soethout and Tangerine Holt

ENABLING FACILITATORS AND TEACHERS

Throughout this chapter we provide some detailed examples of outcomes and resources aimed at enabling facilitators. In Chapter 7 in Part 2, examples of curriculum structure were shared, and in Chapter 15 in Part 4, details of sessions are presented, but here we focus on the needs of facilitators and teachers to support their role with health promotion and public health learning outcomes.

Whatever the curriculum structure, problem-based learning (PBL), PBL hybrid or systems-based approach, the content that reflects on health promotion and public health will be reliant on facilitators and teachers who are non-specialist in either of these fields. The associated learning outcomes may be part of a range of learning outcomes within the context of a case or they may be quite explicit and central to the session. About 76% of UK medical schools have public health content integrated into clinical teaching, and 50% report difficulty in finding teachers.[1] Therefore the briefing notes need to be such that a skilled facilitator and teacher, not specialising in public health or health promotion, can follow and work with. To expect facilitators and teachers to make commitments to additional training sessions can be unrealistic, especially when so much of medical teaching is on a goodwill basis. It is incumbent therefore on the small numbers of public health and health promotion academics to ensure that learning outcomes are explicit, achievable, integrated and relevant. In many ways the fact that material has to be prepared for other non-specialist facilitators and teachers, becomes a safeguard about keeping the level basic and relevant for the core content.[3]

Yet working with material produced by others can be difficult for a number of reasons.

The students themselves may have little interest or engagement with public health and health promotion issues and few express any interest in this field as a specialty when qualified.[4]

According to colleagues in the UK National Network of Medical School Educators of Public Health, students can marginalise the public health content. But the likelihood of this can be reduced with a skilled and enthusiastic teacher, if the content is relevant and accessible, as well as the students being aware of what aspects will be assessed and how.

The challenge, they suggest, is to stimulate student interest, accepting that they are naturally more orientated towards the clinical care of individual patients and this can be helped as follows:

➤ some focus on international public health, electives, global burdens of disease
➤ exploring the impact of politics of health and health inequalities
➤ identifying health protection aspects, what all doctors need to do to fulfil their responsibilities to control communicable diseases
➤ using research and data analysis to improve the quality of clinical care.

We would add that attention should also be paid to the impact of health problems, complaints or diseases on the environment or context of the patient (i.e. school, work), and the impact of public health problems (i.e. infectious diseases) on the health of the individual patient.

The balance between complexity and basic knowledge and skills can be difficult, for both the facilitators and the students.

The intended outcomes related to the public health and health promotion content need to focus on how this enables the doctor being able to practise medicine effectively, to deal with uncertainty and apply clinical epidemiology, as well as doctors having an understanding of their role within the wider context of health and social care.[5]

PUBLIC HEALTH AND HEALTH PROMOTION: EXPLORING DIFFERENCES

Earlier in the book, in Chapter 2, definitions and what differentiates health promotion and public health were considered, but further clarification is offered here. For any teacher working with public health- and health promotion-related outcomes, curriculum designers and the academics involved need to offer working definitions, although the caveat is that there is considerable overlap, a lack of consensus and they are mutually dependent on each other.

Traditionally, public health as a practice discipline was thought to have developed from the concerns of Chadwick about the poor sanitary conditions and the risk these posed.[6] In 1875, in the UK, the Public Health Act made provision for water supply, sewage disposal and animal slaughter. Individuals did not have to be proactive to improve their health as engineers and legislators were the prime drivers for the public's health. By 1988 the 'new public health' included the need to consider implications for health in all public policies.[7] One frequently quoted definition for public health is: 'the art and science of preventing disease, prolonging life and promoting health through the organised efforts of society'.[8]

It remains the function of public health to identify determinants of disease, to look for causal relationships, to study disease patterns and trends and to analyse and interpret data not only directly associated with health and disease but also from wider social sources such as education attainment, income, environment and housing. The science of public health is concerned with the diagnosis of a population's health problem, establishing the causes and effects of this problem and determining effective interventions.[5]

The public health sciences are usually classified as:
- ➤ epidemiology and demography
- ➤ health economics
- ➤ medical statistics
- ➤ sociology, psychology and management.

It is from these that we link tobacco to lung cancer, that social deprivation leads to health inequalities, that we can estimate the cost effectiveness using models based on 'numbers to treat' to test efficacy of interventions, observe trends, monitor mortality and morbidity, explore behaviour as well as predict and manage finite healthcare resources.

It is epidemiology that we are most familiar with as the core science of public health. It comes from the Greek language, with 'epi' meaning around, 'demos' relating to people or population and 'logy' or 'logos' meaning the study of. Although it is especially useful for communicable diseases and infection control, we now use this for exploring risk-related behaviour and predicting the scale of problems, especially for non-communicable diseases (NCD) such as cardiovascular disease and cancers.[9]

Sessions linked to chlamydia and HIV infections may present epidemiological information such as prevalence and incidence, based on notifications, but additional demographic information such as sex, age and geographic location all provide useful data to help with diagnosis and management. These public health data can relate directly to the clinical scenario being presented, the diagnosis and prognosis. In addition, aspects of the legislation and public policy about notification that are in place to protect the wider population can be linked to the scenario if appropriate for the learning outcomes.

So for the most part public health is associated with disease, causation and determinants, impact on populations, prevention and surveillance, health information and data from sufficiently large cohorts and whole population surveys such as census data. The semantics of public health can become integral to a clinical teaching session or facilitating a PBL session. There is a need to decide how much depth is relevant: for example, students being able to critique a paper with chlamydia data or students being asked to analyse data and suggest what additional data are needed.

Health promotion overlaps with some of the above but it is more linked to health and its promotion, associated with intervention rather than data collection. It can offer the clinician the means by which health can be improved either by behavioural change that requires effort from the patient and/or engaging with community-based interventions that enable the easy choice to be the healthy choice as promoted by Tones.[10] The ideals of health promotion are based on the question 'what causes health?' and what factors or determinants are linked to health and which of these are modifiable, and indeed how are they modifiable.

The salutogenic approach to health was explored by Antonovsky,[11] with the question being:

> what keeps us healthy despite the stressors and unavoidable disruptions that we all encounter?' In early work, he presented his theory of 'sense of coherence' (SOC) which he defined as 'a global orientation that expresses the extent to which one has a pervasive, enduring, though dynamic feeling of confidence.[12]

Antonovsky later expanded this theory.[11] There are three factors for SOC as follows: (i) *comprehensibility*, which refers to the extent to which one perceives the stimuli that confronts as consistent, structured and clear; (ii) *manageability*, which is the extent to which one perceives that the resources at one's disposal are adequate to meet life's demands; and (iii) *meaningfulness*, which refers to the extent to which one feels that life makes sense emotionally.[13] The challenge is to move from the theory to the development of interventions that modify health determinants, so enabling people to experience SOC. That also means that health promotion is therefore a multidisciplinary and interdisciplinary field, yet for many health professionals this eclectic field is too broad for core curriculum content unless health promotion is a substantial aspect of the course being studied. Regardless of the amount of curriculum time and space, however, some aspects of SOC have become central to most health promotion teaching, such as the concepts of autonomy and empowerment, patient-centredness and concordance, community involvement, social inclusion and social capital.

Some of these ideas are difficult to translate into learning outcomes and may also be difficult to discuss in teaching sessions, but they can inform professionals about the complex social determinants of health; this in itself is a worthy learning outcome.

A working definition for health promotion that can be pragmatic for both teachers and facilitators, as well as for students, is as follows: '*the study of, and the study of the response to, the modifiable determinants of health*'.[3]

The 'response' refers to the intervention, be it a simple and evidence-based approach to advice-giving or a coordinated and strategic programme, also evidence-based, working with policy directives and incorporating the Beattie model, which has action in terms of professional/expert for the individual, client-centred listening intervention, alongside legislative action and community development.[14] But before the 'response', there should be sound argument that the relevant determinants have been identified and are, in the given context, modifiable. The outcome that facilitators and teachers are aiming to achieve with their students could relate to the 'response', such as evidence base and evaluation, or it could relate to determinants and level of confidence and how strong is the argument that these determinants, in the defined context, are modifiable with the planned response or interventions.

In clinical settings, health promotion will frequently be linked less to health and more to disease and disease prevention in medical and health professional curricula. The facilitator needs to know at what level the students are working, and what outcomes are expected, such as those in the Miller's Pyramid:[15] knows, knows how, shows how and does. There should be clarity as to whether the student has to have knowledge recall, skills, ability to discuss theoretical principles or problem-solve and, most importantly, how far beyond the immediate clinical context is relevant.

Given that much of the health promotion work related to clinical activity is associated with lifestyle issues such as tobacco use, diet, alcohol and the need for behavioural change to improve prognosis, the following example provides a number of opportunities for the facilitator and teacher. Using the example of food, nutrition and obesity, Naidoo and Wills[16] provide a comprehensive framework showing how different disciplinary paradigms can inform our understanding about the determinants involved and where coordinated intervention is needed.

Naidoo and Wills offer a framework of questions that could be explored as follows:
- What is a healthy diet and is this culturally or historically relative?
- Do people know what constitutes a healthy diet?
- How is obesity defined and measured?
- How easy is it to access foods for a healthy diet?
- What influences individual food choices?
- Is what people eat an entirely individual matter or should governments be concerned?
- What accounts for the rise in overweight and obesity? Is this confined to the UK?
- What interventions are effective in promoting healthy eating and addressing obesity?
- What are the economic costs of the rise in overweight and obesity?

Food, nutrition and obesity is associated with history, sociology, organisation and management, economics, ethics and law, politics, epidemiology, social policy, biology, psychology and cultural and anthropology studies.[16] Those providing the briefing notes for facilitators and teachers would need to decide what is appropriate for the students if for example they have a case scenario of a patient, with co-morbidities, trying with little success to reduce body mass index (BMI) from 35 to 30.

These types of questions juxtapose both public health and health promotion learning outcomes and can be adapted to other lifestyle issues. There are, however, some terms that also juxtapose with health promotion and public health and should have further clarification as follows:

➤ prevention – this could relate to the public health evidence and intervention data and is a subsection of public health[17]
➤ screening – often seen within a public health context of early disease detection for better prognosis but health promotion to enable individuals to make informed choices[18]
➤ promoting immunisation – like screening a public health issue but individual decision for action
➤ prophylaxis –the complex risk-assessment process, for example with antibiotic use in patients with sickle cell disorder or advice about anti-malaria medication
➤ risk factors – these are identified and quantified by public health but intervention evidence informs health promotion responses either with individuals or with a targeted population.

In summary, the terms associated with health promotion and public health learning outcomes need to be clear for teachers and facilitators, who also need to be provided with suitable briefing notes and guidance from health promotion and public health academics. These outcomes can be realistic in the context of a relevant clinical teaching session.

The following sections provide examples of learning outcomes for facilitators and teachers.

TRAINING IN HEALTH PROMOTION SKILLS AT THE VU UNIVERSITY MEDICAL CENTRE IN AMSTERDAM: THE PREPARE MODEL

During medical school, and especially during their clerkships, medical students are confronted with many different patients with their various different problems. They learn to solve these problems by means of problem-solving skills. However, these skills mainly focus on clinical problems, and less attention is paid to public health problems, in which prevention and advice are the most important aspects. Public health in this context refers to occupational health and consists of individual and community-based problems.

In the Netherlands, a model was developed in which students are taught in a structured way to solve public health problems. This so-called PREPARE model integrates, stepwise, the skills that are related to communication (presentation of the problem), analysing the determinants of the problem (relevance for public health), presenting the evidence of the effectiveness of interventions and preventive action (evidence), choosing a certain preventive action and advising the different parties involved (prevention and advice, including health promotion), recognising the need for registration (registration) and the applying feedback mechanisms after the action has taken place (evaluation) (*see* Table 13.1). The final assessment of the students is based on a presentation, in which the students can demonstrate their skills in all seven steps of the model.

Key issues

- Public health is a practice discipline.
- It considers implications for health in all public policies.
- It identifies determinants of disease, looks for causal relationships, studies disease patterns and trends, analyses and interprets data not only directly associated with health and disease but also from wider social sources such as education attainment, income, environment and housing.
- It focuses on the diagnosis of a population's health problem, establishes the causes and effects of these problems and determines effective interventions.
- Health promotion is a multidisciplinary and interdisciplinary field.
- Health promotion is linked to health and its promotion, associated with intervention rather than data collection.
- Its focus is on how health can be improved either by patients and community through engagement and education.

Key concepts of health promotion include:
- autonomy and empowerment
- patient-centredness and concordance
- community involvement
- social inclusion and social capital.

Key questions asked include:
- What causes health?
- What factors or determinants are linked to health?
- Which of these are modifiable?
- How are they modifiable?

TABLE 13.1 The seven steps of the PREPARE model

		Step	*Remarks*
1	**P**	Problem	*What is the health problem?* – What is the case?
2	**R**	Relevance	*What is the relevance?* – What are the determinants?
3	**E**	Evidence	*What evidence is there of the effectiveness of intervention and prevention?* – What is the source of this information?
4	**P**	Prevention	*Which preventive actions can be taken, and why?* – Primary/secondary/tertiary (individual/group/society)?
5	**A**	Advice	*Which advice/information can be given?* – Individual/group/society?
6	**R**	Records	*Which written records are necessary, and why?* – Is there a duty to report?
7	**E**	Evaluation	*Is evaluation necessary and if so, why?* – Individual/group/society?

The model is introduced and explained at the start of a public health clerkship, and students use this model to analyse a health problem they encounter during their clerkship. Students can choose a problem themselves, or they can choose together with their clerkship tutor. The latter choice has the advantage of commitment of the tutor in solving the problem and moreover, the tutor will probably also be able to use the results of the structured analysis in future in his or her practice.

The following steps should be analysed by the students (as in Table 13.1).

Step 1: What is the health problem?
The students and their tutor have to discuss the way in which this specific problem is related to health. In other words, is there a relationship between the health problem and human biology (e.g. genetic inheritance), environment (e.g. work or school), lifestyle (e.g. health risks such as smoking) and healthcare organisations (e.g. providers of healthcare) based on the health field concept formulated by Lalonde,[19] the Canadian Minister for Health and Welfare in the 1970s.

Step 2: What is the relevance?
The different determinants of the health problem are analysed and described in more detail according to the four elements of the Lalonde concept.

Step 3: What evidence is there of effectiveness of intervention and prevention?
What is the incidence and prevalence of the health problem in the direct environment (work, school) or nationwide?
Which information can be used (preferably evidence-based) for advice and prevention, including health promotion activities?

Step 4: Which preventive actions can be taken, and why?
Which preventive actions (primary, secondary and/or tertiary) can be taken to prevent this individual health problem in the future, and which community-based preventive actions can be taken (including health promotion activities)?

Step 5: Which advice/information can be given?
Which advice can be given to the individual, and which advice can be given to the environment (e.g. employer, school or society)?

Step 6: Which written records are necessary, and why?
Is it mandatory to report the health problem, for instance in the case of infectious diseases or work-related healthcare problems? Do the health regulations impose any restrictions with regard to revealing patient information to others (e.g. school, employer)?

Step 7: Is evaluation necessary and, if so, why?
What further appointments will be made with the patient with regard to the health problem, and are any other appointments necessary for instance with the employer, school, or healthcare service?

An example of a public health problem and how it might be analysed with the PREPARE model is shown in Table 13.2.

This method of instruction has worked well so far, although we face challenges such as more instructions about the use of model for tutors, and training of students for an adequate description of the health problems and the determinants.

TRAINING IN HEALTH PROMOTION SKILLS: MONASH UNIVERSITY, SCHOOL OF MEDICINE, AUSTRALIA

The Community Based Practice Program (CBP) is an integration of the Community Partnerships Program (CPP) and health promotion curriculum components of the Monash University Bachelor of Medicine/Bachelor of Surgery degree course, as a Year 2 core integrated themes of Personal and Professional Development and Population, Health and Society.

It focuses on developing the personal attributes and qualities needed by medical students and, ultimately, medical practitioners and citizens in a larger societal context. The main goal is for medical students to 'Develop an interprofessional perspective on the social justice, equity and model(s) of health interventions in the community'.

The achievement of this goal is accomplished through specific learning objectives at the end of a 14-day community-based placement. The placements are within community partners, which include welfare agencies, local government, schools and community health centres. These community placements focus on medical students developing personally and professionally by experiencing the socioeconomic context and health determinants of clients from diverse backgrounds and needs who are in some way marginalised in our society. The students develop, in negotiation with their field educators in the agency, a learning plan that includes a personal goal, a field educator's goal of what they expect the medical student to learn from their experience and a contributory goal which focuses on the student giving back to the agency/clients/community through the completion of a health promotion project. Multidimensional

TABLE 13.2 Example of a public health problem analysed with the PREPARE model

		Step	Analysis
1	**P**	Problem	32-year-old male employer in a supermarket with health problems: cough, fatigue and subfebrile temperature during the past months → general practitioner → antibiotics with no results → positive Mantoux test → Municipal Health Service (according to infectious disease regulations) → source and contact research
2	**R**	Relevance	Open tuberculosis: infectious disease 1400 new patients a year in the Netherlands, 20–30 of whom die each year in the Netherlands Risk groups: immigrants, IV addicts
3	**E**	Evidence	Good results of screening and treatment
4	**P**	Prevention	Municipal Health Service: screening of risk groups, and source and contact research Vaccination
5	**A**	Advice	Hygiene and contamination advice coping with treatment (resistant to antibiotics) Regular screening of risk groups
6	**R**	Records	Positive diagnosis → Municipal Health Service according to infectious disease regulations National registration and surveillance
7	**E**	Evaluation	Protocols for outbreak management by Municipal Health Services Surveillance

assessments demonstrate a significant learning on the part of the students about social justice, communication and development of knowledge of the barriers and the social determinants of health. Impressive projects have been undertaken including the establishment of a food cooperative for refugees in a high-rise housing commission block, social issues of bullying, party culture and drugs among high-school students, needs of homeless people and utilising a harm minimisation approach for drug addicted Vietnamese clients who femorally inject.

With over 300 students and a case-based curriculum, large numbers of teachers and facilitators from a variety of backgrounds are involved. For CPP, the partners are the local providers of health and social care, some funded by the statutory authorities, some are not-for-profit organisations and others are charity-based services. Enabling these partners to become effective facilitators involves a number of stages, although each placement is unique.

Although there is increased emphasis in medical education on learning outcomes, still it was found that the establishment of an outcome-based guide may restrict students in the achievement of their learning outcomes.[20] Sometimes the learning context and environment is not conducive to demonstrating the achievement of a particular outcome, but can certainly be linked to other outcomes of continuity in patient care.[21] Given this situation, the establishment of a partnership agreement is an immediate step that reflects the principles of good practice for community-campus partnerships and fosters community-based medical education. The formation of a true partnership with the community is a critical factor in ensuring the realisation of learning outcomes. This agreement predetermines student learning outcomes at an organisational level and defines the processes used to achieve them.

Below is a modified example of a Monash University and Community Partnerships Agreement. It reflects the key components of any such agreement.

THIS AGREEMENT   dated the   day of   20XX.
BETWEEN
   MONASH UNIVERSITY of Wellington Road, Clayton in the State of Victoria ('University')
AND
   PARTNER of Address in the State of Victoria ('Agency')
WHEREAS
A. The University offers courses of study through its Faculty of Medicine, Nursing and Health Sciences pursuant to which students undertake a programme of community service as part of their tertiary education.
B. The University has requested the Agency to permit students enrolled in the courses to attend the Agency for the purpose of undertaking a period of supervised community partnerships placements with staff at the Agency.
C. The Agency has agreed to permit students to attend its premises for the purposes described in Recital B upon the terms and conditions hereinafter contained.

The following aspects of community based medical education are agreed upon:
- Definitions
- Date of commencement and term of agreement
- Students
- Control and discipline
- Agency staffing
- Attire and identification
- Insurance
- Student Learning Plan
- Learning outcomes

On completion of the Community Partnerships project student will have:
- Developed a perspective on issues of social equity and justice, but particularly as they relate to the practice of medicine;
- Developed an understanding of social and public policy and how it impacts on peoples' lives;
- Developed knowledge of the welfare system and its relevance to medicine;
- Developed an appreciation of the operational philosophy and service delivery components of key agencies working in the areas of social action, social justice and advocacy;
- Developed their understanding of the 'whole person' and in particular the social and economic context of health and illness;
- Understood that from their position of responsibility within the community they

> have knowledge and skills which can contribute to the well being of those people who are disadvantaged.

Put simply, community-based medical education has the following requirements.
➤ Expected learning objectives and outcomes determine curriculum content, teaching methods and assessment and should be explicitly stated in the partnership agreement,
  - Communicate to all key stakeholders involved in the educational process:
    — within the university – At Curriculum Management Committee meetings for academic coordinators, orientation workshops for academic advisors/ tutors and for students through delivery of lectures content, discussion through tutorials, and educational resources such as the CBP Guide, CBP website, and Monash University Student Online for students
    — external to the university – Community Partners, agency coordinators, field educators through field educator orientation workshops, agency presentations, CBP guide, CBP website.

Given the change in emphasis from knowledge acquisition and factual recall to more widely embracing learning outcomes such as problem solving, clinical judgement, communication skills, attitudes and professionalism, it is important to design and implement a programme where field educators and academic advisors are knowledgeable about the expected learning outcomes and the methods available, hence the need for adequate preparation and training of community field educators off campus and tutors who serve as academic advisors to students on campus.[22]

The CBP program is a good example of an outcome-based approach to medical education as proposed by Harden, with specific learning objectives, expectations and a framework of learning outcomes which uses a multidimensional assessment.[20] This component describes the application of the CBP approach and process with second-year medical students in Australia. In particular, of the 12 learning outcomes described on the AMEE Guide No. 25[22] in relation to a doctor's performance in the clinical context across the four levels of the Miller pyramid, the following are the outcomes achieved by the CBP program (*see* Table 13.3).

A CBP guide outlines what the programme is about, its goals, objectives, placement parameters, teaching and learning requirements and assessment. It provides a wide range of tools and examples to assess the above learning outcomes on a continuing basis across the 14 days of placement, tutorials and lectures which together span across two semesters. This longitudinal emphasis provides us with an opportunity to assess outcomes at student and community level across development of knowledge, skills and attitudes. However, it is more complex to assess learning outcomes such as attitudes, teamwork and professionalism.

Student performance and feedback provided on the students' personal and professional development and the completion of a health promotion project within a community context are assessed through a multidimensional form of both qualitative and quantitative assessment consisting of the following components:
➤ learning plans and the achievement of their learning goals at various levels
➤ completion of a health promotion project which includes a final team poster, peer-reviewed presentation, final project report

TABLE 13.3 Outcomes achieved by the CBP program, against Association of Medical Education in Europe (AMEE) Guide learning outcomes

AMEE Guide learning outcomes	CBP learning outcomes
Learning Outcome 5: Competence in health promotion and disease prevention	• Understand the application of a range of health promotion (HP) theories of change that are used in the development of HP interventions and what roles doctors can play in this • Participate in the basic HP process of program development, planning, implementation and evaluation through HP Project • Develop and apply a range of critical appraisal skills in health promotion • Demonstrated ability to compare and contrast medical, behavioural, and socio-environmental approaches to health promotion
Learning Outcome 6: Competence in communication	• Develop communication skills, ethical awareness, socio-cultural understanding; professional behaviours with diverse populations
Learning Outcome 8: Approach practice with an understanding of basic and clinical sciences	• Have an overview of the impact of political, economic and social policies on the organisation, staff professional practice and service users
Learning Outcome 9: Approach practice with appropriate attitudes, ethical stance and legal responsibilities	• Develop communication skills, ethical awareness, socio-cultural understanding; professional behaviours with diverse populations
Assessment of personal competences ('The doctor as a professional')	
Learning Outcome 11: Physicians should have an appreciation (understanding) of the doctor's role in the health service	• The way the community organisation works • Professional relationships within and external to the organisation • The users of the services provided and the issues encountered • The relationships between the service providers and the clients/communities served
Learning Outcome 12: Physicians should have an aptitude for personal development	• Reflection

➤ reflective writing
➤ field educator assessment which is based on observation of students on placements, discussion and feedback from staff and clients within an organisation
➤ peer assessment is based on the student's individual and team interactions in the completion of their health promotion project across a number of meetings, discussions and contribution to the health promotion project.

Given the diversity of placements and learning environments across the placements for these students, our strategy has been to use both qualitative and quantitative assessment. Also, it is not possible to rely on a single measure of assessment at a single point of time.[22] As can be seen from the assessment, the use of multiple measures of assessment of the learning outcomes from different sources – namely field educators, academic advisors and students – can corroborate validity and reliability in the assessment, to assessment of higher-order application of knowledge, attitudes and skills resulting in a process of triangulation.

Field educator observations of students have been vital in the ongoing personal and professional development of the students across the learning outcomes previously outlined. As field educators are health professionals from disciplines other than medicine, they are extremely familiar with their learning environment and are able to assess the knowledge, attitudes and skill of medical students from an interprofessional perspective. This feedback to students is often the first that they have received from a different perspective.

Of course to ensure reliability of these assessments, training of all our field educators and academic advisors takes place through the use of examples, inter-rater marking of assignments, discussion and feedback prior to implementation. In order to achieve desired standards of evidence-based practice it is important to have refresher training sessions on a regular basis. Throughout the process of the programme, planning, development and implementation of a programme in medical education, a key focus should be on the end product – are the learning outcomes achieved? For this it is critical to consider the following:

➤ what learners are expected to do in their placements
➤ how it will be learned
➤ when it will be learned
➤ whether it is learned well.

In summary, the CBP program requires, as noted by Harden, 'in addition to identifying, making explicit and communicating learning outcomes to all concerned, that decisions about the curriculum including the teaching methods and learning strategies, the assessment procedures and the learning environment are based on the agreed learning outcomes'.[23]

TRAINING IN HEALTH PROMOTION SKILLS AT LIVERPOOL

Liverpool has a PBL curriculum with four themes:
➤ structure and function
➤ individuals, groups and societies
➤ population perspective
➤ professional and personal view.

It has been noted informally that the students, and frequently their facilitators and teachers, put greater effort into the structure and function theme so the task of ensuring there is sufficient attention to the public health and health promotion aspects of the problem has to be considered. Stimulating and relevant learning outcomes therefore are provided to assist the facilitators and teachers as much as the students.

Aspects of public health and health promotion could be integrated into all of these but the most substantive input is within the population perspective theme. The guidance for students and facilitators alike with each problem is the 'Liverpool Seven Pointers towards a Population Perspective on Health'.[5]

The Liverpool Seven Pointers

1 What public health issues are raised by this problem?
2 How does this problem affect the population?
3 What are the health needs of the population in relation to this problem?
4 How can the burden of this problem be reduced?
5 How should health (and other) services be organised and delivered to address this problem?
6 What are the main research and development issues raised by the problem?
7 What are the main public health policy implications of this problem?

With these seven pointer questions, there is scope for the learning outcomes to be simple and basic or to be deep and complex. This will depend on the guidance for the given problem, the teacher's and facilitator's background knowledge and what is expected at assessment as well as what stage the students are at.

Further domains are also considered, these being health and social services improvement, health improvement, which in essence is similar to health promotion and addressing health inequalities. Traditional aspects of public health are also important for learning outcomes in teaching this. Liverpool uses contemporary examples such as 'Avian Flu' which in turn enables learning to be relevant to both the learners and the facilitators and teachers.[5]

TRAINING IN HEALTH PROMOTION SKILLS: THE CANADIAN EXPERIENCE

The medical schools in Canada are guided by the CanMEDS 2005 Framework which sets out what should be expected of the doctor in terms of being a medical expert, communicator, collaborator, manager, health advocate, scholar and professional.[2] The importance of the Canadian framework is that modern health promotion is very much rooted in Canada and in Ottawa in particular.[24] The CanMEDS framework is also implemented outside Canada, for instance in Denmark and the Netherlands.[25,26] So, the role of health advocate, including health promotion is a role of many future medical doctors. However the importance of the roles depends on the specialty characteristics.[27] Facilitators are provided with many opportunities to explore, with the learners, public health and health promotion within this framework.

In the section on 'medical expert', six key competencies are defined, with the fourth being 'use preventative and therapeutic interventions effectively'. Enabling these competencies is then described as 'demonstrate effective, appropriate and timely application of preventive and therapeutic interventions relevant to the physician's practice'. This very much focuses on the one-to-one clinical encounter. There is no specific health promotion and public health directive within 'communicator' but as for 'collaborator', the key competencies are linked to effective team-working with the healthcare team.

It is within 'health advocate' that the most obvious health promotion and public health learning outcomes are evident. For the facilitator and medical teacher the four key competencies the physician should be able to demonstrate are as follows:

1 respond to individual patient health needs and issues as part of patient care
2 respond to the health needs of the communities that they serve
3 identify the determinants of health of the populations that they serve
4 promote the health of individual patients, communities and populations.

Respond to individual patient health needs and issues as part of patient care
1.1 Identify the health needs of an individual patient;
1.2 Identify opportunities for advocacy, health promotion and disease prevention with individuals to whom they provide care.

Respond to the health needs of the communities that they serve
2.1 Describe the practice communities that they serve;
2.2 Identify opportunities for advocacy, health promotion and disease prevention in the communities that they serve, and respond appropriately;
2.3 Appreciate the possibility of competing interests between the communities served and other populations.

Identify the determinants of health of the populations that they serve
3.1 Identify the determinants of health of the population, including barriers to access to care and resources;
3.2 Identify vulnerable or marginalised populations within those served and respond appropriately.

Promote the health of individual patients, communities and populations
4.1 Describe an approach to implementing a change in a determinant of health of the populations they serve;
4.2 Describe how public policy impacts on the health of the populations served;
4.3 Identify points of influence in the healthcare system and its structure;
4.4 Describe the ethical and professional issues inherent in health advocacy, including altruism, social justice, autonomy, integrity and idealism;
4.5 Appreciate the possibility of conflict inherent in their role as health advocate for a patient or community with that of manager or gatekeeper;
4.6 Describe the role of the medical profession in advocating collectively for health and patient safety.[2]

Because Canada embraced the concepts and ideals of health promotion as a discipline, much of the above language will be familiar to the facilitators and teachers working within medical schools and other health faculties.[24] In addition, there will be many practical examples to draw on as a resource for learning, whether at local or national level, hence making the learning relevant to all protagonists.

TRAINING IN HEALTH PROMOTION SKILLS: KING'S COLLEGE LONDON

Health promotion is integrated at King's College London School of Medicine (KCL) and involves a number of teachers and facilitators. However, below is an example of an explicit aspect that involves health promotion practitioners as facilitators and what is shown here is the documentation in the handbook. The wider context for this is that these students will have had six clinical rotations over two years and the intervention they will be allocated to will have some links to one of those rotations. The allocation process is complex given the number of students so there is very limited student choice. At the same time students do a vertical strand following a woman from late pregnancy to the first three months of the infant's life. At the same time they prepare a portfolio for themselves, in preparation for an overseas elective; about 1000 words of the portfolio is focused on their own health and well-being. There is ample opportunity therefore for students to appreciate the relevance of this health promotion review to their own learning and development.

Facilitators have commented that the briefing notes below, as well as feedback, enable them to be limpid about their role as facilitator rather than teacher.

REVIEW OF HEALTH PROMOTION INTERVENTION

The Health Promotion Review is now established. We have worked with a number of health promotion professionals and consultants in public health in the areas where the students have been allocated to GP teaching practices. It is our aim for the students to see a health promotion initiative in action, study the rationale behind the intervention and look at the ways in which the success of the intervention is measured.

Task

Review the impact of a community-based health promotion intervention on a local/practice population

Note: The students have been reminded that they must work in their PAIRS or GROUPS to complete their health promotion Intervention. This will depend on how they have been allocated.

Key questions
- What are the aims of the intervention?
- What argument/hypothesis/theory/model informs the intervention?
- What evidence/argument/research informs the intervention?
- What is the impact and will it be measured/evaluated?

What exactly will the students do?

(The students need to prepare their questions and email these to the coordinator in advance of their meeting. This will enable their coordinator to prepare appropriate answers and make best use of their time together.)

They will expand on the key questions above to ask their coordinator about the following:

- The aims, objectives, evidence, approach/model, theoretical framework behind the intervention
- Resources/funding
- Where the intervention fits in with the wider picture: strategies/policies/national programmes
- How the success of the intervention is measured – how is it evaluated? What evidence contributes to its evaluation?
- What indicators/evidence informs the target population and primary care team, if any?
- They may get the chance to see the intervention in action. As senior medical students, they will understand if there were ethical reasons which prevent them from doing so
- They may want to contribute – the health promotion coordinator will decide if this is appropriate
- They may want to see/use the coordinator's resources
- They might have personal interests as they will be studying their own health and well-being within the Phase 4 programme

What will the health promotion coordinator do and who are health promoters?

Facilitate – we do not expect the health promotion coordinator to teach or help the students produce their presentations. The students must understand that we are NOT asking coordinators to teach or make any special arrangements but that they share with the students some background information and help address the key questions about the intervention they implement. Their work is very variable as are their hours, time and place of work so it is important for the students to arrange mutually agreeable meetings – for some this will be Friday afternoon. Some coordinators, however, will be involved in youth work and after schools programmes and they may work evenings in community-based settings. We anticipate having about 120 coordinators and a similar number of interventions, so some will fall into the 'out of hours' category.

- We would like the coordinator to attend the presentation if possible, but this is not essential.
- Provide constructive feedback to us about organisation, feasibility, sustainability, value, challenges and opportunities.

Health promotion coordinators are community-based specialists. Some coordinators will have a clinical background. However, this is an eclectic professional group – sometimes coordinators are employed by NHS organisations; others work in the voluntary sector; some work for local authorities. It is very important that the students are aware they have NO contractual obligations to the medical school.

Defining health promotion and the health promotion curriculum content

The students will be using this working definition:

'The study of, and the study of the response to, the modifiable determinants of health (and disease).'

Wylie 2004

The students will have studied health promotion in previous years. They will have been introduced to the Stages of Change model in Year 3. *See* Figure 13.1 below:

Stages of change model – Year 3

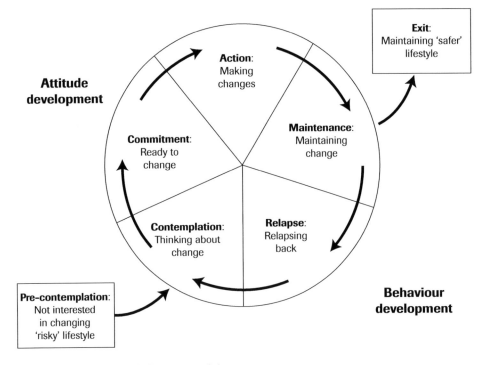

FIGURE 13.1 Stages of change model

The students also look at Beattie's model in Years 3, 4 and 5. See Figure 13.2 below.

In Beattie's model, each quadrant can:

- inform the intervention theory
- identify skills needed
- explore relevant guidance
- inform the argument for identified modifiable determinants.

Beattie's model – Years 3, 4 & 5

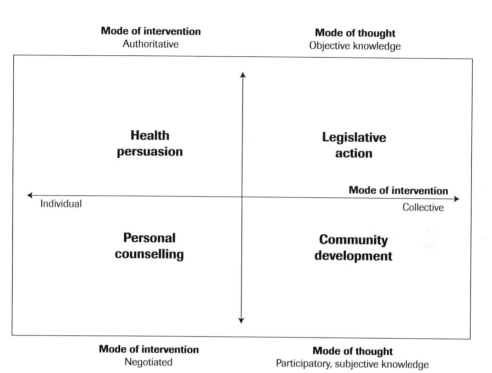

FIGURE 13.2 The Beattie model

Types of evaluation information the students may require
- Evaluation should be designed during the planning of the intervention, and adequate resources should be allocated.
- Input: the resources committed to the initiative
- Process: the activities carried out with the resources available
- Outcomes: the results of these activities (*see* Figure 13.3)

Presentation assessment
- Student pairs or small groups will deliver a presentation – a review of the impact of the intervention – to the practice team late morning on Day 4. The health promotion activity coordinator will be invited to attend and comment.
- A marking schedule will be provided to the practice.
- You will be asked to focus on the students' ability to do a review and present their findings, consider how well the local action matches the national guidelines for example, what are the adaptations and limitations.
- The presentation will make a small contribution to the students' overall assessment mark. However, it is mandatory, and is a 'hurdle' requirement for their entry into Phase 5.

Key indicators of success

Types of indicators:

Input	Process	Outcome

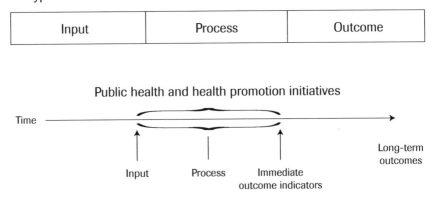

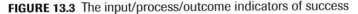

FIGURE 13.3 The input/process/outcome indicators of success

Recommended reading
Students will be advised as follows:
- *A Textbook of General Practice* 2004 (2nd ed) edited by Anne Stephenson (Chapter 11, Health Promotion, Ann Wylie)
- Naidoo & Wills and Ewles & Simnett
- Health Education Research
- Health Promotion International
- Health Education Journal
- And others as relevant
- Websites NICE, WHO, DH etc., White Papers, NSFs
- Please indicate to students what additional specific reading is relevant for the intervention they have looked at.

HEALTH PROMOTION LEARNING OUTCOMES: CONGRUENT WITH FACILITATORS' AND TEACHERS' PRACTICE?

With regard to the examples given above, there is an intention that the learning outcomes and experiences are as close to reality and practice as possible whilst also demonstrating, at an appropriate level, how theory and evidence informs practice. There is also an intention to enable the facilitators and teachers to be active and participatory agents in the development of health promotion curriculum content, through feedback and discussion, either formal or informal.

The gaps between theory and practice can be highlighted in small groups and facilitators need to be skilled to deal with these. For example students may share with facilitators and teachers that they observe 'poor' or inconsistent health promotion practices in clinical settings. Research has also shown this to be the case with approaches to patients who smoke and GPs' decisions about referral to evidence-based services[28,29] as an example. In such cases we must remind ourselves of how 'young' health promotion is, relatively speaking and hence, established clinicians may have had little in the way of formal training and may hold doubts about the discipline and its evidence base. That said, by encouraging more health professionals to be involved in teaching and facilitation, providing good, piloted materials with realistic, pragmatic and relevant learning outcomes, this process itself becomes helpful to those health professionals on their own health promotion learning curve.

Best practice in medical education is what we aspire to but that is dependent on best practice in practice. For health promotion there is progress both within medical education and in clinical practice and this progress will be accelerated by working in partnership, being pragmatic and ensuring defined learning outcomes are relevant to students.

REFERENCES

1 Gillam S, Bagade A. Undergraduate public health education in UK medical schools – struggling to deliver. *Med Educ.* 2006; **40**(5): 430–6.
2 The Royal College of Physicians and Surgeons of Canada. *CanMEDS 2005 Framework.* Ottawa: The Royal College of Physicians and Surgeons of Canada; 2005.
3 Wylie A, Thompson S. Establishing health promotion in the modern medical curriculum: a case study. *Med Teach.* 2007; **29**(8): 766–71.
4 Soethout MBM, ten Cate OJ, van der Wal G. Development of an interest in a career in public health during medical school. *Public Health.* 2008; **122**(4): 361–6.
5 Gillam S, Maudsley G. *Public Health Education for Medical Students: a guide for medical schools.* London: Department of Public Health and Primary Care, University of Cambridge; 2008.
6 Chadwick E. *Report on the Sanitary Conditions of the Labouring Population of England.* London: HMSO; 1842.
7 Ashton J, Seymour H. *The New Public Health.* Basingstoke: Open University Press; 1988.
8 Acheson D. *Public Health in England: report of the inquiry into the future development of Public Health Function.* London: HMSO; 1988.
9 Hocking J, Crofts N. Public health information. In: Moodie R, Hulme A, editors. *Hands-on Health Promotion.* East Hawthorn, Victoria: IP Communications; 2004. pp. 3–15.
10 Tones K, Tilford S. *Health Education: effectiveness, efficiency and equity.* 2nd ed. London: Chapman & Hall; 1994.
11 Antonovsky A. The salutogenic model as a theory to guide health promotion. *Health Promot Int.* 1996; **11**(1): 11–18.
12 Jones L. What is health? In: Katz J, Peberdy A, editors. *Promoting Health, Knowledge and Practice.* Basingstoke: Macmillan; 1997.
13 Eriksson M, Lindstrom B, Lilja J. A sense of coherence and health. Salutogenesis in a societal context: Aland, a special case? *J Epidemiol Commun.* 2007; **61**(8): 684–8.
14 Beattie A, Gott M, Jones L, *et al. Health and Wellbeing: a reader.* Basingstoke: Macmillan; 1993.
15 Miller GE. The assessment of clinical skills/competence/performance. *Acad Med.* 1990; **65**(9 Suppl.): S63–7.
16 Naidoo J, Wills J. Introducing health studies. In: Naidoo J, Wills J, editors. *Health Studies: an introduction.* 2nd ed. Basingstoke: Palgrave Macmillan; 2008. pp. 1–21.
17 Rose G, Khaw K-T, Marmot M. *Rose's Strategy of Preventive Medicine.* Oxford: Oxford University Press; 2008.
18 Raffle A, Gray M. *Screening Evidence and Practice.* Oxford: Oxford University Press; 2007.
19 Lalonde M. *A New Perspective on the Health of Canadians.* Ottawa, ON: Ministry of Supply and Services; 1974.
20 Harden RM. Developments in outcome-based education. *Med Teach.* 2002; **24**(2): 117–20.

21 Khogali Shilab EO, Laidlaw JM, Harden RM. Study guides: a study of different formats. *Med Teach.* 2006; **28**(4): 375–7.

22 Shumway JM, Harden RM. AMEE Guide No. 25: The assessment of learning outcomes for the competent and reflective physician. *Med Teach.* 2003; **25**(6): 569–84.

23 Harden R. Outcome-based education: the future is today. *Med Teach.* 2007; **29**(7): 625–9.

24 World Health Organization. *Ottawa Charter for Health Promotion.* 1986; Geneva: World Health Organization; 1986.

25 Danish Ministry of Health. *The Future Specialist.* Report No. 1385. Copenhagen: Statens Information; 2000.

26 Scheele F, Teunissen P, Van Luijk S. Introducing competency-based postgraduate medical education in the Netherlands. *Med Teach.* 2008; **30**(3): 248–53.

27 Ringsted C, Hanson TL, Davis D, *et al.* Are some of the challenging aspects of the CanMEDS roles valid outside Canada? *Med Educ.* 2006; **40**(8): 807–15.

28 Kerr S, Watson H, Tolson D, *et al.* An exploration of the knowledge, attitudes and practice of members of the primary care team in relation to smoking and smoking cessation in later life. *Prim Health Care Res Dev.* 2007; **8**(1): 68–79.

29 Vogt F, Hall S, Marteau TM. General practitioners' beliefs about effectiveness and intentions to recommend smoking cessation medications: qualitative and quantitative studies. *BMC Publ Health.* 2006; **6**(277). Available at: www.biomedcentral.com/1471–2458/6/277 (accessed 4 November 2009).

PART FOUR

Practical approaches for medical and health professional teachers

INTRODUCTION

Tangerine Holt and Ann Wylie

How does a session defined as health promotion look? Are health promotion models described; are the health promotion aspects identifiable; how accessible and relevant is the session for the learner; how visible are the health promotion aspects within integrated courses; what resources are readily available to enhance this teaching? It seems that both students and teachers need to have clarity about this for a number of reasons.

For teachers and facilitators there could be a directional pull towards the topic or case, especially if the teacher is a clinician working in this field. For example, working with the scenario of a patient with chronic obstructive pulmonary disease (COPD) who is a smoker but requests help to stop, the sessions may well focus on smoking behaviour, smoking cessation and the social support needs, as well as medication, management and prognosis. But is that health promotion or smoking cessation, is it respiratory medicine or chronic disease management, is it a combination of all of the above? Will the students be skilled in approaches to individual behaviour change or perceive they have learnt only about smoking cessation approaches?

Recently at King's College London School of Medicine (KCL), some final-year students claimed they had had smoking cessation teaching but had not had much health promotion teaching. When questioned further on this during a research focus group, they mentioned that they had looked at their own health and well-being for their elective portfolio but had not realised this was health promotion and in their final year, during their eight-week primary care placement, they had not associated immunisations, screening, antenatal and postnatal care, travel health services and self-care with health promotion. However, they had linked chronic illness management with smoking cessation and therefore considered this was part of the health promotion content. Whilst smoking cessation may be the most obvious choice for health promotion teaching within medical and health professional curricula, it can also offer valuable insights to the learner about behavioural change *per se* as well as how the principles of health promotion are relevant and applicable to many other situations.

We have also become more aware of the health promotion opportunities and issues for students themselves, although there is still some questioning of the ethics of intervention while they are at university. If we are enabling future health professionals to be skilled health promoters within their practice, can we not also find acceptable ways within the sessions to enable students to be reflective and responsive to their own health and well-being?

In Part Four we look at some of the practical ways of delivering health promotion sessions, starting in Chapter 14 with healthcare needs and health promotion opportunities for students themselves. In Chapter 15 we have a number of worked examples of health promotion sessions from international contributors. And finally, in Chapters 16 and 17 we take the opportunity to explore the many terms that could also be an alias for health promotion and the resources that can be shared.

Same objectives, different students: the practical challenges of health promotion teaching for the learner

Craig Hassed and Ann Wylie

ARE STUDENTS IN NEED OF HEALTH PROMOTION?

At most medical schools and health courses, as well as in other university courses, there will be students with serious health concerns, either physical or mental. There will inevitably be access to healthcare and student welfare but how easy and acceptable are such services to those on medical courses, do students seek help early enough, what prevents them from or encourages them to take proactive steps to keep healthy, to seek help and advice and in the case of medical students, see themselves as vulnerable in the way the general population are?

We know for instance that alcohol consumption is high amongst the student population but seems to be excessive, and a cause for concern, with medical students.[1]

Students on high-stakes courses, like medical students, can have high levels of stress and experience financial problems, unlike many of their peers who have already entered the workplace some two years earlier with lucrative salaries and good career prospects.

The conundrum, therefore, is why students, especially medical students, seem more vulnerable to engaging in behaviours potentially harmful to health, given they probably would be more aware that these behaviours pose health risks. Will health promotion sessions either directly aimed at them or more likely aimed at skills for improving the health of patients have any impact? Medical students should, by other criteria for health-related behaviour, be less, not more, vulnerable to poor health outcomes, given they have high educational attainment and will enter secure and well-paid posts.

The medical profession, for example, were quick to act on the deleterious evidence associated with tobacco and ill health. In the UK, the medical profession have the lowest rates of tobacco consumption of any professional group.[1] This would suggest factual knowledge is a motivator for health-related behaviour. So why then do we see other harmful or potentially harmful behaviours in medical students and junior doctors?

Alcohol consumption is not in itself harmful; indeed this is an important contrast with tobacco. Alcohol is pleasurable and part of sociable activity. There is even evidence to suggest it may confer health benefits in certain circumstances. Alcohol is readily available, especially to university students, and within medical schools it is frequently provided at social gatherings and occasions.[1] For some students, this easy access to alcohol leads to excessive consumption although we have limited epidemiologic data to demonstrate cause and effect and prevalence.

There have been studies documenting excessive drinking and the experimentation of illicit drugs in medical students.[2] What is difficult is to establish whether this is a phase, as part of university life, or whether it poses a genuine health risk to some individuals and whom those individuals might be. In addition, we need to try and establish if these habits are likely to continue into training when life as a junior doctor may well be more stressful.

The health risks are varied and are also linked to social risks. Students have indicated that they are slightly embarrassed when they need to attend the emergency services at the local hospital, which is also their teaching hospital, following a drinking session that results in accidents and injuries, vomiting or alcohol poisoning. Few say they will refrain next time there is a drinking session and many will drink with tutors and junior clinical staff. Ongoing research with Monash School of Medicine and King's College London School of Medicine (KCL) suggests that students are aware of their drinking habits and some are concerned but anecdotal findings indicate that they see this as part of student life which will be modified on graduation.

Some students have reported sleep difficulties especially as they approach exams, but rarely link this to aftereffects of high alcohol consumption and some have reported using alcohol as a remedy. Others have reported a trend towards binge drinking, a cause for further damage in the future.[3] Students doing special study modules (SSMs) at KCL focused on prevention of obesity have indicated that the calorie content of alcohol may be a contributory factor to weight gain in young adults, including students, but rather than curb their drinking, those who are aware of the calorie content, prefer to reduce their food consumption, with potentially unsatisfactory consequences. Another concern is that although alcohol is relatively inexpensive at university outlets, it nevertheless adds to the financial burden of those consuming large amounts.

An interesting point is to compare the use of alcohol between years. A longitudinal cohort study in Newcastle surveyed students in their second year, fifth year and first year as a pre-registered house officer (PRHO). It found that the overall consumption of alcohol (both male and female) over the four-year period of the survey had increased. However the results in males were still significantly greater.[4] This same study reported that experimentation with illicit drugs had increased from 50% to 63%.

There are negative consequences of alcohol and drug misuse and these could include an increase in morbidity in students and junior doctors if behaviours are unaltered.

We could question what actual knowledge students have about alcohol and harm, their knowledge about the dangers of illicit drug use, poor eating and exercise habits, and question what coping strategies they have for mental and emotional well-being and whether they can relate this knowledge base to themselves.

At KCL, as part of the longitudinal research with Monash School of Medicine about the impact of health promotion curriculum content, we held focus groups with final-year students following their final examinations. They reported finding it difficult to raise specific lifestyle issues with patients other than smoking, but said they were familiar with the process of motivational interviewing, using the five As (Ask, Assess, Advise, Assist and Arrange), and they could quote guidelines for safe or sensible drinking, exercise and nutrition when with patients, if they felt it appropriate. This contrasted with their personal behaviours. For example two students noted that their parents frequently 'drank too much' at home and were gaining weight, becoming less active and concerns about raised blood pressure were expressed. But the students felt unable to 'do anything' as they themselves were heavy drinkers at times of celebrations and weekends. Within days of the focus group these students would graduate and celebrate, which would include copious amounts of alcohol. Their level of exercise had reduced as they progressed to finals, although they were confident they would return to their sports and physical activities within weeks. They had never smoked although they were aware that some medical students did.

As part of the health and well-being aspect of the elective portfolio, these students had indicated that they had been more concerned about avoiding blood-borne virus infections and malaria than improving their health, although they admitted they needed to reduce their weight, improve their diets, improve their overall fitness and/ or reduce, at some stage, their alcohol consumption. They expressed no surprise that some of the survey findings had suggestion a high level of risk-taking sexual activity, by that we meant poor protection against sexually transmitted infections (STIs) and pregnancy. The hedonism of youth and student life normalised this behaviour and the advice they might dispense to patients in their future practice when qualified seemed distant from what they would do themselves. We have yet to fully analyse and publish the findings from this study but would agree with Wallace[1] and Newbury-Birch, et al.[4] that the situation could improve with properly structured educational approaches in curriculum as well as looking at improving school policies related to alcohol which reflect work place policies.

CREATING CURRICULUM OPPORTUNITIES EXPLICITLY: THE MONASH EXAMPLE; PROMOTING THE HEALTH OF MEDICAL STUDENTS AND ITS IMPACT

Introduction and rationale

Students may have little idea about the potentially high risks for morbidity and premature mortality associated with the medical profession and being a medical student. In contrast they may be very familiar with the possibility of a pleasurable and even hedonistic time as a university student. It is therefore at the crucial stage of medical education when students arrive at university that the Monash course endeavours to promote the health and well-being of its students.

As students leave the defined parameters of home life and look forward to the freedoms of university, this course aims to ensure the relevance of its health promotion teaching and starts with some findings from the literature about student health, hence embedding a sound rationale for the subsequent teaching.

The course starts with reference to the health of students based on the literature. Studies have shown that medical students experience high rates of psychological morbidity and that stress becomes increasingly important after the commencement of the medical course.[5] The problems begin from first year, with stress, anxiety, depression and burnout being common and highest in the pre-exam period.[6] Some studies put the prevalence of depression among undergraduates at close to 20% overall, and 25% for some ethnic subgroups.[7]

Factors predisposing students to depression include ethnicity, study demands, being female[5] and performance anxiety.[8] Commonly cited stressors include 'talking to psychiatric patients', 'effects on personal life', 'presenting cases', 'dealing with death and suffering' and relationship with clinical teachers.

Poor mental health has been linked to medical errors[9] and may also affect the high rate of unhealthy behaviours and co-morbidities such as binge drinking and use of illicit substances.[4] High workload affects other aspects of student health and lifestyle, such as reduced physical activity and poor diet.[10] Denial is common among clinical teachers and affects the educational environment into which medical students enter.[11]

Burnout and psychiatric morbidity is common in medical graduates. As many as 75% of interns have reported burnout at eight months into internship, and 73% met criteria for psychiatric morbidity on at least one occasion throughout their intern year[12] and this may affect the ability to deliver compassionate medical care.[13]

For these and other reasons, enhancing the health of medical students is an important part of their personal and professional development and is not only an investment in their own well-being but also that of their patients.

Health promotion for medical students in curricula: the Monash Health Enhancement Program (HEP)

Few comprehensive, integrated student well-being programmes are built into core curriculum.[14] Trials on optional mindfulness-based stress reduction (MBSR) programmes for medical students found reduced anxiety, psychological distress and depression, and increased empathy, control and spiritual experiences.[13] Other evidence suggests that mindfulness facilitates the development of empathy and compassion and better clinical decision making,[15] is associated with emotional intelligence, improves immunity and has effects on neural plasticity.[16] Early training in self-care may provide a foundation for later clinical and professional skills and may reduce the level of medical errors.[17]

The Monash University Health Enhancement Program, having been a significant part of core curriculum since 2002, is the first integrated program of its type in medical education.[18] The HEP is part of the personal and professional development theme and occurs in the second half of first semester of first year. The objectives of the HEP are to foster behaviours, attitudes, skills and knowledge conducive to:

➤ learning personal self-care strategies for managing stress and maintaining a healthy lifestyle
➤ enhancing students' physical health
➤ laying the foundations for clinical skills in stress and lifestyle management
➤ integrating HEP content with biomedical, psychological and social sciences
➤ understanding the mind-body relationship
➤ developing a holistic approach to healthcare
➤ developing a supportive environment among the student body
➤ enhancing performance.

Over and above these objectives, however, it is also intended that the HEP provides an experiential and evidence-based background for the health promotion component of the course, which occurs in second year through the ESSENCE lifestyle program and stress release program (SRP) within the Monash curriculum. The ESSENCE program provides a practical approach to the early theories of Antonovsky about 'sense of coherence' (SOC),[19-21] discussed in the previous chapter.

The mindfulness component has since been incorporated into the optional self-care workshops for Harvard medical students.[7] The mindfulness program was developed in the early 1990s and has been used at undergraduate and postgraduate levels since then.

Eight introductory lectures provide an overview of the HEP covering the evidence-base linking mental and physical health, mind-body medicine, behaviour-change strategies, mindfulness-based therapies, and the ESSENCE lifestyle program (Table 14.1). Lectures are supported by six two-hour tutorials. An example of part of the HEP curriculum is shown in Table 14.2. Tutorial content includes one hour on the stress release programme and one hour dedicated successively to other ESSENCE elements. Face-to-face teaching is supported with self-directed learning.

The stress release program (SRP): a mindfulness-based stress management and cognitive therapy program

Since 1991 the SRP has been used for postgraduate training. It incorporates mindfulness practices and a series of related cognitive strategies which identify some of the processes underpinning stress, negative emotions and poor performance. Students are encouraged to do weekly 'homework' by personally applying the mindfulness strategies. The following week the group discusses their experiences and insights. Class discussion is driven by the questions, issues and insights of the students and support materials include a student manual, course text[22] and a two-CD set.

The ESSENCE lifestyle program

Each week an ESSENCE topic is explored by the group and students examine their own behaviours and motivations in relation to it. The aim is to foster awareness, conscious choice, empathy and effective behaviour-change. Students set their own agenda, rate of progress and goals in applying these strategies to themselves. To enhance the ability of students to make and maintain healthy lifestyle change, a range of behaviour-change and goal-setting strategies are taught.

Throughout the HEP students maintain a journal, which benefits from weekly formative feedback from their tutor. Integration of the experiential components with the biomedical sciences and clinical applications form the basis of the journal content. The approach to self-care and building clinical skills relies heavily on the tutorial

TABLE 14.1 The 'ESSENCE of Health' lifestyle model

Code	Description
E	Education: the importance of knowledge and reflection
S	Stress management: the importance of mental health. Intervention covered in the mindfulness program
S	Spirituality: the role of meaning and/or spirituality on coping, health and illness
E	Exercise: the importance and application of physical activity
N	Nutrition: the role of healthy nutrition and the influences on eating patterns
C	Connectedness: the role of social support for well-being and healthcare
E	Environment: creating a healthy physical, emotional and social environment

TABLE 14.2 Example of HEP Curriculum

Course objectives	Activities	Assessment

• Reinforce and expand on major themes introduced on the transition residential (TR) program
• Improve personal stress management skills
• Raise awareness about our lifestyle choices
• Empower the ability to change behaviours to healthier patterns if desired
• Foster peer support and communication
• Help integrate the relationship between biological science and well-being
• Lay foundations for development of clinical and counselling skills
	• Transition residential lecture and tutorial
	• Health enhancement program (HEP)
	• Eight lectures on stress, lifestyle issues, and mind-body medicine
	• HEP: Six two-hour tutorials on mindfulness-based stress management and the ESSENCE lifestyle model (education, stress management, spirituality, exercise, nutrition, connectedness, environment)
	• Second semester: Three two-hour seminars on mental health, enhancing performance and stress management
	• Integration with wider learning
		• Summative
		  – Written exam questions (multiple-choice, short-answer)
		  – An OSCE station
		• Formative
		  – HEP journal
		  – Weekly learning activities during HEP

working as a support group although the extent of personal disclosure is up to the students. The confidentiality of the groups is emphasised.

The level of personal application is the choice of individual students, although experiential learning is the most effective way to achieve deep learning, integration, empathy and personal benefit. If at any time students identify themselves as having significant mental-health, behavioural, academic or drug problems, whether it be in conversation or through their journal, they are referred to the student support counselling service.

Care is taken to integrate the HEP with all the other elements of the medical curriculum via a number of methods:

➤ an evidence-based lecture series which includes the scientific foundations of mind-body medicine, neuroscience, psycho-neuro-immunology and lifestyle-based interventions
➤ core knowledge is integrated into weekly case-based learning to demonstrate clinical application
➤ assessment is integrated with other components of the medical course.

Although personal application is optional, core content and skills are examinable. Summative assessment of the student's ability to understand and apply core knowledge and skills is covered in all written and observed structured clinical examinations (OSCE) where, for example, a student might role-play a clinician helping a role-playing patient to implement behaviour change, explain the relationship of stress and health, or discuss mindfulness-based stress management.

Outcomes

The outcome of the HEP was reported in 2008.[23] Previously unpublished evaluation data found that on a 5-point scale the HEP was rated as 'somewhat – 3' to 'extremely – 5' enjoyable (90%), useful (84%), instructive (82%), relevant (84%) and interesting (90%) respectively.

We have found an encouragingly high uptake of the mindfulness practice with over 90% of students reporting personally applying them. Student well-being has been measured before (mid-semester) and after the HEP, with the post-course evaluation taking place a few days prior to their midyear exams, a time when it is expected that their well-being should be at its worst. Counter to such expectations we found that by the end of the HEP students reported improved well-being on all scales of the symptom checklist 90-R including the depression, anxiety and hostility subscales, as well as the global severity index. Benefits were also seen for the psychological and physical domains of the World Health Organization (WHO) quality-of-life scale.

Discussion

Our findings are that the HEP has a beneficial effect on students' physical and psychological well-being even during a high stress period, for example prior to exams. The strength of the HEP lies in the fact that it is delivered to all students and that it is integrated with subjects that are seen as core curriculum, such as the biomedical and behavioural sciences as well as clinical practice. Variable compliance in a programme with a heavy emphasis on experiential learning may be affected by a range of factors such as learning style. For example, those with a deep learning style, greater self-awareness and emotional intelligence (EI) are more likely to engage in such an experiential programme than those with surface learning, avoidant coping styles or lower EI. The implementation and application of the HEP content is integral to engaging and motivating students. For example, it is important to make the material relevant to the student's personal needs, be inclusive and respectful of cultural and religious diversity, present material in a non-threatening way, and to avoid imposing material by inviting inquiry and exploration.

The benefits of the programme are likely to be due to the synergistic effects of a range of lifestyle factors and social support including the mindfulness components. These may facilitate beneficial lifestyle habits relating to physical activities with a positive impact upon mental and physical health.

Tutor selection is especially important in a programme where tutors will be serving as role models and they need specialised skills such as mindfulness training. Personal and professional qualities are therefore important in the selection of such tutors.

It should doubtless be the aim of any medical course to have its students graduating healthier and more resilient than when they came into it, at the same time as important knowledge and skills are being imparted. In our experience this is a realistic goal.

CREATING CURRICULUM OPPORTUNITIES IMPLICITLY

The curricular time restraints and the inappropriateness of 'preaching' to adult learners can be a barrier to implementing explicit health promotion programmes for students. There is also a supposition that if medical students learn about sensible drinking for their future patients they will also learn about this for themselves. Such supposition is reasonable given the response of the medical profession to evidence about smoking-related diseases.[28]

Students at many medical schools learn about the behaviour change transtheoretical model and its efficacy,[25] although many practitioners, and hence teachers, have expressed a lack of confidence in approaching patients with lifestyle issues and some are yet to be convinced of efficacy of such interventions.[26,27] We can therefore not assume that students will have equitable learning experiences related to health promotion, given that many of the teachers and facilitators show limited enthusiasm and experience. Conflicting messages of 'do as I say, not as I do' may also limit the value of health promotion teaching as applicable to students themselves when aimed at student health. The arguments that medical schools should provide structured health promotion teaching are well supported but there are few examples about effectively doing this. At KCL the approaches are implicit rather than explicit and ongoing research is focused on establishing impact.

Part of the first year programme, in the context of the lecture 'What is good health?', invites the students to do the simple exercise (*see* Table 14.3) taken from Ewles and Simnett (1990).[28] When complete they compare their individual Column 3 with their neighbour in the lecture theatre. It would be rare, even with more than 400 students, for any two of them to have the exact same result. Usually what follows is a realisation that about three of the final statements relate to their own choices and priorities. In other words they can be empowered to be proactive about their health.

TABLE 14.3 'What is good health?' activity (*adapted from Ewles and Simnett 1990*)[28]

What does being healthy mean to you?

In Column 1, tick any statements which seem to you to be important aspects of your health.
In Column 2, tick the *six* statements which are the most important aspects of being healthy to you.
In Column 3, rank these six in order of importance – put '1' by the most important, '2' by the next most important and so on down to '6'.

For me, being healthy involves:	*Column 1*	*Column 2*	*Column 3*
1 Enjoying being with my family and friends			
2 Living to a ripe old age			
3 Feeling happy most of the time			
4 Being able to run when I need to (e.g. for a bus) without getting out of breath			
5 Having a job			
6 Being able to get down to making decisions			
7 Hardly ever taking tablets or medicines			
8 Being the ideal weight for my height			
9 Taking part in lots of sport			
10 Feeling at peace with myself			
11 Never smoking			
12 Having clear skin, bright eyes and shiny hair			
13 Never suffering from anything more serious than a mild cold, flu or stomach upset			
14 Not getting things confused or out of proportion – assessing situations realistically			
15 Being able to adapt easily to changes in my life such as moving house, changing jobs or getting married			
16 Feeling glad to be alive			
17 Drinking only moderate amounts of alcohol or none at all			
18 Enjoying my work without much stress or strain			
19 Having all parts of my body in good working condition			
20 Getting on well with other people most of the time			
21 Eating the 'right' foods			
22 Enjoying some form of relaxation/recreation			
23 Hardly ever going to the doctor			

By the third year the students at KCL come face to face with hospitalised severely ill patients often with degenerative conditions that are associated with smoking, alcohol abuse, drug dependency or poor healthcare. For some students this is a motivator for their own health-related behaviour change, for others the link between their own behaviour and the conditions they see is not made. Instead, as students progress to senior years they become more anxious, they find their course more demanding and become less able to take steps to maintain and improve their own health, often with poor outcomes as new graduates.[12] Towards the end of their third year, however, KLC students have formal teaching related to behaviour modification and the transtheoretical model. Within this session, scenarios about smoking cessation, weight loss and type 2 diabetes and alcohol are worked through in small groups. The alcohol scenario is as follows:

A young woman has suffered minor head injuries and has been vomiting following a heavy drinking session. As she is sobering up in A & E you are asked to give her some advice about sensible drinking.

For the students the task provokes discussion about their own similar experiences and encounters. They consider the patient's knowledge about alcohol, whether this is a regular experience or the first time, what factors or antecedents preceded the drinking session, what possible dangers or more serious harm could have resulted. So far there is no evidence or suggestion that this session leads to improved behaviour or attitudes to alcohol consumption, but students in focus groups have said it 'hits home', raises awareness and encourages discussion beyond the session.

In the penultimate year at KCL, students need to prepare a portfolio in preparation for an elective, usually taken overseas. One aspect is their 'personal health and well-being' and below is part of the information provided in the student handbook.

This is assessed within the context of the personal health and safety section of the elective portfolio which carries a total of 20% of the mark and is usually a 1000-word essay or using a pro forma/matrix format (*see* Table 14.4). Students are allocated time to specifically explore their health and health-related behaviour at this unique time in their medical education, identifying an issue/health-related behaviour (possibly more than one) that they would like to review and perhaps modify.

Lecture notes/symposium material is presented and students consider questions relating to:

➤ their own fitness to practice reflecting on their health status and how it compares to studies of medical students and that of the medical profession
➤ preparing for the elective: what changes may be needed/advisable
➤ awareness and use of appropriate coping strategies
➤ what behavioural change is desirable for their health now
➤ what action they could take and what challenges do they face
➤ what health and safety issues should be considered for the elective, for example vaccination information, HIV considerations, antimalarial prophylaxis, travel safety, accommodation, foreign and commonwealth office (FCO) advice, financial and emergency contingency and other areas of vulnerability and areas of responsibility.

TABLE 14.4 Proposed framework for assessment of personal health and well-being section of the elective SSM (20% of the elective portfolio mark)

Student name	Student report	Grade/mark
Country planning to visit	Major health risks identified	
FCO advice	What is it, date written, any warnings against travel in the country or within specific regions	
Vaccinations	What is needed, source and date of information, action taken or planned	
HIV risks and other viral infections	Sources and date of information, action taken or planned	
Parasites and malaria	Sources and date of information, action taken or planned	
Guidance for safe travel	Sources and date of information, and action taken or planned	
Guidance for accommodation	Sources and date of information, and action taken or planned	
Personal financial guidance	Sources and date of information, and action taken or planned	
Emergency contingencies	Sources and date of information, and action taken or planned	
Personal health conditions e.g. asthma	Action taken or planned	
Personal health status	Summary of current positive attributes and one area for change and improvement	
What changes are needed	How have these been identified – give information sources	
Will I cope well during elective with changes? What strategies am I adopting/ already have adopted?	Name them and explain	
Identify desirable behavioural change	Name and explain, how do you know?	
Identify action plan for change	Ensure you have identified antecedents, what is modifiable, what re-enforcers will help and short-term goals	

During this module students explore health issues by engaging with some of the following:

➤ identifying relevant agencies
➤ exploring sources of advice and resources to improve or maintain their health
➤ testing out helplines and websites
➤ doing a diary/audit of their health-related behaviour
➤ identifying relevant *antecedents* to poor health-related behaviour

➤ setting out an action plan for change for *modifiable* factors
➤ recognising the potential for relapse
➤ considering what is needed for maintenance of change and identify re-enforcers at times of weakness.

This will be of direct benefit to the student and will also enable them to appreciate the challenges patients face when advised to change behaviour. Some students, for example, will have observed during the Year 4 community study home visits that women who gave up smoking during pregnancy have returned to smoking in the postnatal phase. They may reflect on why this might be and how best to explore relapse as a normal step of working towards behaviour modification.

During their elective preparation students should consider what the public health issues are and what influences health-related behaviours in the countries and communities they visit. For example, the public health indices for Cuba are good yet this is a poor country. Reasons for this include the ongoing rationing of food and lack of 'fast food' outlets and suggestions that this may be a more important factor in weight management than personal choice/behaviour, as well as the need for most people to walk or cycle because of limited public transport and access to cars. More affluent countries that experience good public health indices are democracies such as Sweden and Australia, where individual behaviour and autonomy are highly valued and health-related policies facilitate the 'healthy' choice.

Students are not expected to share personal and confidential information, and guidelines on how to write up this are provided (*see* Table 14.4).

The symposium introduces students to the wider principles of health promotion based on the WHO Ottawa Charter of 1986, and subsequent WHO declarations.[29] They learn the basic theoretical frameworks for community interventions, namely the Beattie model and Tones' healthy public policy theories. The symposium aims to inform the students about the contribution community interventions make to the health of local populations, and how the success of these interventions are measured, that is, evidence and evaluation. We hope that, as future doctors, the students will examine their own health and well-being, and identify any opportunities for change and improvement. Current, albeit limited, data about medical student health-related behaviour is presented.

To date the students have focused more on the prevention of blood-borne virus infections and malaria prevention, as well as the wider public health concerns of the countries they are visiting, than on their own health-related behaviour change in their portfolios. What we have yet to establish as part of our ongoing research is to what extent this actively influences personal reflection and change. Through focus groups so far we have had feedback that students valued the opportunity to review their own health-related behaviour but are hesitant about what to reveal. They have indicated that this also helps them reflect on the challenges patients face when advised to take more exercise or reduce their weight and alcohol consumption. They become more aware of high probability of relapse, based on their own experiences.

Given the level of knowledge these students have about the determinants of disease and the trajectory of risk behaviour to irreversible chronic disease, there is a balance to be considered about how much emphasis and time core curricula should have on their own health-related behaviour and more importantly the difficulties of summative assessment associated with this. Whilst Wallace and Newbury-Birch, *et al.* argue that education about alcohol, tobacco and drugs issues should be part of core curricula[1,4] as a way of reducing these activities within the student population, we have little evidence to indicate whether the focus should be directed at the students themselves or be more implicit and abstract, related to health promotion for patients in the hope that it will have a positive impact on the students.

SUPPORTING STUDENT HEALTH-PROMOTING INFRASTRUCTURES AND STUDENT AWARENESS OF RESOURCES

Students arriving at universities, regardless of the course, can have health-promoting experiences. 'Freshers' week is the time before the formal academic year starts when students orientate themselves, are given advice about facilities, agencies and social issues. They may of course be overwhelmed with choice and even disregard some information as not relevant at this early stage in their university life. In addition the types of student infrastructures at universities that promote and support health and well-being may not be easily recognised as such.

Financial services, welfare services, social services and counselling services can provide students with basic advice and support but also provide help when students get into difficulty. In some universities students themselves provide these services and in the UK about 40 universities offer 'Nightline'.

> Nightline is a listening, support and information service, run by students for students.
>
> Nightline services operate in over 40 universities in the UK and beyond. All of them offer a telephone helpline service – usually all night, every night during term-time – and many also offer a drop-in service and email listening.
>
> We have no political, religious, sexual or moral bias. If you're a student at a university with a Nightline, you can call about anything you like. We won't judge you and we won't tell you what to do, but no matter what it's about, we'll listen.
>
> Nightline is confidential and anonymous. You don't have to tell us anything about yourself – not even your name.
>
> The Nightline Charity is the association of individual Nightlines. It exists to promote, support and develop Nightlines on both a national and local scale.[30]

As well as university-run services, students will also be advised about other similar services such as how their banks can help, external welfare services and listening services such as 'Samaritans'.

Healthcare and occupational health services are available to students as well as advice about sickness and absenteeism regards academic work, disabilities and special needs advice and support, as well as advice about maternity leave, child care and care of dependents.

Universities must, by law, of course comply with health and safety regulations to protect staff and students as well as visitors. Students will be expected to comply with these regulations.

Whilst the above apply more or less to all students there are additional concerns for medical and health professional students that need to be considered.

Financial concerns loom large given the extended time spent at university and the expenses of books, equipment and travel. Medical schools can help by arranging grants, bursaries and awards, and clearly disseminating information about how students can access these. Students sometime complain they had little or no information about such funds or the application process was cumbersome.

The availability of alcohol within medical schools and the social norm of inappropriate drinking could be modified to comply with conventional workplace policies.[1] Access to drugs may also be too lax and a culture of self-medication needs to be proactively discouraged. Students need to know that they can and should seek help as soon as possible if they are unwell, misusing drugs or concerned about alcohol consumption. They should also be advised about what action to take if they are concerned about a fellow student, teacher or clinician. This is, of course, uncomfortable and fraught with potential difficulties, but most universities will have official policies to help guide students thought these processes.

There are practical concerns about student health and well-being regarding infections. First, the student with any kind of infection, however mild, should consider whether or not they should be with fellow students and with patients. There is a balance but in some cases, where the student feels well enough, there is much to be gained from attending scheduled sessions. However, being unwell or having persistent and disabling symptoms may indicate that the student should seek medical advice. Students returning from countries where there are endemic communicable diseases have to consider what risk they pose to others if, for example, they have diarrhoea and vomiting, even if the symptoms have reduced from severe to intermittent. Pyrexia, weight loss, rashes, weeping wounds, unexplained swellings and haemorrhaging are all symptoms for which students should seek help and advice before returning to lectures, seminars or clinical patient-contact sessions. Second, a student found to have a notifiable disease, such as a salmonella infection, will not be able to work in a hospital or clinical setting until the statutory requirements have been met. Third, students are vulnerable to hospital-acquired infections and should be well prepared to protect themselves and others. This is usually related to good aseptic techniques, compliance with hygiene regulations, observing procedures for disposable of waste materials and reporting any incidents such as needle-stick injury.

What may seem obvious to experienced clinicians and medical teachers will not necessarily be obvious to students unless time is set aside to ensure they are well briefed in principle and for the local context in which they are learning and working.

There are other personal health and well-being issues for students in the clinical settings. For example, students need to be advised about being safe, how to be assertive, avoiding potentially violent or dangerous patients and situations, adequate access to refreshments, toilets and breaks. All this has to be an integral aspect of briefing and induction procedures, where adequate time and information is provided to ensure the learning context is not health-harming.

With the introduction of new curricula at many medical schools, the pedagogy itself has become a health-enhancing experience. Concepts such as being student-centred, mixed methods of evidence-based assessments, including formative assessment and the provision of fair and equitable procedures all contribute to the students' health promotion, as well as reviews of curricula, which consider the amount of curriculum content and the quality of the student experience. For example, Monash has been a leader in transition and provides a wide range of resources and activities through its transition residential (TR) program for new intakes of medical students since the inception of the new Monash medical curriculum in 2002. It is a core component of the medical curriculum that addresses many of the issues and problems associated with transition to university in general. The core aims of the TR include:

➤ beginning the process of enculturation into the teaching and learning styles, life, procedures, practices and culture of the university

➤ encouraging students to engage with the university, a particular course, and people at a specific campus

➤ emphasising the need for students to take responsibility for their own learning and have realistic expectations

➤ acknowledging the importance of the support provided by peers, staff and students' families.

There is little question that these aims are accomplished effectively through the TR as indicated by the 2007 evaluation findings. Looking after the well-being of the student body for its own sake and educating competent and compassionate doctors should be the most important aims.

If students are to become health-promoting practitioners, they need to have had their own health-promoting experiences and whilst they may not exactly be role models in all aspects, they should be able to meet the requirements of *The New Doctor*.[31] These requirements include being able to maintain their own health, have a suitable balance between work and personal life and know how to deal with personal illness.

While evidence is still sparse about how best to promote student health, it is important therefore that curricula, explicitly or implicitly, facilitate students in meeting their health needs.

REFERENCES

1 Wallace P. Medical students, drugs and alcohol: time for medical schools to take the issue seriously. *Med Educ.* 2000; **34**(2): 86–7.

2 Howse K, Ghodse AH. Hazardous drinking and its correlates among medical students. *Addict Res Theory.* 1997; **4**(4): 355–66.

3 Pickard M, Bates L, Dovian M, *et al.* Alcohol and drug use in second-year medical students at the University of Leeds. *Med Educ.* 2000; **34**(2): 148–50.

4 Newbury-Birch D, Walshaw D, Kamali F. Drink and drugs: from medical students to doctors. *Drug Alcohol Depend.* 2001; **64**(3): 265–70.

5 Dyrbye LN, Thomas MR, Shanafelt TD. Systematic review of depression, anxiety and other indicators of psychological distress among US and Canadian medical students. *Acad Med.* 2006; **81**(4): 354–73.

6 Dyrbye LN, Thomas MR, Shanafelt TD. Medical student distress: causes, consequences and proposed solutions. *Mayo Clinic Proceedings.* 2005; **80**(12): 1613–22.

7 Rosenthal JM, Okie S. White coat, mood indigo: depression in medical school. *New Eng J Med.* 2005; **353**(11): 1085–8.

8 Chandavarker U, Azzam A, Mathews CA. Anxiety symptoms and perceived performance in medical students. *Depress Anxiety.* 2007; **24**(2): 103–11.

9 Fahrenkopf AM, Sectish TC, Barger LK, *et al.* Rates of medication errors among depressed and burnt out residents: prospective cohort study. *BMJ.* 2008; **336**(7642): 488–91.

10 Ball S, Bax A. Self-care in medical education: effectiveness of health habits intervention for first-year medical students. *Acad Med.* 2002; **77**(9): 911–17.

11 Sexton JB, Thomas EJ, Helmreich RL. Error, stress and teamwork in medicine and aviation: cross-sectional surveys. *BMJ.* 2000; **320**(7237): 745–9.

12 Willcock S, Daly MG, Tennant CC, *et al.* Burnout and psychiatric morbidity in new medical graduates. *Med J Aust.* 2004; **181**(7): 357–60.

13 Rosenzweig S, Reibel DK, Greenson JM, *et al.* Mindfulness-based stress reduction lowers psychological distress in medical students. *Teach Learn Med.* 2003; **15**(2): 88–92.

14 Shapiro SL, Shapiro DE, Schwartz GE. Stress management in medical education: a review of the literature. *Acad Med.* 2000; **75**(7): 748–59.

15 Epstein RM. Mindful practice. *JAMA.* 1999; **282**(9): 833–9.

16 Davidson RJ, Kabat-Zinn J, Schumacher J, *et al.* Alterations in brain and immune function produced by mindfulness meditation. *Psychosom Med.* 2003; **65**(4): 564–70.

17 Epstein RM, Hassed CS. Mindfulness training: from student care to clinical practice. 13th Ottawa International Conference on Clinical Competence; Melbourne; 5–8 Mar, 2008.

18 Hassed CS. Bringing holism into mainstream medical education. *J Altern Complement Med.* 2004; **10**(2): 405–7.

19 Eriksson M, Lindstrom B, Lilja J. A sense of coherence and health. Salutogenesis in a societal context: Aland, a special case? *J Epidemiol Commun H.* 2007; **61**(8): 684–8.

20 Antonovsky A. The sense of coherence as a determinant of health. In: Beattie A, Gott M, Jones L, *et al.*, editors. *Health and Wellbeing: a reader.* Basingstoke: Macmillan; 1993.

21 Antonovsky A. The salutogenic model as a theory to guide health promotion. *Health Promot Int.* 1996; **11**(1): 11–18.

22 Hassed CS. *Know Thyself: the stress release program.* Melbourne: Michelle Anderson Publishing; 2002.

23 Hassed C, de Lisle S, Sullivan G, *et al.* Enhancing the health of medical students: outcomes of an integrated mindfulness and lifestyle program. *Adv Health Sci Educ Theory Pract.* 2009; **14**(3): 387–98.

24 Doll R, Peto R, Wheatley K, *et al.* Mortality in relation to smoking: 40 years' observations on male British doctors. *BMJ.* 1994; **309**(6959): 901–11.

25 Marteau T, Dieppe P, Foy R, *et al.* Behavioural medicine: changing our behaviour. *BMJ.* 2006; **332**(7539): 437–8.

26 King LA, Loss JHM, Wilkenfeld RL, *et al.* Australian GPs' perceptions about child and adolescent overweight and obesity: the Weight of Opinion study. *Br J Gen Pract.* 2007; **57**: 124–9.

27 Vogt F, Hall S, Marteau T. General practitioners' beliefs about effectiveness and intentions to recommend smoking cessation services: qualitative and quantitative studies. *BMC Fam Pract.* 2007; **8**(1): 39.

28 Ewles L, Simnett I. *Promoting Health: a practical guide.* 4th ed. London: Bailliere Tindall; 1999.

29 World Health Organization. *Ottawa Charter for Health Promotion.* Geneva: World Health Organization; 1986.

30 Nightline. Available at: www.nightline.niss.ac.uk/ (accessed 5 November 2009).

31 General Medical Council. *The New Doctor.* Available at: www.gmc-uk.org/education/postgraduate/new_doctor.asp (accessed 5 November 2009).

CHAPTER 15

Health promotion teaching: some examples of sessions and programmes

Tangerine Holt and Ann Wylie

with additional contributions from Albert Lee, Elizabeth Garland, Richard Bordowitz, Craig Hassed, Max de Courten and Dragan Ilic

The universal goal of medical education is to train doctors to develop knowledge, skills and behaviours that translate into advancing the health of the community they serve. As noted by Philips[1] the transmission of content and delivery has shifted, with many schools and accreditation bodies raising the following questions:

➤ What do we want to accomplish/what is the vision of medical education?
➤ Whose vision is it/what are the roles and powers of government, the profession, individual teachers, students and the public?
➤ What is included in the curriculum (the content) and how is it presented (the process)/how do we accomplish our goals?
➤ How is effectiveness measured/how do we assess whether we have succeeded?

Although the Flexner Report in the US shaped medical education, governments, institutions and regulatory bodies have recently begun to recognise that the mission of medical schools together with its defined graduate attributes and outcomes must meet the needs of the community. Furthermore, contemporary medical education is grappling with the development of competency- and outcome-based education (OBE) approaches, with debates taking place across learning objectives, content delivery, assessment and evaluation processes. Harden[2] believes that the problem with medical education is its narrow focus on learning outcomes only and less on the implementation of an OBE approach in practice. For OBE to be successful in medical education, the curriculum has to take on a 'both–and' approach, whereby learning outcomes are clearly defined *and* decisions relating to the curriculum are based on the learning outcomes specified.

From a health promotion curriculum point of view this becomes more critical as the medical education fraternity are beginning to recognise their professional social responsibility to meet the healthcare needs of the community. The developments in learning theory and the content shift in medical education from detailed to essential knowledge embedded in the context of the patients' lives is evidenced by accreditation requirements, guidelines and frameworks developed by the Australian Medical Council, the Association of American Medical Colleges (AAMC), the British General Medical Council, CanMeds Framework, and in Bergen, the European Union, via the Bologna Process.

With the philosophical shift from organs and knowledge to patients and performance as focal points, medical curricula throughout the world are slowly beginning to encompass their professional responsibility in dealing with the patient as opposed to an organ or disease, communication skills, professionalism and the social, economic and cultural aspects determining the significance of social determinants of the patient's health. Furthermore Harden[3] highlights the importance of considering learning outcomes for health promotion and disease, including international dimensions if students are to practise in a global economy.[4] The focus of this chapter is to outline current pedagogical approaches and learning technologies being used at international levels in Australia, Hong Kong, the US, and the UK. It will highlight educational strategies and learning opportunities adopted such as problem-based learning, community-based learning and interprofessional cooperation to match the learning outcomes as delivered, assessed and evaluated in health promotion.

EXAMPLE 1: THE CENTRE FOR HEALTH EDUCATION AND HEALTH PROMOTION (CHEP) AT THE CHINESE UNIVERSITY OF HONG KONG
Albert Lee

Using a 'settings' approach for health promotion
Chronic illnesses account for the majority of the health burden, and a number of risk factors including high cholesterol, high blood pressure, obesity, smoking and alcohol are responsible for most of the chronic disease burden.[5] Research by Yusulf, *et al.* concluded that abnormal lipids, smoking, hypertension, diabetes, abdominal obesity, psychosocial factors, consumption levels of fruits, vegetables and alcohol and lack of regular physical activity accounted for most of the risks of myocardial infarction worldwide in both sexes and at all ages in all regions.[6] Health promotion and disease prevention is possible when sustained actions are directed both at individuals and families; as well as the broader social, economic and cultural determinants of non-communicable diseases.[7] Many leading causes of mortality and morbidity are related to health risk behaviours which are often established during youth and extend to adulthood; and those diseases might not be curable but preventable.

Healthcare systems provide a mechanism for the management of illnesses, but there is no specific system to address health promotion, particularly tackling the broader determinants of health. The World Health Organization (WHO) has actively pursued a 'settings' approach to promote health, as the Ottawa Charter for Health stated that 'health is created and lived by people within the settings of their daily life: where they learn, work, play and love'.[8] The Bangkok Charter for Health emphasised investment in sustainable policies, actions and infrastructure to address the determinants of health, and capacity building for policy development, leadership, health promotion practice, knowledge transfer and research and health literacy.[9]

Most of the health risk behaviours adopted by adolescents will have the greatest health impact later in their life, but the impact has been underestimated so a 'Life

Course' approach to promote healthy behaviours should begin early in life. Effective health promotion must take place in the context of people's everyday life and therefore opportunities for health to enter different settings such as schools, workplaces, communities are very important. The first and widely known example of the settings-based health promotion approach was the 'Healthy Cities' project which occurred in many countries from the late 1980s, with parallel initiatives in settings such as schools, workplaces, hospitals, neighbourhoods, villages and prisons.[10] The concept of a Health-promoting School (HPS) was first identified at the WHO conference in the early 1980s and has been strongly supported as it embodies a holistic, whole-school approach to personal and community health promotion in which a broad health education curriculum is supported by the environment and ethos of the school.[11] Such a comprehensive approach has been widely accepted by school health professionals as an effective and important method of implementing school health.[12,13] The essential elements of HPS include improvement in the school's physical and social environment, active promotion of the self-esteem of all pupils by demonstrating that everyone can make a contribution to the life of the school, development of the education potential of the school health services beyond routine screening towards active support for the curriculum, and development of good links between the school, home and the community.[14]

'Healthy setting' approaches such as HPS can therefore address the determinants of health, particularly the social, cultural and political aspects, and facilitates organisations and institutions to create a culture for health improvement. A positive culture for health would facilitate higher levels of health literacy, helping individuals to tackle the determinants of their own health better as they build up the personal, cognitive and social skills which determine the ability of individuals to gain access to, understand and use information to promote and maintain good health.[15] Schools are essential in helping students to achieve health literacy.[16]

The Centre for Health Education and Health Promotion (CHEP) at the Chinese University of Hong Kong launched the Hong Kong Healthy School Award in 2001, building on the concept of HPS to create better health for students and supporting them in improving the quality of their lives.[17] The scheme was modelled on the WHO Western Pacific Regional Office HPS framework covering six key areas (health policy, physical and social environments, community relationships, personal health skills and health services) which was designed to assist schools in addressing particular health issues strategically.[18,19] Each key area has a number of components and a set of indicators, based on extensive literature and documentary reviews, that are relevant, adaptable and achievable, with a contextualisation specific to Asia-Pacific countries.[20-25] The concept of HPS can therefore help to ensure sustained positive changes and encourage schools to address the interlinked social, educational, psychological, and health needs of school children.[26] It has been suggested that well developed school health promotion programmes are more effective than the traditional information-giving approach in encouraging children to adopt health-enhancing behaviours and reduce health-compromising behaviours.[27]

Evidence has shown that the whole-school approach using the HPS framework is effective in health improvement ranging from physical activities and healthy eating to emotional health.[28,29,30] There is also evidence to show that schools adopting the HPS framework have better school health policy, higher degrees of community participation, and a more hygienic environment.[31] Students in schools that had adopted the HPS framework had a more positive health behaviour profile than those in non-HPS schools.[32] The concept of HPS is therefore seen as an effective way to teach health in a holistic way and improve standards of health literacy.[33]

How would one introduce the concept to medical curriculum so the medical professionals perceive it directly relevant to clinical practice?

Linking the health and education sectors is essential to promote the concept of HPS.[34] The approach for undergraduate medical education is quite different from postgraduate. For the undergraduate medical curriculum, a module on management of common adolescent health problems in primary care paves the way for the future medical doctors to understand that successful management of adolescent health problems needs to go beyond the health sector. Addressing the principles and practice of health education introduces the concept of healthy settings to promote better health.

Undergraduate level
MANAGEMENT OF ADOLESCENT HEALTH PROBLEMS IN PRIMARY CARE AND PRINCIPLES AND PRACTICE OF HEALTH EDUCATION

The lesson on adolescent health in primary care first started with data of a local study showing that a high proportion of adolescents presented to primary care physicians with non-specific complaints and a very low proportion of adolescents received health promotion advice on common health issues such as safe sex, avoidance of alcohol, healthy diet, management of emotional problems, accident prevention.[35] Barriers perceived by adolescents seeking help from primary care were discussed. Students were taught practical tips for communicating with adolescents. Special skills in understanding the cognitive and social development of adolescents and their social context of behaviours were also emphasised. For young people to gain maximum benefit from health services, age-appropriate health services should be available, with collaboration between schools and communities. Data from a local study was shown to illustrate that the uptake rate of preventive health services drops as students get older, despite the availability of student health services for a very low cost.[36]

The work on the principles and practice of health education used the example of the outbreak of SARS to demonstrate how a school would step up measures in coping with epidemics of infectious disease.[37] The lesson discussed how the healthy setting movement could provide a framework for an integrated and holistic approach to public health. The approach could also lead to intersectoral action and community participation in identifying and solving priority problems by addressing the physical and social health determinants of health.[38] The concept of a 'hygiene charter' was introduced, putting forward suggestions and guidelines on hygiene practices for individuals, management and businesses and organisations over 10 different sectors. The charter would facilitate the development of public health policies as it involved different sectors, and would also strengthen community action to create and sustain a supportive environment for health.[39,40]

Using examples of adolescent health and public health crises, students develop an insight that many health issues are beyond the control of healthcare providers. There is no one solution to the health problems of childhood and adolescence. Intervention should be aimed at changing the 'systems' within which people are embedded, rather than at changing the individual. Continuity of programming must be maintained across development stages. Successful partnership and collaboration with other sectors are essential. The healthy setting approach would offer a solution for wider community participation, capacity building and creating a positive health culture. Some groups of medical students conducted selective study modules on health promotion topics such as prevention of childhood obesity, helping adolescents in weight control, and a self-management programme for asthma.[41]

Postgraduate level (Master of Family Medicine)

THE ROLE OF FAMILY PHYSICIANS IN CHILD AND ADOLESCENT HEALTH:
FIELD EXPERIENCE OF SCHOOL HEALTH

At postgraduate level, the need for a reorientation of school health services was discussed. Assessment of students' health needs was stressed, as routine health data might not capture all the information on the health of school children, especially their medical consultation patterns and health-risk behaviours.[42] The course participants were introduced to the concept of the Hong Kong Healthy School Award scheme building on the concept of HPS, which conducted a comprehensive assessment of schools covering different areas related to the health of students.[43] Youth health surveillance was conducted to establish a community diagnosis of youth health problems.[44] The youth health surveillance in 1999, 2001 and 2003 all revealed that a substantially high proportion of our young people did not have healthy eating habits, were not performing exercise regularly and also were emotionally disturbed.[45,46] Therefore school health services should contain core services such as emotional and behavioural problems, nutritional advice, physical activities, and should maintain a close link with primary care health services.

Coordinated school health programmes can provide a range of services addressing health needs:

➤ core services only
➤ core services plus expanded health services
➤ services through school-based or school-linked health centres.

The school health team should consist of professionals from various disciplines such as family physicians, nurses, counsellors, psychologists and allied health professionals such as physiotherapists, occupational therapists and dietitians. There are increasing numbers of schools expressing interest in developing expanded services through school-based or school-linked health centres. This can be done in partnership with local health departments, community health centres and other community agencies.

A high-quality core student health services model would be a good option if the community assessment demonstrated students having access to healthcare from community providers. If many students were found to have difficulty accessing community providers, the 'core-plus' expanded school health services model would become the choice, with identification of the health problems and referral to appropriate health professionals. An integrated primary healthcare team would provide the necessary services when needed. Some schools would consider school-based health centres to provide a minimum of on-site, primary and preventive healthcare, emotional health counselling, health promotion, referral and follow-up services for selected groups of young people. School-based centres could be part of a larger organisation such as a primary healthcare group. A health centre beyond school property serving a group of schools as school-linked centres would provide a variety of primary healthcare services ranging from preventive, screening and treatment. Such a centre would accept referrals from schools, provide priority appointments for young people, market their services meeting youth needs, and offer classroom health education on specific topics.

In the Master of Family Medicine programme, the elective module on child and adolescent health also discusses the integration of school health services and other school health programmes. This would involve:

➤ formation of a health-promoting school team with representation from across the school (overall school health coordinators, teachers, coordinators of each component of the school health programme, administrators, students, parents), as well as community healthcare providers and government

➤ establishment of an interdisciplinary school health services team, which is a subcommittee of the health-promoting school team.

The following action steps in implementing school health services are discussed:

➤ identify a school health services coordinator amongst the interdisciplinary team

➤ link the work with other components of the coordinated school health programme

➤ map healthcare resources and the availability of primary healthcare services meeting youth needs

➤ using results of mapping to identify the most appropriate school health services configuration.

The postgraduate students of Master of Family Medicine taking the 'child and adolescent' module also need to propose a health-enhancement program for children or adolescents (or for their parents). They need to discuss briefly which issue they would choose and why. The program can be in any form such as exhibitions, talks, small-group activities etc. The students need to outline the aim of the program, the target group, the location, the activities and so on and also describe how coordinators/facilitators and participants are recruited. They need to show how a family physician can be involved in this program.

How would 'healthy setting' notions have a significant place in the medical curriculum?

Although 'healthy setting' is an effective strategy to address the socio-political, economic and environmental determinants of health, it is not easy for medical students to appreciate the importance. Using adolescent health as an example stimulates them to think about what kinds of skills are needed for the health management of young people. Some of the skills would be best handled not only by non-medical but also by non-healthcare providers such as educators and social service providers specialising in youth services. Students can also think about effective ways to influence the health-promoting behaviour of adolescents. The culture and context of their everyday life would have greater effect than simple delivery of health information. This should lead them to explore how 'healthy setting' strategies could make a difference.

It is important to include 'healthy settings' in postgraduate curriculum for family physicians as they are the front-line physicians in the community. If family physicians have a clear concept of healthy settings, they can reorient their services to better meet the needs of the community.

City health profiles include information about the residents on:

➤ health status
➤ healthcare services utilisation and satisfaction
➤ lifestyles
➤ personal safety
➤ exercise level
➤ quality of life.

Family physicians can make use of this information to work in partnership with other sectors to improve the health of residents, acting across the three levels of prevention described in Figure 15.1.

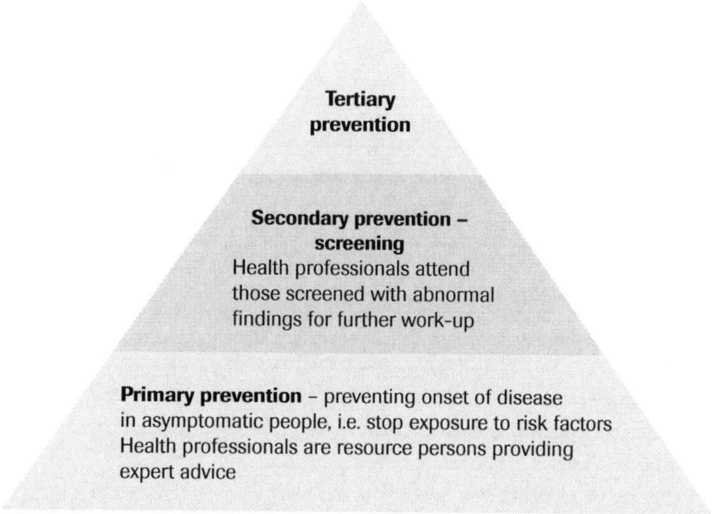

Tertiary prevention

Secondary prevention – screening
Health professionals attend those screened with abnormal findings for further work-up

Primary prevention – preventing onset of disease in asymptomatic people, i.e. stop exposure to risk factors
Health professionals are resource persons providing expert advice

FIGURE 15.1 Three levels of prevention for health professionals

The school health profile would serve a similar purpose. Family physicians would facilitate the development of the necessary infrastructure. During the community-based attachment, students are not exposed to community initiatives in health promotion, but family physicians also share their experience of how they can make use of the concept of 'healthy setting' in the deployment of health resources aimed at promoting, maintaining and improving health and protecting members of the community from harm, illnesses and injuries. Closer integration of primary healthcare and healthy setting approaches would solve the problem of essential services not being delivered to the population groups with the greatest needs.

EXAMPLE 2: MOUNT SINAI SCHOOL OF MEDICINE (MSSM) GENERAL PREVENTIVE MEDICINE RESIDENCY PROGRAM
Tangerine Holt, Elizabeth Garland and Richard Bordowitz

Earlier, Chapter 7 outlined the purpose, programme goals and the mapping of the American College of Preventive Medicine's published competencies for its programme goals and objectives against the MSSM residency program in relation to the Masters

Degree in Public Health. In this chapter we will describe how the programme is delivered through a snapshot of the educational components for postgraduate residents in General Preventive Medicine. The two-year residency program includes concurrent academic and practicum phases, each equivalent to one full year. Candidates for the residency program must have completed at least one full year in an Accreditation Council for Graduate Medical Education (ACGME)-accredited clinical program with six months of direct patient care. All incoming residents must supply proof of successful completion of the ACGME six core competencies from their clinical year (or years) from their prior residency program.

The resident meets with the residency director at the start of the programme to develop an educational plan and then biannually, to discuss goals and identify suitable sites and projects for achieving them (*see* Table 15.5, presented at the end of this section). While still encouraging residents to identify an area of interest to pursue in depth, all residents entering the program are required to diversify their experience, devoting no less than 10% of the practicum experience to each of the core areas. The core areas are learned in a variety of settings at the Mount Sinai Medical Center and its affiliated institutions. Required and recommended rotations include:

➤ Seminar in Applied Preventive Medicine (required) (APM)
➤ The Division of Environmental and Occupational Medicine (required)
➤ The Education Unit
➤ Journal Club for Health Professionals
➤ American Cancer Institute Society
➤ New York City Department of Health and Mental Hygiene
➤ HIP – A managed care organisation in the New York area; a practicum site for activities in health and administration
➤ Health Bridge Program
➤ The East Harlem Community Health Committee
➤ The Asthma Working Group, Inc.

Within the Department of Community and Preventive Medicine (DCPM) at the MSSM, activities are available in several of the divisions and units. In addition, residents are required to perform no less than 10% of their practicum activities at a community-based organisation and to develop a community project. Furthermore, the rotation at the New York City Department of Health and Mental Hygiene serves as the residents' required practicum for the Mount Sinai Master of Public Health Program.

Table 15.1 gives an outline of required and optional conferences and seminars which residents attend.

Practicum experience

Practicum activities are varied and reflect individual residents' clinical experiences and fields of interest. Not only are the faculty in the Department of Community and Preventive Medicine available as preceptors, but the Departments of Pediatrics, Internal Medicine, Health Policy, Surgery, Geriatrics, Pathology and Psychiatry have also mentored preventive medicine residents. Special relationships have been developed with the AIDS Center/AIDS Scholars Program, the Adolescent Health Center, the Mount Sinai School Health Program, The Diabetes Center of Excellence, Narcotic Rehabilitation Center, community-based organisations and the East Harlem Community Health Committee, among others. The practicum placement is designed collaboratively

TABLE 15.1 Conferences and seminars for general preventive medicine residents

Required	Optional
• Applied Preventive Medicine; weekly • Journal Club; biweekly • Health Policy Grand Rounds; biweekly • Careers in Preventive Medicine Seminars • Environmental Journal Club; monthly • Community Medicine Grand Rounds; monthly • Citywide GPM Journal Club; three per year • Domestic Violence lectures; annually • New York State Dept. of Health Conference; annually • Master's Thesis Presentations; annually	• Occupational Clinic lectures; weekly • AIDS Institute, New York State Dept. of Health; weekly • Clinical Grand Rounds; weekly • Geriatrics/Health Policy Grand Rounds; weekly • Women's Faculty Group; biweekly • Schwartz Ethics Rounds • Medical Education Grand Rounds; biweekly • Biometry; monthly • Asthma Working Group; monthly • East Harlem Community Health Committee; monthly • Ethics Grand Rounds; monthly • New York Academy of Medicine Conferences; monthly • Complementary Alternative Medicine Conferences at Columbia • Children's Environmental Health Conferences; quarterly

with the director of the program, field practicum mentors and General Preventative Medicine (GPM) residents.

A brief overview of selected practicum rotations and their activities, including goals and objectives for required rotations are provided below to showcase the breadth of teaching and learning opportunities at the postgraduate level in health promotion by practising preventive medicine.

Selected examples of required and recommended rotations

SEMINAR IN APM (REQUIRED)

APM holds a two-hour weekly conference; attendance is required for residents. The Resident Chair chooses a preventive medicine theme each month, and organises guest speakers or residents to give presentations. The Resident Chair rotates on a monthly basis. It offers residents the opportunity to participate in the development, implementation and evaluation of new models of health services delivery in community-based settings, including the development of consortia among healthcare institutions and planning for interinstitutional shared patient data cases. Residents collect information from health departments and other public sources for the purpose of providing geographic and epidemiologic analyses of disease prevalence in the local catchment area of Mount Sinai (East Harlem) and at state, national and international levels. Themes in past years have included nutrition/obesity, bioterrorism, public health law, international health, mental health and integrative medicine.

The goals and objectives of the APM seminars are shown in Table 15.2.

TABLE 15.2 Goals and objectives of mandatory APM seminars for GPM residents

Goals	Objectives
• Communicate to target groups and to the media in a clear and effective manner, both orally and in writing, the levels of risk from potential hazards and the rationale for selected interventions	• The resident will chair the seminar at least two months of the year
• Communicate to health professionals in a clear and effective manner, both orally and in writing, the findings and the rationale for selected interventions	• The resident will design a theme for the month such as maternal child health, public health law, etc.
• Prepare and critique a proposal for program resources	• The resident will review and synthesise literature pertinent to the topic from MMWR, NYCDOH, relevant journals etc.
• Order priorities for major projects and/or programs according to definable criteria	• The resident will present the topic to fellow residents, faculty and students attending the seminar utilising PowerPoint and other computer modalities
• Use computers for specific applications relevant to preventive medicine	• The resident will arrange for guest speakers expert in the chosen topic
• Interpret legal and regulatory authority relating to protection and promotion of the public's health	• The resident will perform an academic exercise in which he/she picks a health problem pertinent to East Harlem using DOH statistics to evaluate the epidemiology of the problem and design a potential program for the solution
• Identify ethical, social and cultural issues relating to policies, risks, research and interventions in public health and preventive medicine contexts	• The resident will create a community health project to improve a health issue
• Identify the processes by which decisions are made within an organisation or agency and their points of influence	
• Identify and coordinate the integrated use of necessary and sufficient resources to improve the community's health	
• Design and conduct an epidemiologic study	
• Design and operate a surveillance system	
• Select and describe limitations of appropriate statistical analysis as applied to a particular data set	
• Translate epidemiologic findings into a recommendation for a specific intervention to control a public health problem	

THE DIVISION OF ENVIRONMENTAL AND OCCUPATIONAL MEDICINE (REQUIRED)

GPM residents complete a minimum one-month required rotation with the Division of Environmental and Occupational Medicine. Practicum experience includes clinical occupational medicine at the Irving B. Selikoff Occupational Medicine Clinic, with emphasis on taking an occupational history with management of a wide variety of occupational illnesses. Residents are involved in weekly case presentations, quarterly Children's Environmental Center Conferences, radiology conferences, environmental journal clubs, workmen's compensation surveys and educational outreach and screenings for union workers.

The goals and objectives of this rotation are shown in Table 15.3.

TABLE 15.3 Goals and objectives of GPM residents' rotation at the Division of Environmental and Occupational Medicine

Goals	Objectives
• Assess individual risk for occupational/ environmental disorders using an environmental and occupational history • Identify potential occupational and environmental hazards in defined populations, and assess and respond to identifiable risks	• The resident will perform clinical evaluations of patients in the occupational medicine clinic and the World Trade Center clinic and learn how to manage occupational injury and exposures • The resident will receive the legal, ethical and societal impact of occupational disease through didactics during the rotation

NEW YORK CITY DEPARTMENT OF HEALTH AND MENTAL HYGIENE (REQUIRED)

Mount Sinai GPM residents are required to do a one-month public health practice rotation at the NYC Department of Health and Mental Health (NYCDOHMH). The NYCDOHMH arranges a schedule that includes exposure to most health department activities, including programmes, clinics, home visits, restaurant inspections and laboratory activities. Opportunities exist to do more extensive projects in outbreak investigations, tuberculosis control, surveillance activities and other public health activities.

The goals and objectives of this rotation are shown in Table 15.4.

HEALTH BRIDGE

This is a funded program through the DCPM, which provides medical care to pregnant women living in single-occupancy hotels in New York City. These women are HIV-positive or at-risk for infection and have histories that include substance abuse, child abuse, domestic violence, prostitution and poverty. Home visits are made twice weekly and there is a coordinating support group meeting at Mount Sinai weekly. Residents accompany a department faculty member at least once and participate in the weekly Helping After Neonatal Death (HAND) support group meetings.

TABLE 15.4 Goals and objectives of GPM residents' rotation with the New York City Department of Health and Mental Health

Goals	Objectives
<ul><li>Monitor health status and identify community health problems</li><li>Diagnose and investigate health problems and health hazards in the community</li><li>Inform and educate populations about health issues</li><li>Mobilise community partnerships to identify and solve health problems</li><li>Develop policies and plans to support individual and community health efforts</li><li>Enforce laws and regulations that protect health and ensure safety</li><li>Ensure a competent public health and personal healthcare workforce</li><li>Evaluate the effectiveness, accessibility and quality of personal and population-based health services</li></ul>	<ul><li>The resident will choose a bureau of the department of health where he/she will participate in ongoing community projects and research</li><li>The resident will conceive and implement a sustainable project such as patient education, physician education and data analysis or policy protocol</li><li>The resident will participate in restaurant inspections</li><li>The resident will participate in lead abatement</li><li>The resident will participate in an infectious disease conference</li><li>The resident will participate in a pertinent DOH meeting</li><li>The resident will participate in grand rounds</li><li>The resident will have the opportunity to participate in an outbreak investigation</li></ul>

The goals and objectives for residents in this rotation are to:
➤ identify ethical, social and cultural issues relating to policies, risks, research and interventions in public health and preventive medicine contexts
➤ identify and coordinate the integrated use of necessary and sufficient resources to improve the community's health
➤ monitor health status to identify health problems
➤ link people to needed personal health services and ensuring provisions of healthcare when otherwise unavailable
➤ evaluate the effectiveness, accessibility and quality of personal and population-based health services
➤ acquire an understanding of primary, secondary and tertiary preventive approaches to individual and population-based disease prevention and health promotion
➤ develop, implement and evaluate the effectiveness of appropriate clinical preventive services for both individuals and populations.

THE EAST HARLEM COMMUNITY HEALTH COMMITTEE

This is a consortium of health providers, community-based organisations, Department of Health, School Health, political and spiritual leaders, consumers and anybody interested in the health of the East Harlem population. The committee has been meeting for over 25 years. The paediatric/child health subcommittee and the Diabetes Center for Excellence are among the most dynamic, as are the substance abuse and the health policy subcommittees. Many faculty members in the Departments of Community Medicine and Health Policy at Mount Sinai serve on the board, are chairs of subcommittees, or are active members. Residents attend monthly meetings and report on the progress of their East Harlem projects. There is a longstanding history of collaborative relationships to study immunisations, paediatric asthma, referral networks, substance abuse services, diabetes and congestive heart disease.

The goals and objectives for residents in this rotation are to:
➤ monitor health status and identify community health problems
➤ diagnose and investigate health problem and health hazards in the community
➤ inform and educate populations about health issues
➤ mobilise community partnerships to identify and solve health problems
➤ develop policies and plans to support individual and community health efforts
➤ evaluate the effectiveness, accessibility and quality of personal and population-based health services.

THE ASTHMA WORKING GROUP, INC.
This is a consortium of health providers, community-based organisations, Department of Health, School Health, political and spiritual leaders, consumers and anybody interested in the prevention of asthma in East Harlem. An outgrowth of the East Harlem Community Health paediatrics subcommittee, the group has been meeting monthly since 1996.

The goals and objectives for residents in this rotation are the same as those for the East Harlem Community Health Committee rotation above, but in this context specifically targeting the disease of asthma.

Assessment of residents

At the beginning of the programme the programme director and resident complete a GPM competency-based planning chart (*see* Table 15.5) as part of the incoming assessment. At the end of each practicum activity, or at six-month intervals (*see* Table 15.6), whichever comes first, each resident is assessed by his or her preceptors. The programme director is provided with a copy of the written evaluation by the supervisor or preceptor for review and inclusion in the resident's file. The programme director meets individually with each resident twice a year, at 6 months, 12, 18 and 24 months, or more if needed, to review the resident's practicum and academic performance. At these times, a written evaluation of each resident's progress will be included in his or her file. At the conclusion of 12 and 24 months the programme director reviews each resident's achievement of the GPM competencies. If the performance has not been satisfactory, goals and a timetable for improvement in performance and reevaluation will be established and provided to the resident in writing. An exit interview is conducted with all residents and a written assessment placed in his or her chart. In-service exams are required in each year of the programme and are offered in August by the American College of Preventive Medicine.

Programme evaluation

At MSSM, programme evaluation is based on the GPM resident, the learning activities and the learning environment and is an ongoing process that is discussed in a transparent and professional manner by residents and faculty. One example is at the conclusion of each practicum activity, or at six-month intervals, each resident evaluates their practicum activity on its strengths, weaknesses and the quality of the faculty guidance.

Another example is the annual meeting of GPM residents for the purpose of evaluating the programme. Together they complete a confidential programme evaluation form, which includes questions on the academic curriculum, clinical experience, research opportunities, practicum activities, the programme director's leadership and overall atmosphere in the Department of Community and Preventive Medicine.

Upon completion of the residency program, each resident may submit a written evaluation of the entire programme to the residency director. Such comments by the residents will be reviewed by the programme director, kept on file, and responded to in writing. A meeting with the programme director may be requested by any of the residents at any time to express opinions regarding the quality and appropriateness of any component of the programme.

At a faculty level, the evaluations of the programme and recommendations for improvement are discussed at regularly scheduled teaching committee meetings, GPM steering committee meetings or may be submitted by faculty members at any time. The programme director will review the evaluations, keep them on file, and respond in writing to the faculty member. The programme director will provide the chair of the residency advisory committee with copies of all evaluation materials at least once a year.

TABLE 15.5 Competency-based planning chart

Competency	Goals		Objectives (resident plans for achieving this competency) (What activity? When?)
Generic preventive medicine competencies			
1 Communicate to target groups and to the media in a clear and effective manner, both orally and in writing, the levels of risk from potential hazards and the rationale for selected intervention	a	Participate in writing a press release	
	b	Participate in writing material intended for release to the general public or to a specific audience	
	c	Attend seminar on public affairs	
	d	Handle a press call on an issue you have been involved with	
2 Communicate to health professional in a clear and effective manner, both orally and in writing, the findings and the rationale for selected interventions	a	Present at Journal Club	
	b	Present at Masters course	
	c	Present at Health Services Research & Development Meeting	
	d	Present at conference	
3 Prepare and critique a proposal for programme resources	a	Assist with development of a programme proposal or grant application	
	b	Assist in evaluation of requests for funding, e.g. responses to a request for proposal (RFP)	
4 Order priorities for major projects and/or programmes according to definable criteria	a	Develop a community needs assessment	
	b	Develop goals and objectives for specific project	
5 Use computers for specific applications relevant to preventive medicine	a	Participate in analyzing data set	
	b	Design data set for Master's thesis	
6 Interpret legal and regulatory authority relating to protection and promotion of the public's health	a	Attend meetings on development of Immunisation Registry	

(continued)

TABLE 15.5 *(cont.)*

Competency	Goals	Objectives (resident plans for achieving this competency) (What activity? When?)
7 Identify ethical, social, and cultural issues relating to policies, risks, research, and interventions in public health and preventive medicine contexts	a Work on a plan or program targeting specific social groups for public health b Present a research proposal to the Institutional Review Board (IRB), or attend a meeting of the IRB as an observer	
8 Identify the processes by which decisions are made within an organisation or agency and their points of influence	a Attend staff and planning meetings in at least one practicum site b Attend staff meetings at as many levels as possible in the organisational structure, and compare content and type of discussions	
9 Identify and coordinate the integrated use of necessary and sufficient resources to improve the community's health	a Attend East Harlem Community Health Committee Meetings and one of the subcommittees b Attend Asthma Working Group meetings	
Epidemiology and biostatistics competencies		
1 Design and conduct an epidemiologic study	a Work on an epi study, leading to a report, abstract, or thesis	
2 Design and operate a surveillance system	a Participate in the evaluation and/or modification of an existing surveillance system b Participate in designing a new surveillance system	
3 Select and describe limitations of appropriate statistical analysis as applied to a particular data set	a Select appropriate statistical methods for analysing a data set you are working with, and explain why you chose those methods b Discuss limitations of a published study in a written or oral presentation	

Competency	Goals	Objectives (resident plans for achieving this competency) (What activity? When?)
4 Translate epidemiologic findings into a recommendation for a specific intervention to control a public health problem	a Include a discussion section in the written report, abstract, or publication above	
Management and administration planning		
1 Formulate policy for a given health issue		
2 Develop goals and objectives for a given health issue		
3 Design an implementation plan to address goals and objectives		
4 Conduct an evaluation and/or quality assessment based on measurable criteria (process and outcome)		
5 Manage the operation of a program or project, including human and fiscal resources		
Clinical preventive medicine competencies		
1 Develop and refine screening programs for groups to identify risks for disease or injury, and opportunities to promote wellness	a Identify a problem that warrants widespread screening Explain why, what the target group should be, and how the screening should be carried out b Critique an existing or proposed screening programme. Does it meet the criteria for a worthwhile screening programme? Was the target group chosen appropriately? Is it cost-effective?	

(continued)

TABLE 15.5 *(cont.)*

Competency	Goals	Objectives (resident plans for achieving this competency) (What activity? When?)
2 Implement screening programs for groups and individuals	a Learn about screening programmes sponsored by the health department, and observe one in action at the community level b Participate in implementation of a screening programme	
3 Implement individual and community-based interventions to modify or eliminate identified risks for disease or injury and to promote wellness	a Select appropriate statistical methods for analysing a data set you are working with, and explain why you chose those methods b Discuss limitations of a published study in a written or oral presentation	
4 Diagnosis and management of diseases/injuries/conditions of significance within general preventive medicine and public health	a Occupational medicine clinic b City health department clinic – STD, TB, prenatal c Primary care to high-risk populations	
Occupational and environmental health competencies		
1 Assess individual risk for occupational/environmental disorders using an environmental and occupational history	a Respond to public inquiries related to environmental or occupational risks b Participate in clinical activities at the Occupational Medicine clinic	
2 Identify potential occupational and environmental hazards in defined populations, and assess and respond to identified risks	a Assist with an environmental investigation at the city health department, e.g. lead poisoning investigation, restaurant or summer camp inspection	

TABLE 15.6 Competency assessment

Competency	Activity	Level Key: I: Independent P: Participated O: Observed	Date	Initials
Generic preventive medicine competencies				
1 Communicate to target groups and to the media in a clear and effective manner, both orally and in writing, the levels of risk from potential hazards and the rationale for selected interventions		I P O		
2 Communicate to health professional in a clear and effective manner, both orally and in writing, the findings and the rationale for selected interventions		I P O		
3 Prepare and critique a proposal for programme resources		I P O		
4 Order priorities for major projects and/or programmes according to definable criteria		I P O		
5 Use computers for specific applications relevant to preventive medicine		I P O		
6 Interpret legal and regulatory authority relating to protection and promotion of the public's health		I P O		
7 Identify ethical, social and cultural issues relating to policies, risks, research and interventions in public health and preventive medicine context		I P O		
8 Identify the processes by which decisions are made within an organisation or agency and their points of influence		I P O		
9 Identify and coordinate the integrated use of necessary and sufficient resources to improve the community's health		I P O		
Epidemiology and biostatistics competencies				
1 Design and conduct an epidemiologic study		I P O		
2 Design and operate a surveillance system		I P O		

(continued)

TABLE 15.6 (cont.)

Competency	Activity	Level Key: I: Independent P: Participated O: Observed	Date	Initials
3 Select and describe limitations of appropriate statistical analyses as applied to a particular data set		I P O		
4 Translate epidemiologic findings into a recommendation for a specific intervention to control a public health problem		I P O		
5 Design and/or conduct an outbreak/cluster investigation		I P O		
Management and administration planning				
1 Formulate policy for a given health issue		I P O		
2 Develop goals and objectives for a given health issue		I P O		
3 Design an implementation plan to address goals and objectives		I P O		
4 Conduct an evaluation and/or quality assessment based on measurable criteria (process and outcome)		I P O		
5 Manage the operation of a programme or project, including human and fiscal resources		I P O		
Clinical preventive medicine competencies				
1 Develop, implemented and refine screening programmes for groups to identify risks for disease or injury and opportunities to promote wellness		I P O		
2 Design and implement clinical preventive services for groups and individuals		I P O		
3 Implement individual and community-based interventions to modify or eliminate identified risks for disease or injury and to promote wellness		I P O		
4 Diagnose and manage diseases/injuries/conditions of significance within general preventive medicine and public health		I P O		

Competency	Activity	Level Key: I: Independent P: Participated O: Observed	Date	Initials
Occupational and environmental health competencies				
1 Assess individual risk for occupational/environmental disorders using an environmental and occupational history		I P O		
2 Identify potential occupational and environmental hazards in defined population, and assess and respond to identified risks		I P O		

EXAMPLE 3: THE BACHELOR DEGREE IN MEDICINE, MONASH UNIVERSITY, AUSTRALIA

Craig Hassed

The Monash health promotion project which is embedded within the student's community placements and the health enhancement program component of personal and professional development were outlined in Chapter 7. In this section some of the tutorial activities will be described. These are aimed at providing the students with generic knowledge and skills which they can reinforce by applying them to their particular HP projects.

The tutorials take place in average group sizes of 17 students per group. These groups will constitute anywhere from five to eight HP projects, with the tutor also acting as the students' project supervisor (academic advisor).

Outlined below are four of the five tutorial plans for first semester, which are aimed at supporting the students' project work. There are a total of five two-hour HP tutorials in each semester. The fifth tutorial in first semester is focused on international health topics and was designed in conjunction with 'Ignite', which is the medical student organisation promoting international health.

Tutorial 1: Health promotion principles and practice
Context and background
To this point there has been delivered a HP lecture series covering basic HP principles and affirming the aim that HP is a process that enables individuals or communities to have increased control over and to improve their health, and to provide individuals and communities with the knowledge, expertise and skills to attain a state of complete physical, mental and social well-being. HP can be seen to be taking place in a number of different settings (one-on-one practitioner-patient interactions; with specific target groups; community-wide interventions) and is based on different conceptual models which correspond with those settings:

➤ biomedical
➤ behavioural
➤ socio-environmental.

There have also been lectures covering some basic research methods (including study design and data types) and research ethics.

This tutorial links with health promotion project work but more broadly to research, ethics, health psychology and population health. It is important that at the outset of undertaking the HP project work that students have a good grasp of the relevance and context within which this activity sits.

Session plan example
At first the tutor will get to know their students as they will be seeing a lot of each other throughout the year. Then the tutorial is split into three parts.

1 See that the students are clear about:
   a the course requirements for the year, in particular their project work
   b what they hope to achieve from Health Promotion and Knowledge Management (HPKM)
   c look over the project proposal template and discuss with them what is needed in

each section of this document. This will be their first assessed task for the year, and while many groups will not have settled on a project topic as yet, go through the form and explain what sorts of information should be included in each section of it.

   d ask the students to consider their teamwork strategy and goals.

2 Next the students consider the various ways that doctors can promote health; as practitioners, researchers, advocates, policy makers, administrators etc.

3 A 'quiz' session is drawn from previous OSCE and written exams.

PART 1: COURSE REQUIREMENTS AND TEAMWORK

Students have an initial project proposal due by the end of first semester (see handbook for details). This is to be submitted on a HP modified Standing Commitee of Ethics Research for Humans (SCERH) form, not because these will be submitted as research projects, but because we want them to understand the ethical issues involved in what they are doing. The requirements are laid out in detail in the CBP handbook.

Some groups may not have any idea yet of what they want to do in their project although they may well have already had discussions with their community placements about potential projects. For those groups who do have an idea of what topic they want to cover, we want them to start planning their projects early rather than late.

Goals for HPKM and group work

In previous years, working within the group has posed the most problems for students during their studies for HPKM. As such, this year we want all groups to produce for themselves a one-page document outlining a set of combined goals and objectives, and a written guide of what they are expected to put in, in terms of time, commitment and work ethic. This document should also include a written description on how the group plans to resolve any conflicts that may arise throughout the year. This document will then be signed off on by all the group members and the tutor and will be used if necessary during the year. It is basically a 'contract' between the students to ensure that everyone is aware of what is expected of them right from the start. As a starting point:

a Get them to write goals/objectives for themselves individually – what they hope to achieve throughout the year. A good tool for developing sound objectives is to ensure they are **SMART**:
    i Specific
    ii Measurable
    iii Attainable
    iv Realistic
    v Timely

b Then ask them to discuss these with their other group members and come up with a list of goals and objectives that they will attempt to achieve through HPKM (these should be acceptable to all group members and must be achievable).

c What is expected in terms of time and commitment to the project?

d What expectations do group members have for the marks they wish to achieve?

e What will be the process for dispute resolution? (e.g. majority vote, group leader decides, tutor decision, 'flip of a coin' . . .).

Students will then be required to sign that document, and provide a copy to the tutor at the next tutorial.

PART 2: HEALTH PROMOTION: WHAT DOES THIS MEAN FOR DOCTORS?[47,48]

1 The students then explore the key concepts of:
   a ADVOCACY: means representing the interests of disadvantaged groups and may mean speaking on their behalf or lobbying to influence change (e.g. policy)
   b ENABLEMENT: allowing people to achieve their full health potential by increasing knowledge, understanding and individual health/coping strategies
   c MEDIATION: Liaising, coordinating and cooperating with many health agencies or sections, to provide or gain evidence or advice.
2 Students are asked to provide examples of how they could implement these three ideas into their future work.
3 The three steps to carrying out the process of health promotion are DEVELOPMENT (planning); IMPLEMENTATION (intervention), and EVALUATION. Students explore why it is important that these are not done in isolation, but rather that all three are completed for each project.

Quiz: students participate in a quiz on health promotion content delivered so far in lectures and tutorials.

Facilitators

Facilitators are tutors are drawn from the medical faculty teaching staff. They need to have the following experience and qualifications:
1 experience in health promotion
2 experience with small group teaching
3 experience with project supervision
4 a research background
5 personal commitment and enthusiasm.

Support resource

The Victorian Department of Health's publication: *Planning for Effective Health Promotion Evaluation* (*see* www.health.vic.gov.au/healthpromotion/downloads/planning_may05.pdf).

Tutorial 2: Health promotion projects in community settings

Max de Courten

Context and background

Community action aims to encourage and empower communities to build their capacity to develop and sustain improvements of their social and physical environments that are conducive to improved health outcomes.[49] A discussion on the use of appropriate evaluation frameworks to assess community-based health promotion projects to document the process, and impact and outcomes will take place.

Although most medical practitioners will find themselves working as medical practitioners within general practices and hospitals, it is an important objective of health promotion teaching for students to realise that health promotion takes place largely within community settings.

Typically, community-based initiatives involve multicomponent interventions that are implemented with diverse target groups across a range of community settings. Assessing the process of programme implementation is critical in order to capture and document the realities of programme planning and implementation.

Comprehensive evaluation approaches adopted for such projects should be based on a model which gives equal emphasis to process and outcome evaluation and seeks to relate the realities of programme implementation to intended programme outcomes. Process evaluation is used to monitor and document programme implementation and can aid in understanding the relationship between specific programme elements and programme outcomes.

Suggested elements for process evaluation plans include fidelity, dose (delivered and received), reach, recruitment and context.

Key words/phrases: multicomponent interventions, logic model research paradigm, community definition, process evaluation plan.

Session plan example

PART 1: HEALTH PROMOTION IN COMMUNITIES

Aims and objectives

1   Understand the different components of a community definition in the health promotion (HP) context.
2   Understand the application of different evaluation components to assess community-based interventions.

Making a case for communities

The Global Consortium on Community Health Promotion created in 2003 as a collaborative initiative of the US Centers for Disease Control and Prevention (CDC) and the International Union for Health Promotion and Education (IUHPE) defines community health promotion as a participatory empowering equity-focused process – one that regards community participation as being essential to every stage of health-promoting actions as well as one that leverages community assets and knowledge to create the necessary conditions for health.

However, not all health-promoting policies and actions conform to this definition. Lessons learnt from the evaluation of Healthy Municipalities, Cities and Communities initiatives in the Americas relate their modest impact to the fact that most of these initiatives had not appropriately taken into account what are now recognised as key health promotion principles, such as intersectoral collaboration and community participation.

A recent article by Baum[50] illustrates the implications of not doing so by referring to health-promoting policies and actions in Australia: demonstrating a significant impact at the population level across a range of health outcomes, but having remained unsuccessful in addressing inequities and reducing the existing gradients. Such experiences underscore the need to design health promotion policies and actions with a strong equity lens, and it is here that the need to combine top-down political commitment and policy action with bottom-up action from communities and civil society groups assumes importance.

Understanding the role of the communities is therefore critical to health promotion. The role of the community in health intervention projects can be seen as fourfold:
➤ setting for interventions
➤ target of change
➤ agent with developmental capacity
➤ resource with a high degree of ownership and participation.

These categories are proposed to (a) define better the aim of community action; and (b) illustrate the difficulties in summarising results across the array of community-based projects.

The *characteristics of community-based health promotion programmes* can be described as being integrated and comprehensive programmes, not limited to health-care settings, using multiple interventions, targeting change among individuals, groups and organisations, while incorporating strategies to create policy and environmental changes.

In health promotion, *community action* is the participation of community members and groups in advocacy and action for social and environmental change. It aims to encourage and empower communities (both geographical areas and communities of interest) to build their capacity to develop and sustain improvements in their social and physical environments that are conducive to improved health outcomes.

Examples would be community-led advocacy and programmes to improve safety in certain neighbourhoods; employee groups acting to improve work conditions in their workplace etc.

The *concept of empowerment* has been championed by the 'new health promotion movement' that emerged in the early 1980s and focused on achieving equity in health and increased public participation in health programme decision making and culminated in the WHO's Ottawa Charter in 1986.[8]

In effect, two seemingly different health promotion approaches have evolved and coexist. The conventional approach focuses on lifestyle management or, in the case of infectious disease, vector control to prevent diseases. The more 'radical' approach emphasises social justice through community empowerment and advocacy. Each approach has different and distinct characteristics which make them somewhat exclusive, at least in theory or as 'classic types', and often problematic in practice for health promoters (*see* Table 15.7).

Such top-down programmes follow a predetermined cycle. Cycle stages and terminology may differ between agencies but generally consist of the following elements: overall design, objective setting, strategy selection, strategy implementation and management and programme evaluation. Examples of top-down health promotion programmes include the North Karelia Project on cardiovascular disease in Finland, the US Multiple Risk Factors Intervention Trial (MRFIT), the US Community Intervention Trials for Smoking Cessation (COMMIT) and numerous other chronic disease prevention programmes.

In bottom-up programming, the outside agents act to support the community in the identification of issues that are important and relevant to their lives, and enable them to develop strategies to resolve these issues. The programme design and management is negotiated with the community and there is, or should be, a much longer time frame. Much of the work in this area remains anecdotal or unpublished, and includes community development initiatives ranging from anti-poverty or housing development projects, to community gardens and policy advocacy support.

Health promoters have conventionally viewed community empowerment and the resulting strengthened community capacity as the key feature of the bottom-up approach. The tension they experience in practice is how they might include the concerns and issues of the community in a top-down implementation approach that usually characterises their own job descriptions or funding mechanisms. The dichotomy between top-down disease prevention/lifestyle change and bottom-up community

TABLE 15.7 Key differences between top-down and bottom-up approaches (based on Laverack and Labonte)[51]

Feature	Top-down approach	Bottom-up approach
Underlying concept	Individual responsibility	Empowerment
Approach	Weakness, deficit	Strength, capacity
Operational focus	Solve problem	Improve competence
Definition of problem	By outside agent such as government body	By community
Primary vehicles for health promotion and change	Education, improved services, lifestyle	Building community control, resources and capacities toward economic, social and political change
Role of outside agents	Service delivery and resource allocation	Respond to needs of community
Primary decision makers	Agency representatives, business leaders, 'appointed community leaders'	Community forum, indigenous appointed leaders
Community control of resources	Low	High
Community ownership	Low	High
Evaluation	Specific risk factors Quantifiable outcomes and 'targets'	Pluralistic methods documenting changes of importance to the community

empowerment approaches is not as fixed as it is described here. Many health promoters, in their community work, shift between the options of marketing and managing lifestyle programmes, and efforts to organise and support community efforts to change more systemic health risks in their physical and social environments.

PART 2: EVALUATING COMMUNITY PROGRAMMES

Debates about appropriate methodology for the evaluation of community health projects point to the fact that the evaluation of complex community initiatives presents as much of a challenge as their actual design and implementation. There is a general consensus that traditional experimental approaches may not be appropriate for the evaluation of community health promotion initiatives. The need for more flexible approaches to evaluation and a greater emphasis on evaluating the process of implementation have also been highlighted.

The complexity of multifaceted community programmes presents a particular challenge in programme evaluation, both in terms of the methodologies applied and the role of the evaluator. Brown identifies the following as particular challenges for evaluators of comprehensive community initiatives: broad multiple goals dependent on an ongoing process of synergistic change programmes that are purposively flexible and responsive to local needs and conditions; the centrality of principles of community empowerment, participation and ownership; longer-term community change requires longer time frames than more narrowly defined approaches; and initiatives produce impacts at different levels in different spheres.[52]

At a more general level, and in the spirit of a community approach, evaluators must work with practitioners and the community when adapting their designs and evaluation techniques to fit the local context and needs. This calls for a move away from traditional evaluation approaches to one characterised by partnership with key players. Community programmes must take account of the needs of different stakeholders such as the local community, funders, workers and health professionals and use an evaluation design that can respond to their differing goals. The evaluation also needs to address and capture the individuality of the specific community contexts. Dynamic community programmes require a continual flow of information from formative and process evaluation in order to fine-tune programme interventions and to respond to changing circumstances. Evaluation is, therefore, less of a discrete activity and becomes more of an integral part of the project's core activities, and outcomes need to reflect the goals of a broad range of stakeholders.

Community empowerment can be a long and slow process, and is one that, almost by definition, never fully ends. Particular outcomes in the community empowerment process may not occur until many years after the time frame of the programme implementation has been finished. Thus, evaluation of community empowerment within the limited time frame of a programme more appropriately assesses changes in the process rather than particular outcomes. In effect, the process becomes the outcome.

To evaluate the process of community empowerment, health promoters need then to question, and answer, how programmes are implemented, looking for outcomes such as:
➤ improves stakeholder participation
➤ increases problem assessment capacities
➤ develops local leadership
➤ builds empowering organisational structures
➤ improves resource mobilisation
➤ strengthens stakeholder ability to 'ask why'
➤ increases stakeholder control over programme management
➤ creates an equitable relationship with outside agents.

Evaluations of community health promotion can thus underestimate the gains that an intervention might make in a community if the outcomes reported are limited to aggregates of changes in health behaviour or attitude made at an individual level. Even those evaluations that report policy changes or descriptive forms of evaluations detailing how communities became involved often fail to capture the improvements a community intervention can make on the problem-solving capacities of a community and its competence in tackling the issues which face it. The essence of what some interventions achieve can, therefore, be missed.

Tutorial 3: Project proposal submissions
Context and background
This tutorial is aimed at students being able to successfully submit their health promotion project proposals. It aims at providing an understanding of generic principles of the health promotion cycle – development, implementation and evaluation – and the ability to apply those principles to their particular project ideas.

The facilitator will require a knowledge of health promotion, research ethics and methodology.

Session plan example

AIMS AND OBJECTIVES

The purpose of this part of the tutorial is to have students thinking about how one health issue/topic could be approached in many different ways, and how each of those methods will have advantages, disadvantages and ethical constraints. It is a vital part of the support required by the students in order for them to complete their project work.

PART 1: PROJECT DESIGN AND METHODOLOGY

Four different scenarios related to different health promotion or prevention projects are provided. To ensure relevance, these scenarios are drawn from current research activity in Victoria.[53,54]

1 Divide the students into four groups with each to consider one of the scenarios. At the end of having discussed their scenarios each group will be asked to report back on their responses to the following questions to the other students in the class.
2 Discuss the following issues:
   a what *phase of the health promotion cycle* (development, implementation or evaluation) this project relates to and why
   b encourage debate and discussion about how they might go about actually doing this project. Use your own knowledge of epidemiology and methods to point out problems or good ideas when they are circulated. We want them to think about the *study type* (design – randomised controlled trial (RCT), cohort, clinical trial, etc.) – they have not had a lot of training in this, so may not know the names, but just see if you can tease out how they would do it; *methodology* (quantitative or qualitative, interviews or questionnaires, and so on); *time frame* required, *resources* that might be required; the *sample* (who they are going to be and where they are being sourced from)
   c what *ethical issues* might be involved in doing the project and how might they be overcome?

There are no specific right or wrong answers for the questions for each scenario. Students are asked to use their knowledge of what might work and what wouldn't and the tutor is asked to facilitate this discussion.

Scenario 1

A longitudinal study that extends on a previous VicHealth-funded epidemiological study into the identification, prevention and treatment of osteoporosis. It will provide comprehensive data across the entire adult female age range and relate bone density and size to fracture risk in the Australian population.

Scenario 2

Available evidence suggests that if infants fail to acquire sufficient iron during pregnancy, they may have a long-term developmental disadvantage. This study will assess the hypothesis that maternal iron supplementation during pregnancy improves developmental outcome of the offspring.*

Scenario 3

This study aims to determine the extent to which attendance at a smoke-free compared with a smoking-permitted nightclub might reduce cigarette consumption by young people.†

Scenario 4

In 1999 the Active Script Program (ASP) was established to increase the number of Victorian GPs who deliver physical activity advice to their patients in a consistent, appropriate and effective manner. To maximise GP participation, a programme was developed to (a) train and support the GPs in advising sedentary patients, and (b) to develop tools and resources to assist GPs. In 2002, it was decided that the success and cost-effectiveness of this programme need to be assessed.‡

PART 2: MODIFIED ETHICS (PROJECT PROPOSAL) FORM

In the second half of the tutorial the tutor spends time going over the project proposal submission form with project groups. These are modified 'low impact research' forms from the website of the Monash University Standing Committee for Ethics and Research on Humans. Explanation of what is required in each section is provided and questions are dealt with. Groups may have a draft of their project proposal by this stage in which case tutors can look over relevant sections and provide feedback. If any issues arise within individual projects that are of general importance then they are brought to the whole group's attention.

Questions to be addressed include:

1 Who, if anyone, should they talk to about it?
   a identify key stakeholders (organisations, the target group, government, students, etc.)
2 What is the rationale for the project? Remember this is about 'selling' the programme.
   a Is this an important health issue/problem? Why?
   b What is the potential significance of their project?
3 How would you determine the rationale for the project?
   a Needs assessment – available data already or do you need to get that (e.g. are they in the development or implementation or evaluation stage)?
   b What would be the merits of their project (increased awareness/knowledge, attitude change, behaviour change, improvement in well-being/health, etc.)?
   c What other programmes of a similar type or in a similar setting have been conducted?

---

* The information provided to students with Scenarios 1 and 2 was adapted from various chapters of the text: Naidoo J, Wills J. *Health Promotion: foundations for practice.* 2nd ed. Sydney: Bailliere Tindall; 2000.

† For Scenario 3, students are also asked to look at the document: Round R, Marshall B, Horton K. *Planning for Effective Health Promotion Evaluation.* Melbourne: Victorian Government of Human Services; 2005.

‡ For Scenario 4, students are also asked to consider the article: Saunders RP, Evans MH, Joshi P. Developing a process-evaluation plan for assessing health promotion program implementation: a how-to guide. *Health Promot Pract.* 2005; 6(2): 134–47.

  d What would be the most important information for the key stakeholders and how could that best be obtained?

4 What are the aims of their project?

5 How feasible is your idea?

6 What resources would you need to carry it out?

7 Are those resources available to you? If not, how will you modify your project to be achievable with the available resources?

Tutorial 4: Literature appraisal and evaluation
Dragan Ilic

Context and background
Literature searching and appraisal is a generic skill required by the medical course, which is reinforced through the HP project work.

Session plan example
AIMS AND OBJECTIVES
After this session students should be able to:
➤ list information sources relevant to health professionals
➤ identify the benefits and limitations associated with information sources
➤ formulate an answerable question (using the 'patient problem, intervention, comparison, outcome' or PICO framework)
➤ construct a search strategy for MEDLINE/PubMed
➤ rationalise the benefits/limitations of studies using the evidence hierarchy.

SCENARIO
Students are introduced to the following scenario which forms the basis of the activities designed for this tutorial.

  Quit Victoria*recently released a report detailing the smoking habits of Victorian students (*see* Table 15.8). Whilst the rate of student smoking has decreased over time, the decrease in smoking cessation is not as significant for 16- to 17-year-old students when compared to the 12–15 years age group. Quit Victoria is considering developing a new smoking cessation health promotion initiative specifically targeting the 16–18 years age group of Victorian students.

PART 1: SOURCES OF INFORMATION
Part 1 aims to generate discussion about the various information sources that are relevant to health professionals and the benefits and limitations associated with information sources. Students are asked to complete the following two activities.

  Beginning with the developmental phase of the health promotion cycle, Quit Victoria would like to identify any previous literature that could be relevant in assisting the development of the new initiative.

---

* Quit Victoria is a joint initiative of the Cancer Council of Victoria, Department of Human Services, the National Heart Foundation and VicHealth. Quit Victoria is dedicated to eliminating the pain, illness and suffering caused by tobacco.

TABLE 15.8 Current smoking among Victorian school students (%) (1984–2002)

Age group	Year	1984	1987	1990	1993	1996	1999	2002
12–15 years	Male	22	15	15	16	18	16	12
	Female	22	17	20	20	20	17	13
	All	22	16	17	18	19	17	13
16–17 years	Male	30	29	23	32	29	30	26
	Female	34	34	31	33	37	33	30
	All	32	31	27	33	33	32	28

Source: Quit Victoria

Activity
List what sources of information could be used to inform a broad literature review on the topic.

Sources of information could include:
- Medical/healthcare databases
  - The Cochrane Library
  - MEDLINE/PubMed
  - AMED (Allied and Complementary Medicine)
  - CINAHL – Cumulative Index to Nursing and Allied Health Literature
  - PsycINFO
- Google
- Wikipedia
- Health professionals, policy makers, researchers, other stakeholders
- Textbooks
- Conference proceedings

Activity
Discuss the potential benefits and limitations of your chosen information sources. (Sample responses appear in Table 15.9.)

PART 2: SEARCHING THE LITERATURE
Part 2 is designed to provide the students with an opportunity to practise constructing an answerable question (using the PICO framework), which they could then use to assist with their search on the Cochrane Library or MEDLINE. Remind students that any question should be specific, and should contain the PICO mnemonic. As such, there will be more than one question that they may be able to construct. Stress to the students that 'alternative' terms are especially useful when searching databases.

As one of the community-based practice partners, Quit Victoria has identified that the developmental phase may be an ideal project for second-year MBBS students undertaking their HPKM unit. As such your group is required to undertake a comprehensive search of the literature using the Cochrane Library and MEDLINE.

TABLE 15.9 Potential benefits and limitations of various information sources

Information source	Benefits	Limitations
• Medical databases • Google • Wikipedia • Health professionals, policy makers etc. • Textbooks • Conference proceedings	• Index of peer-reviewed articles • Quick return of results • Personal opinion • Quick, general information • 'Latest' information, usually unpublished	• Accessibility (only PubMed is freely available) • Combination of 'good' and 'bad' quality information • Time-consuming (in terms of sorting potentially useful information) • Lack of peer review • Personal opinion (can be biased for/against) • Potentially out of date • Not necessarily peer-reviewed material • Difficult to access • Usually offers very specific information, sometimes not completed

Activity

Using the following table (Table 15.10), construct an answerable question to guide your search strategy.

TABLE 15.10 PICO framework for construction of answerable questions prior to literature search

PICO phase	Term(s)	Alternative term(s)
Patient	Adolescent Secondary school students Smokers?	Teenagers
Intervention	Education	Specific education interventions may include: • education (school, family, community) • mass media • peer support • self-help • internet (Students may also wish to consider other methods of delivery)
Comparison	No comparison *or* other behavioural interventions	
Outcome(s)	Smoking cessation	Decrease in smoking Behaviour change Psychosocial change Knowledge increase Uptake of smoking cessation interventions

Answerable question(s)

A few examples may include:

In teenage school children who smoke (P), are education interventions (I) more effective than behavioural interventions (C) in promoting smoking cessation (O)?

In adolescent school children (P), are mass media campaigns (I) effective in increasing the uptake of smoking cessation interventions (O)?

In secondary school children aged 16–18 (P), are peer-support smoking cessation campaigns (I) more effective than self-help interventions (C) in reducing smoking (O)?

Activity

List what filters you may use when conducting your search on MEDLINE. Discuss the level of their appropriateness for your search.

When conducting the hypothetical search, students could adopt the following limits (*see* Table 15.11) to filter their results to a manageable number. Highlight to the students that searches should always begin broad, with limits used to filter the results to a manageable list of returns.

TABLE 15.11 Appropriateness of various filters used to search on MEDLINE

Filter	Appropriateness
1 Age group/s	1 Relevant to adolescent population that we are interested in
2 Human	2 Obviously interested in studies that relate to smoking cessation in the human population
3 Publication year	3 May only be interested in studies from 1984 onwards (as detailed in our scenario)
4 Full-text	4 Full-text could be used so that students do not need to 'chase up' the articles. However, it should be noted that some articles may not be available via full-text, but will be available through the Monash University online library system. So students should be aware that using full-text may limit their search results unnecessarily

5 Publication types	5 Will link to the next activity (Part 3). Using this limit students can choose to identify:
	  a reviews (systematic and narrative)
	  b RCTs
	  c cohort studies etc.

PART 3: CHOOSING AN APPROPRIATE STUDY DESIGN

Part 3 is designed to provide the students with an opportunity to revisit their understanding of the levels of evidence and the benefits/limitations associated with different study types. It is essential that students understand what the strengths and weaknesses of different study types are when drawing upon such studies to inform their literature review.

The National Health and Medical Research Council (NHMRC) has defined an evidence hierarchy detailing the 'levels of evidence' of various study designs (*see* Table 15.12). You will need to identify the strength of the evidence on which you will base your literature review, which will in turn inform the development of the intervention.

Activity
List the levels of evidence relating to quantitative study designs.

TABLE 15.12 NHMRC hierarchies of study design and levels of evidence

Study design	Level of evidence
Systematic review of all relevant randomised controlled trials (RCT)	I
Properly designed RCT	II
Well-designed pseudo-randomised controlled trial (e.g. alternate allocation)	III-1
Comparative studies (or systematic reviews of such studies) with concurrent controls and allocation not randomised, cohort studies, case-control studies, or interrupted time series with a control group	III-2
Comparative studies with a historical control, two or more single arm studies or interrupted time series without a parallel control group	III-3
Case studies, post-test or pre-test/post-test, with no control group	IV

Source: National Health and Medical Research Council. *How to Use the Evidence: assessment and application of scientific evidence.* Canberra: AusInfo; 2000.

Activity
Ask students to complete the following table (Table 15.13) then lead a discussion on the benefits/strengths of the different study types.

Discuss the potential benefits and limitations associated with each design study as it relates to the proposed Quit Victoria project.

TABLE 15.13 Benefits and limitations of different study types

Study design	Benefits	Limitations
Systematic review	• Synthesis of best available evidence • Explicit methodology used including: (i) search strategy, (ii) appraisal of studies, (iii) synthesis/pooling of results	• Information may not be generalisable to a broader question
RCT	• Best level of experimental evidence • Control for a variety of methodological biases • Useful for assessing effectiveness of interventions	• Not ethical to conduct in some situations • Potentially long time-frame required for conducting a RCT • Results may be limited to a specific population (due to explicit inclusion/exclusion criteria)
Cohort study	• Feasible when a RCT is not appropriate	• Susceptible to bias (due to non-randomisation) • Results may be limited to a specific population (due to explicit inclusion/exclusion criteria)
Case-control	• Feasible when RCT/cohort studies are not appropriate • Useful in exploratory data gathering (i.e. first perform a case-control study to ascertain whether it is worthwhile performing a cohort or RCT)	• Susceptible to bias • Limited validity
Case series	• Feasible to gather exploratory pilot data	• Susceptible to bias • Limited validity

REFERENCES

1 Phillips SP. Models of medical education in Australia, Europe and North America. *Med Teach* 2008; **30**(7): 705–9.
2 Harden RM. Outcome-based education: the ostrich, the peacock and the beaver. *Med Teach*. 2007; **29**(7): 666–71.
3 Harden RM. International medical education and future directions: a global perspective. *Acad Med*. 2006; **81**(Suppl. 12): S22–9.
4 Ibid.
5 World Health Organization. *The World Health Report 2002: reducing risks, promoting healthy life*. Geneva: World Health Organization; 2002.
6 Yusulf S, Hawkens S, Ounpu S, *et al*. Effect of potentially modifiable risk factors associated

with myocardial infarction in 52 countries (the INTERHEART study); case-control study. *Lancet*. 2004; **364**(9438): 937–52.

7 Mant D. Principles of prevention. In: Jones R, Britten N, Culpepper L, *et al.*, editors. *Oxford Textbook of Primary Medical Care*. Oxford: Oxford University Press; 2004. pp. 369–72.

8 World Health Organization. Ottawa Charter for health promotion. *Journal of Health Promotion*. 1986; **1**: 1–4.

9 World Health Organization. *The Bangkok Charter for Health Promotion in a Globalized World*. Geneva: World Health Organization; 2005.

10 Ashton J. Healthy cities and healthy settings. *Promot Educ*. 2002; **9**(1 Suppl.): 12–14.

11 Nutbeam D. The health promoting school: closing the gap between theory and practice. *Health Promot Int*. 1992; **7**: 151–3.

12 Seffrin JR. Why school health education? In: Wallace HM, Patrick K, Parcel GS, *et al.*, editors. *Principles and Practice of School Health*. Vol. 2. Oakland, CA: Third Party Publishing Company; 1992.

13 Nutbeam D. Health literacy as a public health goal: a challenge for contemporary health education and communication strategies into the 21st century. *Health Promot Int*. 2000; **15**(3): 259–67.

14 St Leger L, Kobe LJ, Lee A, *et al.* School health: achievements, challenges and priorities. In: McQueen D, Jones C, editors. *Global Perspectives on Health Promotion Effectiveness*. New York: Springer; 2007.

15 St Leger LH. Schools, health literacy and public health: possibilities and challenges. *Health Promot Int*. 2001; **16**(2): 197–205.

16 Lee A. Helping schools to promote healthy educational environments as new initiatives for school based management: the Hong Kong Healthy Schools Award Scheme. *Promot Educ*. 2002; **9**(1 Suppl.): 29–32.

17 St Leger, Schools, health literacy and public health, op. cit.

18 Lee A, St Leger L, Moon AS. Evaluating health promotion in schools: a case study of design, implementation and results from the Hong Kong Healthy Schools Award Scheme. *Promot Educ*. 2005; **12**: 123–30.

19 Lee A, Cheng F, St Leger L. Evaluating health-promoting schools in Hong Kong: development of a framework. *Health Promot Int*. 2005; **20**(2): 177–86.

20 Rogers E, Moon AV, Mullee MA, *et al.* Developing the 'health-promoting school': a national survey of healthy school awards. *Public Health*. 1998; **112**(1): 37–40.

21 Moon AM, Mullee MA, Rogers L, *et al.* Helping schools to become health-promoting environments: an evaluation of the Wessex Healthy Schools Award. *Health Promot Int*. 1999; **14**(2): 111–22.

22 Centers for Disease Control and Prevention, National Center for Environmental Health, Division of Environmental Hazards and Health Effects. *Environmental Public Health Indicators Project*. Atlanta: CDC, NCEH, EHHE; 2002. pp. 2–3.

23 Pattenden J. First workshop on practice of evaluation of the health promoting school: models, experiences and perspectives, 19–22 November 1998, Switzerland. Bern/Thun: ENHPS; 1998. (Executive summary, pp. 39–41).

24 Piette D, Roberts C, Prevost M, *et al. Tracking Down ENHPS Successes for Sustainable Development and Dissemination: the EVA2 project, final report*. Brussels: ENHPS; 2002. p. 24.

25 St Leger LH. Developing indicators to enhance school health. *Health Educ Res*. 2000; **15**(6): 719–28.

26 Lee A, Lee SH, Tsang KK, *et al.* A comprehensive 'healthy schools programme' to promote school health: the Hong Kong experience in joining the efforts of health and education sectors. *J Epidemiol Commun H*. 2003; **57**(3): 174–7.

27 Hawkins JD, Catalano RF. Broadening the vision of education: schools as health promoting environment. *J Sch Health*. 1990; **60**: 178–81.

28 Dobbins M, Lockett D, Michel T, *et al. The Effectiveness of School-Based Intervention in Promoting Physical Activity and Fitness among Children and Youth: a systematic review.* Canada: Ministry of Health; 2001.

29 Bell A, Swinburn B. What are the key food groups to target for preventing obesity and improving nutrition in schools? *Eur J Clin Nutr.* 2004; **58**(2): 258–63.

30 Timperio A, Salmon J, Ball K. Evidence-based strategies to promote physical activity among children, adolescents and young adults: review and update. *J Sci Med Sport.* 2004; **7**(1): 20–9.

31 Lee A, Cheng F, Fung Y, *et al.* Can health promoting schools contribute to the better health and well-being of young people: the Hong Kong experience. *J Epidemiol Commun H.* 2006; **60**: 530–6.

32 Lee A, Wong MCS, Cheng F, *et al.* Can the concept of health promoting schools help to improve students' health knowledge and practices to combat the challenge of communicable diseases? Case study in Hong Kong. *BMC Public Health.* 2008; **8**: 42.

33 Lee A. Health promoting schools: evidence for a holistic approach to promoting health and improving health literacy. *Appl Health Econ Health Policy.* 2009: **7**(1): 11–17.

34 Lee, *et al.*, A comprehensive 'healthy schools programme' to promote school health, op. cit.

35 Lee A, Tsang KK, Lee SH, *et al.*, Healthy School Research Support Group. Older school children are not necessarily healthier: analysis of medical consultation pattern of school children from a territory-wide school health surveillance. *Public Health.* 2000; **115**(1): 30–7.

36 Ibid.

37 Lee A, Cheng F, Yuen H, *et al.*, Healthy Schools Support Group. How would schools step up public health measures to control spread of SARS? *J Epidemiol Commun H.* 2003; **57**: 945–9.

38 Lee A, Abdullah ASM. Severe acute respiratory syndrome: challenge for public health practice in Hong Kong. *J Epidemiol Commun H.* 2003; **57**: 655–8.

39 Ibid.

40 Lee A, Chan KM. Hygiene Charter: laying down the spirit of Healthy City. Gallery paper. *J Epidemiol Commun H.* 2005; **59**: 30.

41 Lai KY, Lam KKL, Lam SC, *et al.* Exploring parents' understandings and concerns on self management of childhood asthma. *Hong Kong Pract.* 2005; **27**(5): 172–8.

42 Lee A. Re-orientating school health services. Invited plenary paper. Asia Pacific Conference on Health Promoting Schools, 13–17 November 2006, National Taipei University of Education, Taiwan.

43 Lee, *et al.* Evaluating health-promoting schools in Hong Kong, op. cit.

44 Lee A, Tsang KK. Healthy Schools Research Support Group. Youth risk behaviour in a Chinese population: a territory-wide youth risk behavioural surveillance in Hong Kong. *Public Health.* 2004; **118**(2): 88–95.

45 Lee A, Lee N, Tsang CKK, *et al.* Youth risk behaviour survey, Hong Kong (2003–04). *Journal of Primary Care and Health Promotion.* 2005: Special issue; 1–47.

46 Lee A, Cheng F, Au G, *et al. Health Crisis of our New Generation: surveillance on youth risk behaviours.* Hong Kong: Centre for Health Education and Health Promotion, School of Public Health, The Chinese University of Hong Kong; 2002.

47 Naidoo J, Wills J. *Health Promotion: foundations for practice.* 2nd ed. Sydney: Bailliere Tindall; 2000.

48 Round R, Marshall B, Horton K. *Planning for Effective Health Promotion Evaluation.* Melbourne: Victorian Government of Human Services; 2005.

49 Saunders RP, Evans MH, Joshi P. Developing a process-evaluation plan for assessing health promotion program implementation: a how-to guide. *Health Promot Pract.* 2005; **6**(2): 134–47.

50 Baum F. Cracking the nut of health equity: top down and bottom up pressure for action on the social determinants of health. *Promot Educ.* 2007; **14**(2): 90–5.

51 Laverack G, Labonte R. A planning framework for community empowerment goals within health promotion. *Health Pol Plann.* 2000; **15**(3): 255–62.

52 Brown P. The role of the evaluator in comprehensive community initiatives. In: Connell JP, Kubisch AC, Schorr LB, *et al.*, editors. *New Approaches to Evaluating Community Initiatives: concepts, methods, and contexts.* Washington, DC: The Aspen Institute; 1995. pp. 201–25.

53 VicHealth. *Research.* Available at www.vichealth.vic.gov.au/en/Research.aspx (accessed 8 November 2009).

54 Sims J, Huang N, Pietsch J, *et al.* The Victorian Active Script Programme: promising signs for general practitioners, population health, and the promotion of physical activity. *Br J Sports Med.* 2004; **38**(1): 19–25.

CHAPTER 16

Topics or principles: health promotion under other names

Ann Wylie and Tangerine Holt

LOCATING HEALTH PROMOTION

With the move to modern integrated curricula which, in essence, starts with the patient, the patient's context and concerns and with a greater emphasis on interprofessional and self-directed learning, many specific disciplines traditionally associated with medical education may not be easily identified. In contrast, some newer themes and skills take on a more prominent presence with the rationale that 'excellent care cannot be separated from communication skills, professionalism, ethics, advocacy and accountability'.[1]

It maybe that health promotion, despite also being a newer theme, may be more obscure and elusive to the learner, teacher and assessor as well as to curriculum committees, than communication skills and ethics. In part, this is because of the nature of health promotion itself. Yet there is a requirement that curricula enable students to promote the health of their future patients and the communities in which they work, and to maintain their own health.

In Chapter 2, and to some extent in Chapter 13, the challenges of defining the discipline of health promotion, and how it differs from public health, were explored. In this chapter, there is an exploration of the possibilities of how curricula can achieve the goal of enabling students to gain basic knowledge and skills for promoting health, without having had exposure to explicitly defined health promotion content.

Health promotion is eclectic, drawing on many research and practice paradigms, with interventions being based on a synthesis of evidence and skills. By accessing some of these paradigms, as they relate to the 'cases' or 'patients', students are working with aspects of health promotion, albeit implicitly. Returning to the working definition of health promotion for this book 'the study of, and the study of the response to, the modifiable determinants of health and disease', integrated curricula could inform and relate to one or more of the three essential aspects of the definition.

These three aspects are further explained in Table 16.1.

Throughout this chapter these three aspects of this working definition of health promotion will be referred to as a way of identifying where and how health promotion could be addressed, albeit with different terminology in some instances.

TABLE 16.1 Definition of health promotion and its three aspects

Aspect	Description
Response or intervention	Referring to planned action, intervention and/or strategy which should be evidence-based insofar as evidence exists, given that evidence will be from multiple sources. The response could be with an individual, community or population
Modifiable	Referring to what, given the context, could be modified, with regard to existing skills, knowledge, resources, support and sustainability. Short-term modifiable determinants or long-term modifiable determinants need to be considered and these may align with public health goals but may not. The evidence to support the argument that the modifiable determinants have been identified needs to be presented
Determinants	The determinants are those factors that have been shown to have an influence on health and disease, usually though scientific studies, demonstrating associations, cause and effect. They may also include risk factors, behaviours, psycho-social factors, biological and genetic factors, environmental factors, political and economical factors

By starting with a 'case' or 'patient', scenarios may be specifically focused on the clinical needs for the individual and to a greater or lesser extent all aspects are ostensibly health-promoting, the proximal tasks being to diagnose, relieve pain and symptoms, enable the patient to manage their lives and to maintain or improve their health. Whilst the pain relief medication may require sound pharmacological knowledge, patient education about the cause of the pain, what steps the patient can take to reduce the likelihood of recurrance, how and when to take the medication, the possible side effects of the medication, if done on an evidence-based best practice approach, could all be considered effective health promotion. But such an example may also be associated with overall clinical skills, history taking, communication skills and clinical reasoning as well as professionalism. How much explicit reference there is to the discipline of health promotion will determine how far the students are demonstrating health promotion skills. In this situation students may be drawing on their knowledge of the determinants of the patient's presenting problems, they may be able to establish what is modifiable and may then be able to apply evidence-based skilled interventions.

Knowledge of probable determinants and associated risk factors will increase as the student progresses and more complex scenarios are presented. For example a patient with a cough seeks some medication. The history-taking process, as well as the clinical examination, will provide the student with a number of possibilities about cause – a viral or bacterial infection is probable and the cause could be exposure to airborne microbes. But why is this patient vulnerable, how serious is this, will this recur, how effective will treatment be and does the patient need medication are further questions to be considered. Determinants of the patient's illness may now expand to consider the following:

➤ social and workplace environment
➤ congenital or genetic factors
➤ existing morbidities
➤ presence of resistant pathogens.

For the students to consider the above they will have drawn on aspects of public health and epidemiology, possibly workplace health and safety policies, biomedical sciences, microbiology and pharmacology. The patient's ability to modify determinants associated with the above is limited so the health promotion elements are restricted to identifying determinants.

On further inquiry, as part of history taking and with the application of effective communication skills, additional determinants associated with the patient's cough are considered as follows:

➤ smoking status and exposure to tobacco
➤ exercise and levels of physical activity
➤ weight and body mass index
➤ use of medication, prescribed or over the counter
➤ use of illicit drugs.

Students following this course of inquiry are looking at risk factors as determinants of disease, and the evidence to support the assertions that smoking is a factor for respiratory problems, as is being overweight. That poor healthcare and inappropriate use of medication can be harmful and that illicit intravenous drug use may also indicate infectious diseases such as tuberculosis also need to be considered.

For students to appreciate the relevance of considering these determinants they will have drawn on public health data and demographic data, health psychology about behaviour and possibly healthcare services regarding procedure for notification of communicable diseases and health protection. To obtain the patient's history they will have drawn on theories and skills associated with communication and applied psychology.

Having to work with the patient and address their presenting problems, the students would now need to consider their appropriate response, but with a good overview of the determinants, they are now in a position to consider what aspects are modifiable.

Modifiable determinants of health and disease may be acted upon as follows:

➤ medical and pharmacological intervention
➤ reference to implementation of policy – such as health and safety regulations in the workplace
➤ screening others also likely to be at risk
➤ motivational interviewing to establish patient's knowledge, skills and attitudes
➤ providing appropriate patient advice, education and referral.

Each one of the above have further aspects to be considered related to health promotion and linked to the notion of determinants being modifiable.

Table 16.2 summarises how these determinants might be modified and the sources of evidence to substantiate the modification.

Students may now be confident about what action they could take, what the limitations are, related to their own skills deficit, as well as the patient's context, and how they would define success or effective intervention in this scenario.

This scenario uses the patient's symptoms as the starting point rather than a defined disease or medical speciality and avoids focusing on specific disciplines within medical and health professional education.[1] It also has the potential to enable students to demonstrate they have generic competencies to act in the patient's best interest, drawing on the discipline of health promotion as well as other fields without any specific discipline or disease dominating.

TABLE 16.2 Modifying determinants

What is modifiable	In what way	Sources of evidence
Medical and pharmacological	Prescribing treatment that is indicated, cost-effective and with high probability of patient compliance	Medical, scientific and pharmacological journals as well as behavioural sciences, public health and health promotion journals
Policy implementation	Clean air, safe environments, trading standards and licensing, policies for health protection	Public health and health promotion journals, environmental health and local authority journals, occupational health and community health journals
Screening	Early disease detection for early intervention, or to identify those posing risks and intervene with prophylaxis and immunisations	Public health and health promotion journals, thorax and tobacco control journals as well as medical journals
Motivational interviewing	To ascertain patient's knowledge, skills and attitudes as well as readiness to change	Health-related journals and psychology journals, health promotion journals and medical journals
Patient education	To equip patients with appropriate information and skills to improve their health by taking planned action to reduce risks	Health-related and health promotion journals, psychology and healthcare journals and medical journals

HEALTH PROMOTION IN BASIC MEDICAL SCIENCES: POSSIBILITIES

Whether basic medical sciences are presented in a didactic format or integrated, whether there are taught sessions and assessments that relate to the basic medical sciences, the students will need to engage with them. Regardless of curriculum structure students will be required to demonstrate their critical thinking, which involves 'systematic evaluation of information preceding any professional decision and action' and as part of this they should be able to evaluate scientific text.[2]

Given that requirement, the links between health promotion and basic medical sciences can be considered.

Some potentially modifiable determinants of disease and health can become explicit within the context of basic medical sciences and are therefore further explored and some examples given.

➤ *Anatomy and physiology*: the basic medical sciences can provide students with information about optimum body functions, exercise and weight, fluid balance, the consequences of insufficient and inappropriate physical activity, from bone health to cardiovascular disease.

➤ *Microbiology*: communicable diseases, personal hygiene, food and water safety, sanitation, immunisation.

➤ *Biochemistry*: mode of action of toxins and carcinogens, role of micronutrients, role of food additives (e.g. folic acid) and water additives (e.g. fluoride).
➤ *Histology*: precursors for cancer, early signs and options.

In the above examples intervention could be linked to individual behaviour change or public health interventions.

The possibility that students can become aware of these health determinants, as well as many others, and how they can be modified, will depend on how and when students explore these basic sciences. This could be integrated with case-based scenarios or as discrete sessions with defined learning outcomes.

HEALTH PROMOTION IN SOCIAL AND BEHAVIOURAL SCIENCES

The term behavioural science is far reaching and may include health promotion, explicitly or implicitly. The fields usually included are as follows:
➤ sociology
➤ psychology
➤ anthropology
➤ political sciences.

Although these fields have established a full and rich literature and research paradigms, there is a limit to which medical and health-related course can engage with them, yet the increased visibility of the behavioural sciences in medical and health professional vocational courses enables students to become aware of a wide range of determinants of health.

'Do we not always find the diseases of the populace traceable to the defects in society' is the famous comment by Virchow that remains as relevant today as when he wrote it.[3] In addition this statement is quoted in the opening of the 2007 report from the representatives of the Civil Society to the Commission on Social determinants of Health of the World Health Organization.[4]

The behavioural sciences, like the basic medical sciences, may be presented to students in integrated curricula, case-based scenarios or in discrete sessions.

For the most part the behavioural sciences offer insights into the determinants of health, rather than what is modifiable or how, but below are some examples as to how they can explored.
➤ *Sociology*: demographic data, such as social class, income, educational attainment and housing, e.g. variables in life expectancy.
➤ *Psychology*: how individuals behave and why, health belief models and locus of control, e.g. smoking behaviours.
➤ *Anthropology*: how specific groups with common identities may behave, react and respond to situations, e.g. asylum seekers, intravenous drug users.
➤ *Political sciences*: although a full and rich discipline in its own right, within the behavioural sciences as they relate to health this could include the impact of statutory change, such as smoking policies and fiscal change on health inequalities.

Looking at a 'case' to examine these collective behavioural sciences, a mother is concerned about her infant's weight, which she claims is low and her family are suggesting she uses formula feed rather than continue with breastfeeding.

Students may familiarise themselves with the suckling frequency and techniques for successful breastfeeding as well as considering the infant's weight and health. Without any obvious physical problem, the students need to explore other determinants that may be influencing the mother's concerns.

Breastfeeding is considered to be mediated by cultural factors. Despite that the breast and the milk are biological and functional, breastfeeding decisions cannot be separated from complex social values and beliefs.[5] Cultures that perceive breastfeeding as a complex social activity, will facilitate mother and child to overcome difficulties, but for some women the breast as a focus of sexuality and femininity may inhibit successful breastfeeding. Grandmothers may also exercise influence on infant feeding and their advice may be followed even if conflicting with that of health professionals. For example, some newborn babies for their first feed were given honey, and some within two weeks were receiving semisolid foods such as cereals.[6,7]

How the students proceed will be based on their ability to explore what factors are influencing this mother's worries and what is actually possible given her circumstances. What is known is that women can feel shame and grief if they are considered unsuccessful breastfeeders. Others struggle with the dilemmas between being a good mother and being an attractive, desirable woman, while some are influenced by other significant carers. The factors that influence breastfeeding can be identified when students are aware of and familiar with the behavioural sciences so as to inform their history-taking and communication skills. Having identified the determinants of health, what is modifiable, and how, is not as obvious and sometimes more difficult.

By exploring these aspects of health determinants students may also be provided with opportunities and even incentives, depending on how these are linked to assessment, to look at what could be modified and how to critically assess the evidence and consider the role of the medical and health professionals in policy development, be it national, regional or global.

Further opportunities for exploring and critiquing social determinants of health can be found at the Social Medicine portal, a project developed by faculty members of the Department of Family and Social Medicine of the Albert Einstein College of Medicine in New York (www.socialmedicine.org).

HEALTH PROMOTION IN HUMANITIES

Human rights and ethics teaching offer further ways of exploring health promotion. Enshrined in laws and declarations of the human rights, for people in need of healthcare as well as for those providing care, this field offers a wealth of opportunities to consider respect and dignity issues, social justice, funding for healthcare, balance between the individual's needs and society's needs, as well considering the needs of the population at large for health-promoting policies and environments.

Core curriculum for medical ethics and law

One of the changes to modern UK medical education core curricula in 1998 was that of the introduction of a model for medical ethics and law.[8] The 12 areas to be covered are outlined below.

1 *Informed consent and refusal of treatment*: why respect for autonomy is so important; adequate information; treatment without consent; competence; battery; and negligence.

2 *The clinical relationship: truthfulness, trust, and good communication*: ethical limits of paternalism; building trust; honesty, courage, and other virtues in clinical practice; narrative and the importance of communication skills.

3 *Confidentiality*: clinical importance of privacy; compulsory and discretionary disclosure; public versus private interests.

4 *Medical research*: ethical and legal tensions in doing medical research on patients, human volunteers, and animals; the need for effective regulation.

5 *Human reproduction*: ethical and legal status of the embryo/foetus; assisted conception; abortion, including prenatal screening.

6 *The new genetics*: treating the abnormal versus improving the normal; debates about the ethical boundaries of and the need to regulate genetic therapy and research.

7 *Children*: ethical and legal significance of age to consent to treatment; dealing with parental/child/clinician conflict; child abuse.

8 *Mental disorders and disabilities*: ethical and legal justifications for detention and treatment without consent; conflicts of interests between patient, family, and community.

9 *Life, death, dying, and killing*: the duty of care and ethical and legal justifications for the nonprovision of life-prolonging treatment and the provision of potentially life-shortening palliatives; transplantation, death certification; and the coroner's court.

10 *Vulnerabilities created by the duties of doctors and medical students*: public expectations of medicine; the need for teamwork; the health of doctors and students in relation to professional performance; the General Medical Council and professional regulation; responding appropriately to clinical mistakes; whistleblowing.

11 *Resource allocation*: ethical debates about 'rationing' and the fair and just distribution of scarce healthcare; the relevance of needs, rights, utility, efficiency, desert and autonomy to theories of equitable healthcare; boundaries of responsibility of individuals for their own health.

12 *Rights*: what rights are, and their links with moral and professional duties; the importance of the concept of rights, including human rights, for good medical practice.[8]

Any or all of these 12 could be linked to case-based scenarios, as students progress and expand the complexity of their understanding and application of patient-centredness approaches.

Each medical school in the UK will approach ethics teaching to suit their curriculum, and the extent to which they align this with health promotion will vary. What is important is that there is scope, within this core teaching, to consider the determinants of health from humanities perspectives, which of those determinants are modifiable, in what circumstances and how. With case-based scenarios and patient-centred approaches, the degree of complexity can be adjusted to suit the situation.

Humanities may also offer opportunities to examine a variety of topics such as:

➤ history of medicine
➤ art and medicine
➤ music and medicine
➤ literature and medicine.

Each of these may examine the determinants of health such as tuberculosis and poverty, drug abuse and breakdown of families, communicable diseases as well as crime and social justice. The scope is extensive, but it is likely that these health promotion learning opportunities will be in special study options and special study modules rather than in core curricula.

Philosophical aspects of health and health promotion may also be within the medical humanities and linked to exploring the determinants of health and the role of healthcare professionals. Lifelong learning is an accepted professional task as well as adapting to changing health issues and political climates. For example, Foucault argued that the reduction in morbidity and premature mortality was a benefit to society 200 years ago,[9] when regulation was necessary to protect the public from quacks. But what of modern society? What do we expect from doctors and other health professionals, from healthcare provision whether wholly or partially public-funded, and who makes such decisions? These are key questions. In the UK, debates about what medication can be available at taxpayers' expense frequent the media headlines, as well as discussion about sexual health and the success, or otherwise, of interventions.

➤ What is the best way (and best for whom) to use finite resources, that is, for treatment or prevention?
➤ Can the public make informed choices – how accessible and informative is the information?
➤ What are the goals of herd immunity – are they always preferable?
➤ What is the role of healthcare professionals, defining clinical parameters?
➤ How do we value complementary and alternative medicine?
➤ Can we distinguish between social care, social need and healthcare?

Although this book cannot explore these questions further, they are linked to the determinants of health and may also be covered in teaching related to healthcare management, politics and health economics. More specifically, The National Institute for Clinical Excellence (NICE) issues guidelines for a number of topics, some disease-related and other concerned with prevention. Within these guidelines some of the philosophical questions can be explored. For example, the guideline 'Falls: the assessment and prevention of falls in older people'[10] suggests that 'all healthcare professionals involved in helping people avoid falls should have been taught about assessing a person's risk of falling and the ways of preventing falls'. This includes the healthcare professional's ability to assess home hazards and devise an exercise programme. In addition the person should be able to discuss with the healthcare professional, whether a doctor or not, the barriers, if any, to change.[10] This still adheres to Foucault's assertion that the medical profession should be active in reducing morbidity and premature mortality, but is an example of how far from the strictly clinical parameters contemporary medical practice can be and yet still be regulated.

HEALTH PROMOTION IN CLINICAL SKILLS AND SPECIALITIES

During clinical work students need to attend to personal and patient hygiene, display aseptic techniques, communicate appropriately with the patient, fellow students, teachers and colleagues and consider the impact of any of these activities on the well-being of the patient. This is less likely to be seen as health promotion but rather as harm reduction and good practice with vulnerable people.

In the clinical context the student's focus may be dominated by tasks to be demonstrated to the medical teacher, such as history taking to plan further investigations, clinical examinations to establish provisional diagnosis and indicate further diagnostic tests, or technical skills such as blood pressure measurements or taking a blood sample. During this time the student needs to be engaged with the patient, even if the patient is a professional 'simulated' patient, to communicate effectively what they are doing and why as well establishing the patient's consent. Such procedures, if done well, are health-enhancing, providing the patient with vital information, explaining the situation and checking with the patient if they are satisfied. The student and indeed the clinician need to work with the patient and/or the carer. The care and management regime will depend on a collaborative arrangement, a workable and acceptable plan, fostering the likelihood of patient concordance. Given that the situation may require some discomfort for the patient and carer, some changes such as financial loss or reduced independence, as well as an unpleasant medication requirement, students will need to be skilled in considering the proposed interventions and what challenges the patient faces. Students need to consider how quickly the patient and carer can adapt, indeed whether they can adapt, what could be realistic in the short term, what additional help may be useful and of course available. From the initial consultation, to acceptance of diagnosis and prognosis, to successful self healthcare, these are stages that all patients with chronic diseases go through; and students, as well as healthcare professionals, can explore in what ways the discipline of health promotion can inform practice and influence this trajectory.

For some clinical specialities, health promotion is dominant. For example, cardiology, respiratory medicine, gastroenterology, obstetrics and gynaecology, paediatrics, general practice and psychiatry are all specialities that frequently encounter patients with health-related problems and risks that are more likely to improve if lifestyle changes can be implemented and social circumstances improved. The problems of obesity in obstetric and reproductive health have been documented. Fertility and gynaecological concerns associated with the increased prevalence of obesity include subfertility and polycystic ovarian syndrome. In pregnancy there are many concerns including hypertension, venous thromboembolism, increased risk of pre-eclampsia, increased risk of operative delivery and complications. The infant is also at risk of neonatal complications and long-term obesity problems.[11] There are problems for obese men as well, including erectile dysfunction. Ramsay, *et al.* do, however, offer some suggestions for management, including advising pregnant women to increase their physical activity and improve their diets.[11] These modifiable health behaviours can be explored by students as follows:

➤ What type of interventions will enable such behaviour change?
➤ How can they be targeted?
➤ What skills are needed by health professionals within the clinical context to enable them to successfully motivate change?
➤ Do clinicians have a role in prevention?

HEALTH PROMOTION IN PRACTICE: SEMANTICS AND JARGON

In the above sections we have considered how health promotion opportunities could be mapped out by curriculum designers and developed from being implicit to more explicit content. Within the broad field of practice occupied by health promotion and public health specialists and allied practitioners, a number of terms to describe their role may be in common use, with a limited number of the incumbents holding professional health promotion or public health credentials. Below is a list of some occupational titles related to health promotion work that we frequently encounter:

➤ health improvement manager, health development manager, health gain coordinator
➤ smoking prevention strategist, smoking cessation manager, smoking cessation advisor, smoking cessation counsellor
➤ drug and alcohol team manager, drug and alcohol counsellor
➤ teenage pregnancy project manager, sexual health outreach coordinator, sex education team leader
➤ school nurse manager, specialist school nurse, community public health nurse, rehabilitation nurse
➤ fall prevention manager
➤ nutrition and healthy eating project manager, community MEND coordinator, school nutritional advisor (MEND = Mind, Exercise, Nutrition . . . Do it! programme targetting childhood overweight and obesity)
➤ exercise referral scheme manager, health walks facilitator
➤ Sure Start director (Sure Start = early childhood protection programme)
➤ health inequalities policy implementer.

In most cases the post holders will have a professional qualification, such as pharmacist, occupational therapist, nurse, nutrition specialist and dietician, but how well they engage with the principles and practice of health promotion may be variable. It is therefore possible that the semantics and jargon from their primary profession are used more fluently and confidently that those of health promotion. So how do we define or guide the health promotion aspects of their work, and more importantly how can students learn from them about health promotion practice, rather than limit their learning to a specific topic such as, say, smoking cessation?

The five approaches to health promotion practice, (*see* Table 16.3) described by Ewles and Simnett, have been helpful for such a diverse group, especially when briefing those who may work as facilitators and teachers with medical and healthcare professional students.[12] By linking the health promotion content of their work to one or more of the five approaches, these professionals can help explain the aims and activities associated with their health promotion work, as well as what indicators of success are pragmatic to students.

The move to integrated curricula, as well as the increase in the prevalence of chronic illness, has provided many opportunities for curriculum designers to include basic health promotion skills and knowledge. Whilst it is recognised that single disciplines are no longer central to modern curricula, some are relevant across many aspects of curricula but may remain difficult to integrate. Health promotion may well fall into that category but by considering the examples given in this chapter, medical and health professional educators may be able to map out increased and more explicit health promotion teaching opportunities.

The next chapter provides information about the wide range of resources available to medical educators, teachers and facilitators that could assist in the planning and implementation of health promotion teaching.

TABLE 16.3 The five approaches to health promotion

Approach	Aim	Health promotion activity	Important values	Comment
Medical	Freedom from medically defined disease and disability	Promotion of medical intervention to prevent or ameliorate ill-health	Patient compliance with preventive medical procedures	Success linked to improved morbidity or reduced risk
Behavioural change	Individual behaviour conducive to freedom from disease	Attitude and behaviour change to encourage healthier lifestyle	Healthier lifestyle as defined by health promoter	Success linked to sustained behaviour change
Educational	Individuals with knowledge and understanding enabling well informed decisions to be made and acted upon	Information about causes and effects of health-demoting factors. Exploration of values and attitudes. Development of skills required for healthy living	Individual right of free choice. Health promoter's responsibility to identify educational content	Success linked to demonstration of learning objectives achieved rather than health improved or behaviour change
Client-centred	Working with clients on the client's own terms	Working with health issues, choices and actions which clients identify. Empowering the client	Clients as equals. Client's right to set the agenda. Self-empowerment of client	Improved self-esteem and internal locus of control implicit in successful intervention
Societal change	Physical and social environment which enables choice of healthier lifestyle	Political/social action to change physical/social environment	Right and need to make environment health-enhancing	Health public policy making the healthy choice the easy choice

REFERENCES

1 Phillips S. Models of medical education in Australia, Europe and Canada. *Med Teach.* 2008; **30**(7): 705–9. Available at: http://dx.doi.org/10.1080/01421590802061134 (accessed 5 November 2009).

2 Hilgers J, DeRoos P, Rigby E. European core curriculum: the students' perspective. *Med Teach.* 2007; **29**(2): 270–5.

3 Virchow R. *Collected Essays on Public Health and Epidemiology.* Cambridge: Science History Publications; 1848.

4 Representatives of the Civil Society to the Commission on Social Determinants of Health of the World Health Organization. Civil Society Report to the Commission on Social Determinants of Health. *Soc Med.* 2007; **2**(4): 192–211.

5 Burch S. Cultural and anthropological studies. In: Naidoo J, Wills J, editors. *Health Studies: an introduction.* 2nd ed. Basingstoke: Palgrave Macmillan; 2008. pp. 185–220.

6 Fikree FF, Ali TS, Durocher JM, *et al.* Newborn care practices in low socioeconomic settlements of Karachi, Pakistan. *Soc Sci Med.* 2005; **60**(5): 911–21.

7 Bentley M, Gavin L, Black MM, *et al.* Infant feeding practices of low-income, African-American, adolescent mothers: an ecological, multigenerational perspective. *Soc Sci Med.* 1999; **49**(8): 1085–100.

8 Doyal L, Gillon R. Medical ethics and law as a core subject in medical education. *BMJ.* 1998; **316**(7145): 1623–4.

9 Foucault M. *The Birth of the Clinic: an archaeology of medical perception.* London: Tavistock; 1973.

10 National Institute for Health and Clinical Excellence. *Falls: The Assessment and Prevention of Falls in Older People: NICE guideline CG21.* London: NICE; 2004. http://guidance.nice.org.uk/CG21

11 Ramsay JE, Greer I, Sattar N. Obesity and reproduction. *BMJ.* 2006; **333**(7579): 1159–62.

12 Ewles L, Simnett I. *Promoting Health: a practical guide.* 5th ed. London: Bailliere Tindall; 2003.

CHAPTER 17

Health promotion resources for teaching

Tangerine Holt and Ann Wylie

WHY DO WE NEED RESOURCES?

Most of us will have reference books and recommended reading lists for learners that we also frequently rely on to check detail, refresh our knowledge base and to question. We are likely to prepare sessions with reference to current literature, key seminal works, and academic or clinical debates. We make decisions about the knowledge content and how to pitch it, depending on what stage the students are at and how the topic fits into their wider learning. For example, a junior student, taking a sexual health history from a patient complaining of a discharge, may include communication skills, an assessment of the patient's concerns and may elicit a description of the symptoms and the duration of symptoms. The recommended reading and approach to this session would be based in or around the current communication skills material, with less emphasis on microbiology, therapeutics and clinical examination.

A student about to qualify may also be expected to be able to demonstrate they are able to advise the patient appropriately about risk reduction to herself and partners, explain what investigations should be done and know how to approach asking her consent, that is, taking a high vaginal swab. The student would also be expected to inform the patient as to when to expect the results and what a treatment plan might be, explaining the importance of continuing and complying with the prescribed medication. How does the student do this, what resources will help and how do we teach and assess the student? The patient may have other concerns and the decision about how, when and if to address these is not straightforward.

Being in a genito-urinary medicine (GUM) clinic or sexual health clinic doesn't negate the need to consider the patient's wider health issues. Co-morbidities – for example asthma, sickle cell disease, diabetes – as well as poor social circumstances and risk behaviours such as drug taking, binge drinking and smoking may not sit well with students, or their clinical teachers, doing a sexual health rotation. Should the student in a patient- or case-focused problem-based learning (PBL) course be able or expected to identify and address the additional and possibly modifiable determinants of health? Maybe not, but this would also to be a lost opportunity to enable the patient to address and improve her health.

Because health promotion and medical education are eclectic fields with multiple research paradigms, supporting both teachers and students, this type of scenario requires a review of the health promotion resources and approaches and what is deemed 'good practice' as well as what is 'good practice' regarding teaching approaches.

Factual knowledge can be checked both by students themselves and by teachers, but what type of leaflet would be advisable to give the patient; would a leaflet be appropriate, and how do learner and teacher decide? What is the best way to engage with the patient and do we know how students can best be taught? In this chapter we see how health promotion and medical education juxtapose their respective challenges of deciding what is best practice and how resources may be accessed and used to facilitate this.

By resources we now mean a variety tools and books, models and equipment, virtual learning materials and interactive programmes. For health promoters the term resources is widely understood and many in the field will be familiar with accessing well tested and reliable resources for use with professionals and the public alike. There is no credit for 'inventing' your own materials when high-quality resources are available; rather there is merit in using such resources in the appropriate context and/or adapting to suit the circumstances.

In health promotion work, factual knowledge is important, for example about what constitutes a healthy diet or the type of sexually transmitted infections (STIs) that are common, easily contracted and their symptoms as well as possible consequences if untreated. How this knowledge is conveyed, indeed whether this is needed by the recipient or client group, has to be considered, but more important usually for the health promoting aspect is the intervention to enable healthy eating or promote sexual health. If factual knowledge was a sufficient motivator for healthy living, we would not be seeing the levels of chronic illness and obesity that currently prevail!

We must therefore ensure that medical students and their teachers do not assume that having informed the patient that they should lose weight or use condoms that such action, worthy as it may be, equates to health promotion.

Away from the clinical one-to-one setting, students may also need to engage with the local community or a specific group such as young people about to leave school. Again the notion that people will come and listen to a talk and then, armed with 'new' factual knowledge, be able to improve their lives is misleading and unrealistic. We have seen students, and in some cases doctors, prepare fine lectures and talks, making them entertaining even with gimmicks and 'fun' activities, but if the central aim remains to convey factual knowledge they will have missed the opportunity for health promotion intervention. So what can 'resources' do and how can they be assessed and accessed?

The parallels with medical education are similar – we have very articulate and intelligent students and providing them with factual knowledge is essential, or indeed enabling them to access factual knowledge. However our task as medical educators and teachers is also to enable them to apply this knowledge, to be skilful in their work with patients and the public so as not to harm but to work for and with the patient's best interests insofar as these can be identified and realised.

HEALTH PROMOTION RESOURCES AND QUALITY

Health promotion resources are frequently considered as leaflets, audiovisual materials, models and teaching packs, but today there is much more. For example, one item is rarely a stand-alone and if a leaflet is seen as suitable to give a patient with or at risk of contracting an STI, the information on that leaflet needs to be checked out and relevant, such as leaflets inviting readers to call telephone helplines or to look up web pages. Can the client use these services and how will they be helpful? Does the leaflet have a recognisable logo and a credible source; is it part of a wider strategic approach linking promotion to services? Has the leaflet been produced with clear aims and objectives and has the reading level been tested? Is this the best leaflet for this circumstance and this client? What harm could the leaflet do, if any? What good could it do, if any? Is it sensitive and likely to be helpful? These are important questions for professionals, but additionally how, when and from whom does the patient receive it and is additional information needed?

Most health promotion resources require similar kinds of interrogation with users, in order that teachers, students and health practitioners can demonstrate how best to use and when not to use them.

The balance between vetting a number of resources for this chapter and giving some guidelines has been considered and as such we have decided that guidelines are more appropriate.

Ewles and Simnett[1] devote a chapter to this very task and outline eight essential questions to ask when vetting resources for use in health promotion activities.

➤ It is appropriate for achieving your aims? The Public Health Agency website www. healthpromotionagency.org.uk/work/Sexualhealth/publications.htm provides a range of materials but the task for the clinician is to have the appropriate one for the client given the context. The needs of a young person not yet sexually active may be to develop assertiveness skills whereas a sexually active adult may need to know how and where to access sexual health advice and clinical services.
➤ Is it the most appropriate kind of resource? Is a leaflet sufficient, can the client read it; would a model or DVD be more suitable?
➤ Is it consistent with your values and approach? Could this resource be considered patronising, authoritarian or scare-mongering? It should avoid victim blaming *per se*, but especially when ill health is rooted in poor social circumstances.
➤ Is it relevant for the people you are working with? The age, ethnicity and social and economical circumstances of the client group need to be reflected in the material, and be in line with their concerns and issues.
➤ Is it racist or sexist? Resources should reflect our multiracial society, avoid assumptions about sexual orientation and should not be demeaning in any way to either gender. For example, we usually advocate the nouns 'women', 'patients' or 'clients' and discourage material referring to 'ladies' or 'girls' when we mean adult women.
➤ Will it be understood? Is it plain English, is it available in Braille or large type, does the DVD have sign language inserts, what languages are available, is it sensitive to those with limited literacy skills or learning needs?
➤ Is the information sound? Is it up to date, accurate and from a reputable source? How does it portray contested and controversial issues, is it biased?
➤ Does it contain advertising? Wherever possible, health promoters should avoid materials that are associated with drug companies and commercial companies such as baby food suppliers. The use of such materials by healthcare professionals can promote the client's health but will also be giving endorsement to a product and company, which may not be appropriate. That said, there are good examples of companies working with health promoters in partnership. The additional

caveats are that the product and the company must be ethically acceptable – and, Ewles and Simnett argue, environmentally friendly – ruling out associations with tobacco and confectionary companies. What advertising is present should also be low-key.

The above eight points refer to all health promotion resources but additionally there are quality issues related to the various types of resources, some of which are noted here, as well as how they are used.

Leaflets are undoubtedly the most common form of health promotion resource, and a vast range are available from the Department of Health in the UK and similarly from Victoria's Health Promotion Service in Australia. The 'publications' websites for these two bodies are:

➤ www.dh.gov.uk/en/Publicationsandstatistics/Publications/DH_074291
➤ www.health.vic.gov.au/doh/publications

Despite these being reliable sources, each leaflet has to be considered is terms of relevance for the client and the context. My own experience of health promotion leaflets reinforces the advice the given by Ewles and Sinmet[1,2]

➤ Engage with the potential client or client group to establish what their needs or concerns are before issuing any leaflet.
➤ Consider the layout, colour, size of print, amount of information, the font size of print and is it appropriate?
➤ Readability testing. There is a need to meet the reading age of the majority and readability tests are linked to sentence length, word choice, passive or active sentences, as well as limited use of jargon, technical and medical terms. Slang is also to be avoided most of the time, especially when working with young people who may have different understanding of the slang terms compared to the professional. Further advice can be obtained from the Plain English society (www.plainenglish.co.uk) for those who want to produce leaflets or written material.
➤ Translated leaflets. A great deal of time and money in my experience has been wasted in creating verbatim leaflets written in English initially and then translated into other languages. But doing it well pays off. If health promoters and practitioners cannot speak the client's language, the issuing of a well translated leaflet could be very helpful and informative. There are four factors to be considered. First, the clients for whom the leaflet is intended may have limited literacy skills in their first language. Second, some words have differing meanings or don't exist in the translated language. Third, some translations can be misleading and are more complex when the issues are contested or controversial. Fourth, some lifestyle issues may be considered not relevant, too difficult or uncomfortable to address and the tone of the leaflet may even be disempowering.
➤ Those who produce reliable leaflets will also have piloted and evaluated them, updated them and indicated their purpose.

Other written materials such as posters, booklets and press releases should be subject to similar scrutiny. However, a media headline may mislead or give more coverage of the counterargument, leading to confusion or reduced credibility. The debate associated with the reporting of the Wakefield, *et al.* paper in the *Lancet*[3] is perhaps an extreme example of how a so-called reliable source, the *Lancet*, published a paper that the media reported on which resulted in a grave impact on the immunisation rates in the UK for measles, mumps and rubella (MMR). There were many lessons learned, and the media also became the prime investigator in challenging the paper, the science and the principal author, Wakefield, with journalist Brian Deer at the fore. (See http://briandeer. com/mmr-lancet.htm for further information.)

Practitioners who sought to help parents make informed choices about consenting to MMR found that the leaflets issued by statuary agencies were having little impact. Doubt and fear about risks of autism were dominating parental decisions and eventually new leaflets to try to address these concerns were produced. The situation was complex, and demonstrated for many in health promotion that the 'simple' message is never really quite so simple, that people have their own understanding and priorities, which may differ from health professionals, and factual reasoning may be of limited value.

There are too many books on health and health promotion-related issues to detail but in essence the same guidance holds in that if, as a professional, you are to recommend a book to a patient or to the public, it must have credibility and be suitable for the person and their context. Books more easily date, and advice and information from one edition to the next may vary, limiting their use. Books may be too general or too specific and be limited to those committed and motivated to reading them. Two UK books, *The Pregnancy Book*[4] (www.dh.gov.uk/en/Publicationsandstatistics/Publications/ PublicationsPolicyAndGuidance/dh_074920) and the *Birth to Five Book*[5] (www. dh.gov.uk/en/Publicationsandstatistics/Publications/PublicationsPolicyAndGuidance/ DH_074924) are regularly updated and available online, but hard copies are provided free to UK first-time mothers.

Other UK Government publications such as *Healthy Weight, Healthy Lives: a cross government strategy for England*[6] provide the public with factual information and suggested ways of improving health. This too can be quickly updated as the situation changes.

Of course, for some, government publications may be unacceptable, seemingly the top-down rather than bottom-up approach, and hence the plethora of health books on the shelves. The various patients' societies and charities such as the British Heart Foundation (www.bhf.org.uk/publications.aspx), the Terrence Higgins Trust (www.tht. org.uk/informationresources) and the American Diabetes Association (http://store.dia- betes.org/) are all a credible source of resources, including books, that are acceptable to the patient and health professional alike.

DVDs and videos are popular formats for health promotion. The following factors need to be considered:

➤ what is the likely attention span of the intended audience?
➤ is this DVD at the appropriate level, is it engaging, is it the right length and quality?
➤ where will it be viewed, for example, in a public waiting area, as part of a part of a public awareness event, with a client or client group in a closed session or for private home use?

Advice on DVD materials can be found at various health promotion websites such as www.bhps.org.uk, but as with written material the generic principles apply, such as produced by a reliable and credible source, current and accurate information, with clear and realistic aims.

Online access to resources, for those with facilities, are the newer ways of informing and enabling people to improve their health. However it is here where scrutiny is
needed before making any recommendations. Advertising and commercial interest may
be more explicit and websites can appear 'official' or genuine, yet mislead. For example,
there are numerous websites associated with weight loss and most potential users would
benefit from guidance. Foucault indicated that the rise of regulated medical practitioners 200 years ago was, in part, to protect the public from quacks and bogus claims.[7] In
many ways the rise of the internet has benefited most of us but left some vulnerable
people exposed again to the quacks, with the need for professionals to be cautious about
recommendations and provide informed advice. This field is rapidly developing, with
interactive options that will be appealing to many. Research into effectiveness is limited;
however the *Journal of Medical Internet Research* is leading the field.

Finally, health promotion materials frequently provide telephone helplines. It is
important to consider how these might help. Do they provide 24-hour services, is it a
recorded message, what are the costs, what kind of advice and support is offered, will
it be appropriate for the client and do these helplines support non-English speaking
users? These are all key questions to be considered.

MEDICAL EDUCATION RESOURCES AND QUALITY

Medical education journals report on research, but the journal *Medical Teacher* in collaboration with the Association for Medical Education in Europe (AMEE) have also
produced a series of guides for teaching and set up BEME – Best Evidence Medical
Education. More than 30 AMEE guides have been published, although some earlier
guides are now out of print (www.amee.org). Following is a quote from the website
(accessed September 2008):

Welcome to the new series of AMEE Guides
- The AMEE guides cover important topics in medical and healthcare professions
  education and provide information, practical advice and support. We hope that
  they will also stimulate your thinking and reflection on the topic.
- The guides have been logically structured for ease of reading and contain useful
  take-home messages. Text boxes highlight key points and examples in practice.
- Each page in the guide provides a column for your own personal annotations,
  stimulated either by the text itself or the additional quotation.
- Sources of further information on the topic are provided in the reference list and
  biography.
- The guides are designed for used by individual teachers to inform their practice
  and can be used to support staff development programmes.
- For each guide, supplements will be prepared that provide additional examples
  and contributions relating to the topic.

'Living guides'
An important feature of this new guide series is the concept of supplements, which
will provide for you a continuing source of information on the topic. Published supplements will be emailed to those who have purchased the guide and they will be
included in the text of future issues.

The authors of these guides are established medical educators with a special area of interest and now, with the supplements, they will encourage readers to give constructive feedback. These supplements will take the form of selected constructed feedback about the guides.[8]

Nine BEME reviews have been published so far, with 15 currently in progress. Following is a quote from the BEME website (www.bemecollaboration.org/ accessed September 2008):

> Welcome to BEME
> The BEME Collaboration is a group of individuals or institutions who are committed to the promotion of Best Evidence Medical Education through:
> - the dissemination of information which allows medical teachers, institutions and all concerned with medical education to make decisions on the basis of the best evidence available
> - the production of appropriate systematic reviews of medical education which reflect the best evidence available and meet the needs of the user, and
> - the creation of a culture of best evidence medical education amongst individual teachers, institutions and national bodies.

These two developments have become the main providers of accessible information regarding quality in medical education but to date no specific guide or review had been dedicated to the field of health promotion *per se*. That in itself is not a problem given the range of topics covered.

The Association for the Study of Medical Education (ASME) produces a series of booklets *Understanding Medical Education*, with 24 in print and a further 6 in progress. The authors, like those of the AMEE guides, are established medical educators with a specialist interest in a specific aspect of medical education.

Medical education conferences with peer-reviewed abstracts provide up-to-date information and research findings on many and varied aspects of medical education. In addition, these conferences, usually international in nature, provide a platform for workshops, debates and special interest groups, as well as informal networking enabling medical and health professional educators to share best practice and current research.

The virtual developments for medical educationalists are a growth area but much still needs to be done. The electronic virtual highway is relatively young, with vast possibilities. But so far we have seen password-protected sites with restricted access, we have seen website addresses published only to find they are not available for any length of time and we have limited information about quality.

That said, there are some reliable sources. The first of the virtual medical school sites with resources was possibly IVIMMEDS (www.ivimeds.org). The institutions contributing to this, and those accessing this site and the resources, have a wealth of information, and the freedom to give feedback. However membership is through fully subscribing institutes.

The MedEd portal (http://services.aamc.org/30/mededportal/servlet/segment/mededportal/information/) is less restrictive and has an American focus, with a wide variety of resources and information presented in collaboration with the Association of the American Colleges. To date there is limited health promotion information.

In the UK the British Medical Association (BMA) has also developed a protected virtual learning site(http://learning.bmj.com/learning), but there is limited access and a wide range of topics.

The British Medical Journal, also part of the BMA, has a series called 'ABC of learning'. Spencer, for example, considers the needs of learners and teachers in a practical approach to clinical teaching.[9] In addition this series, more than 40 publications are freely accessible and cover aspects of both teaching and learning as well as clinical management, with related health promotion issues. Mitchell, for example, reports on STIs and vaginal discharge, noting that there are increased rates of bacterial vaginosis occurring in certain groups of women, such as black African women, lesbians and smokers.[10] The approach regarding smoking cessation that a clinician may take can be explored through the ABC series, for example, in Coleman's paper.[11] Both Mitchell and Coleman provide additional resources, freely accessible for teachers and learners. As an example, Mitchell provided an adapted flowchart for management of vaginal discharge (bimanual, speculum and microscope) adapted from World Health Organization guidelines.[10]

INTERNATIONAL RESOURCES FOR TEACHING AND LEARNING ABOUT HEALTH PROMOTION AND PREVENTIVE MEDICINE

The following list, while not exhaustive, provides a wide range of online sources of information that may assist readers in seeking out resources in their local area, or even from other countries of interest.

Australian Curriculum Framework for Junior Doctors
www.cpmec.org.au/Page/acfjd-project

Royal Australasian College of Physicians
www.racp.edu.au/page/physician-ducation/curriculum

ACT Department of health, Australia
www.healthpromotion.act.gov.au

Australian Health Promotion Association
www.healthpromotion.com.au

Australian Institute of Health and Welfare
www.aihw.gov.au

Department of Health, Western Australia
www.health.wa.gov.au

Drug Info Clearinghouse (2006) for useful fact Sheets on Community Development and Health Promotion, Australia
www.druginfo.adf.org.au

HEALTH*Insite*, Australia
www.healthinsite.gov.au

Healthway, Australia
www.healthway.wa.gov.au

HP 101 Health Promotion online course, Canada
www.ohprs.ca/hp101/main.htm

Planning Tools, Australia
http://som.flinders.edu.au/FUSA/SACHRU/PEW/index.htm

Public Health Association of Australia
www.phaa.net.au

Theory at a Glance: A guide for Health Promotion Practice (2nd ed)
www.nci.nih.gov/PDF/481f5d53–63df-41bc-bfaf-5aa48ee1da4d/TAAG3.pdf

World Health Organization
www.who.int

VicHealth, Australia
www.health.vic.gov.au/healthpromotion

Agency for Healthcare Research and Quality (AHRQ), USA
www.ahrq.gov

Association of Teachers of Preventive Medicine, USA
www.atpm.org

Health Resources and Services Administration, USA
www.hrsa.gov

Alliance for Academic Internal Medicine, USA
www.im.org/Pages/default.aspx

Alliance for Clinical Education, USA
www.allianceforclinicaleducation.org/

Ambulatory Pediatrics Association, USA
www.ambpeds.org/

American Academy on Physician and Patient, USA
www.physicianpatient.org

Association of Professors of Gynecology and Obstetrics, USA
www.apgo.org/index.htm

American Medical Student Association, USA
www.amsa.org

Association for Surgical Education, USA
www.surgicaleducation.com

Association of Preventive Medicine Residents, USA
www.acpm.org/apmr.htm

Clerkship Directors in Internal Medicine, USA
www.im.org/About/AllianceSites/CDIM/Pages/Default.aspx

Put Prevention into Practice (PPIP), USA
www.ahrq.gov/PPIP/

Society of Behavioral Medicine, USA
www.sbm.org/

Society of Teachers of Family Medicine, USA
www.stfm.org

Guide to Community Preventive Services, USA
www.thecommunityguide.org

All of the online resources described or listed above have both merit and limitations, and it is hoped that within a year a dedicated health promotion and medical and health professional website will be operational.[12] (*See* 'An active-feedback consortium and development process' later in this chapter.) A transparent peer-review process will be in place to provide users with guidance about resources, research papers, books, current concerns such as inequalities and the WHO report on the social determinants of health[13] and how the debates about such reports are developing.[14]

CONTEXT, CONTEXT AND CONTEXT!

Medicine is practiced, and taught, at a very local level. The need to ensure that students and teachers relate to local resources and social context is paramount to enable health promotion to be effective. Public transport, leisure facilities, average income and educational attainment, language for the majority and access to food and other material essentials need to be assessed, with professionals having cognisance of what is good and pragmatic advice, for example.

It has been seen that some communities can experience various levels of health and well-being regardless of material wealth.[15] Yet, equally, an apparently wealthy community can have people living in privation, poorly resourced and out of kilter with the overall population's health promotion needs. The agencies and charities that work with the underserved are frequently an excellent source of information for professionals, learners and teachers on the needs of the communities they serve, and can work in partnership with professionals.

In Melbourne, Monash Medical School's Community Partnership Program (CPP) is a significant provider of educational experiences for medical students, and the designated tutors that supervise students whilst on placements undertaking various projects, themselves become more aware of the needs of local people.[16] For many students, working with the homeless, with refugees, with people with addictions and reflecting on their health needs is a new and enlightening experience. Students can explore:

➤ why an individual might be in this situation
➤ the antecedents and determinants
➤ the barriers to change
➤ the options to improve health
➤ the role of healthcare professionals in these circumstances.

The opportunities for students in other medical faculties may be less sophisticated and involved than the CCP, yet in the public hospitals and the primary care clinics, students will encounter patients whose circumstances require a social history and a more thoughtful approach to any health promotion action.

AN ACTIVE-FEEDBACK CONSORTIUM AND DEVELOPMENT PROCESS

A proposed new website, www.med.monash.edu.au/hpipe/index.html will be hosted by Monash University in partnership with King's College London, with a small working party setting it up. It will have a section for educators, institutions and students. In the resources section there will be:

➤ health promotion repository
➤ education
➤ research
➤ links
➤ news.

There will be a section on partners and one for contributors, including the options to contribute, to be a peer reviewer and to be a member. The quality and value of the site will be part of a shared development process; it will be open and inclusive, with clear criteria for those contributing and clear information for users about resources, research and other materials. The partners intend to provide members with free access to teaching resources such as a multimedia smoking cessation and behavioural change teaching pack, with the anticipation that users will also provide constructive feedback on aspects of the resource. Finally we hope to use the BEME model to guide us in the development process.

Such a venture is urgently needed as many health professional courses and medical schools will be increasing their health promotion input in response to the current health priorities and to enable future professionals to be skilled and knowledgeable in health promotion, seeing it as relevant to their professional role.

REFERENCES

1 Ewles L, Simnett I. *Promoting Health: A Practical Guide*. 5th ed. Edinburgh: Bailliere Tindall; 2003.
2 Wylie A. Health promotion in general practice. In: Stephenson A, editor. *A Textbook of General Practice*. 2nd ed. London: Arnold; 2004.
3 Wakefield AJ, Murch SH, Anthony A, *et al*. Ileal-lymphoid-nodular hyperplasia, non-specific colitis and pervasive developmental disorder in children. *Lancet*. 1998; 351(9103): 611–2.
4 Department of Health. *The Pregnancy Book*. London: Department of Health; 2007.

5 Department of Health. *The Birth to Five Book*. London: Department of Health; 2007.

6 Department of Health. *Healthy Weight Healthy Lives: a cross government strategy for England*. London: Department of Health; 2008.

7 Foucault M. *The Birth of the Clinic: an archaeology of medical perception*. London: Tavistock; 1973.

8 Gibbs Trevor J. 'Time to have your say': AMEE Guide supplements. *Med Teach*. 2008; **30**(4): 345–6.

9 Spencer J. ABC of learning and teaching in medicine: learning and teaching in the clinical environment. *BMJ*. 2003; **326**(7389): 591–4.

10 Mitchell H. Vaginal discharge: causes, diagnosis and treatment. *BMJ*. 2004; **328**(7451): 1306–8.

11 Coleman T. Cessation interventions in routine health care. *BMJ*. 2004; **328**(7440): 631–3.

12 Holt T, Wylie A, Soethout MBM. Implementing a virtual international network of health promotion in interprofessional education (HPIPE). *Conference proceedings at the AMEE Conference*. 2008 Sep 2; Prague; 8AD.

13 Representatives of the Civil Society to the Commission on Social Determinants of Health of the World Health Organization. Civil Society Report to the Commission on Social Determinants of Health. *Soc Med*. 2007; **2**(4): 192–211.

14 Davey Smith G, Krieger N. Tackling health inequities. Editorial. *BMJ*. 2008; **337** (Sep 3): a1526.

15 Marks N, Sims A, Thompson S, *et al*. *The Happy Planet Index: an index of human well-being and environmental impact*. London: New Economics Foundation; 2006.

16 Holt T, Goodall J, Jones KV, *et al*. Community-based medical professionalism: learning by doing. In: *Proceedings of the 13th International Ottawa Conference on Clinical Competence*; 2008 Mar 5–8; Melbourne, Australia: pp. 469–72.

PART FIVE

Assessment and pragmatism: relevance to wider learning, student needs and equitable opportunities

INTRODUCTION
Brian Jolly

This book is about health promotion as a core component of competence for all health professionals. This section deals with the assessment of this area of competence.

In many ways 'the doctor', at least in Western hierarchically organised healthcare systems, is regarded as having potentially the most influence over us, the public, in helping us take more responsibility for our own health. So doctors need to take health promotion seriously. The traditional means to address the importance of any curriculum content has been through emphasising its presence in the assessment regime, usually in a system of examinations designed to reflect the state of students' minds at critical points in the course (*see* Chapter 9). However, effective health promotion, as we see in earlier chapters, is a long, complex and, necessarily, team-focussed process that does not lend itself easily to encapsulation in an examination, especially at the top (performance) end of Miller's pyramid (*see* page 255).

Traditionally, health promotion content has been delivered in elective, selective or optional parts of the curriculum, and this further complicates its assessment. For example, as Rigby and Boursicot point out in Chapter 18, whilst 'special study modules' (SSMs) in UK undergraduate medical education generally receive positive feedback, emphasis on the assessment can distract students from the learning experience. And, as Mehta and Wylie point out in Chapter 19, for this reason, it is prudent to ask why we are asking students to learn about health promotion before planning the assessment regime. Externally developed SSMs can deliver generic skills that might be helpful even beyond health promotion boundaries, but students see them as time-consuming and inhibiting their attention to other parts of the curriculum.[1,2]

In my view, the process of blueprinting the assessment to the objectives and outcomes of the course would help considerably here.[3] However the results of this process are not likely to be a written examination framework, or even an objective structured clinical examination (OSCE). It would probably result in identifying project reports, fieldwork analyses and interventional studies as the most sensible additions to the assessment strategies; in fact precisely the sort of work that takes health promotion experts many months and years to accomplish. Relying on examinations and OSCEs may adequately assess a few of the subskills required (and perhaps some of the positive attitudes required to encourage engagement in health promotional activities), but will not reflect the essential expertise required. The OSCE can reflect the extent to which a student can incorporate an appropriate orientation to health promotion within aspects of clinical activities such as history taking, physical examination and informed consent, but it probably will not get to the heart of the matter.

So what will? As Mehta says in Chapter 21:

> Giving students the time and space to critically evaluate the project they have studied will allow them to draw wider conclusions about the discipline and will draw future generations of doctors into the debate.

This will require some considerable change to curricula which the traditional disciplines will resist, at least until the evidence emerges that health promotion is the most cost-effective way to reduce healthcare burdens, and that teaching health promotion to professionals as undergraduates is an effective way to prepare them for this role. And although this evidence may never become clear, given the complexity of doing these types of research, increasing emphasis on health promotion may become a political imperative once governments realise that it is actually considerably cheaper than interventions for chronic disease management.

This section uses a great many examples of educational and assessment innovations from the UK experience. It is therefore pertinent to ask how these ideas can be utilised in areas of the world that need them most, at both undergraduate level and beyond. For example, the UK health promotion community should take a lead and look carefully at the impact that students can have on health problems in a coordinated, team-based way. For example, using interprofessional assessed electives or selectives,[4] long-term projects and assessed themes through the curriculum for a student subgroup, all motivated and intent on delivering appropriately designed assessment outcomes, may be one way forward, even if it allows the majority of students only a cursory glance through the glass darkly. Building specialty interests at postgraduate level in health promotion issues has already had some success outside the traditional academic environments, usually through charitable trusts such as the British Heart Foundation and Andrology Australia. It is a question of harnessing these opportunities to move forward, both in assessment and in curriculum.

REFERENCES

1 Murdoch-Eaton D, Jolly B. Undergraduate projects: do they have to be within the conventional medical environment? *Med Educ.* 2000; 34(2): 95–100.

2 Yates MS, Drewery S, Murdoch-Eaton D. Alternative learning environments: what do they contribute to professional development? *Med Teach.* 2002; **24**(6): 609–15.

3 Hamdy H. Blueprinting for the assessment of health care professionals. *Clin Teach.* 2006; 3(3): 175–9.

4 Jolly B. A missed opportunity. *Med Educ.* 2009; 43(2): 104–5.

CHAPTER 18

Assessment in high-stakes vocational courses: some principles and problems

Emily Rigby and Kathy Boursicot

THE APPROACHES TO ASSESSMENT

Although a number of educational programmes have non-examinable assessment procedures, most vocational programmes, especially in healthcare, will have substantial weighting on formal examinations. Such weighting shifts in line with modern educational theory and evidence about reliability and validity, as well as other factors such as cost and capacity.[1]

Examinations such as objective structured clinical examinations (OSCE)[2] are costly for medical schools and health professional faculties yet since they were developed and introduced they have become applied in a highly reliable manner to test skill and clinical competence.[3-5]

Computer-marked short answers and multiple-choice questions have also become reliable formats and are an efficient and cost-effective way of examining knowledge. Because of the large volume of questions and students taking these examinations, reliability tests can be done to explore how students compare and which questions should be retained or omitted for future examination papers.

In addition to examinations, students will have other forms of assessments, often referred to as in-course assessment and/or hurdle requirements as students are required to reach a satisfactory standard in each of the assessment components to progress. Most schools have log book sign-ups, which indicate the student has demonstrated a specific skill, professional behaviour or has been observed doing clinical work to a satisfactory level. The challenge here is consistency between clinical teacher assessors and having acceptable procedures in each school for auditing and checking the log books. Long essays, portfolios and presentations continue to form part of the overall approach to assessment but like the log book are subject to greater variability dependent on a large number of assessors often seeing a small number of assignments. Second marking and moderating are the usual ways of assessing consistency and reliability. Yet these forms of assessment are central to the student demonstrating higher level knowledge, skills and attitudes, complex concepts and critical reflection and analysis. Within the field of health promotion assessment will be both via formal examinations and in-course assessment.

Assessment within vocational courses ultimately enables students to progress to their future career. In the case of medicine, final examinations certify competence as a doctor. These exams must be rigorous and fit for purpose as passing an incompetent student could have a disastrous effect on patient safety. Additionally, they must also be a just and fair judgement of abilities as students have dedicated up to six years and tens of thousands of pounds to their study.

The judgement of what is necessary to have competence as a medical practitioner within the UK is determined by the General Medical Council (GMC).[6] Medical schools undergo inspection and review to ensure that the education delivered supplies able doctors for service.[7] Standards for undergraduates are outlined in *Tomorrow's Doctors*, and achieving these set outcomes is deemed essential for *good medical practice* throughout a future career. Whilst the GMC is legally responsible for verifying the competence of doctors, there are pressures and assumptions that are made from several areas.

The public rightly assume a competence of their doctors. Over recent times, patients have increasing expectations of what should be included in their healthcare – including attitudes and approach in addition to drugs and interventions. Education must be appropriate to enable practitioners to adapt to provide the care that individual members of the public expect and require.

Medicine is a rapidly changing field and there are many diverse aspects competing for priority and funding. The education of these subjects is similarly competitive. Certain aspects of medical education are considered as 'core' skills, which are essential for competence as a licensed clinician. However, other specific knowledge or skills, whilst desirable, are not essential *per se*, or can be acquired through an assortment of experiences. All doctors will have a variety of different additional skills, which add to the diversity and aid in progress in the field overall.

The GMC has accounted for these additional skills through the introduction of student selected components (SSCs) whereby students can investigate areas of interest and hone skills outside the dictated curriculum. Acceptable standards are still expected within SSCs; they contribute to the medical degree and therefore assessment of competence as a doctor, but their exact content will be different for each individual.

In addition to the national requirements that are enforced by the GMC, there is a growing international dimension to medical education. Legislation exists (93/16/CEE) which enables any individual awarded a medical degree within the EU to work anywhere in the EU. Thus, the standards considered appropriate by one country have to automatically be accepted by other European countries. Initiatives exist which are attempting to unite education throughout Europe. For example:

➤ The Bologna Process – a pledge by European countries to reform higher education in a convergent way
➤ The Tuning project – a competency framework
➤ The World Medical Federation for Medical Education: Global Standards for Medical Education – standards of medical education and quality improvement standards.

Students study for many years at an increasingly high cost and therefore expect an education which is adequate in securing future employment – both in the UK and further afield.

Once the curriculum is decided, it must be appropriately assessed. Assessment must be rigorous – both reliable and valid. This is necessary to validate the licensing of competent practitioners. Examinations at the end of undergraduate medical courses are supposed to guarantee that competent students graduate and are then granted a licence to practise by the GMC. The purpose of such examinations is to allow those who are fit to enter clinical practice and prevent those not yet fit to practise from causing harm. Final examinations in particular are therefore important, high-stakes examinations for students, and false negatives, or failing the competent, need to be avoided. Similarly, false positives or passing the incompetent, are clearly unacceptable when aiming to provide safe, effective patient care. Examinations must be reliable, demonstrating precision and reproducibility in assessing students' abilities. They must also be valid, accurately demonstrating students' competence in clinical practice.

Miller proposed a framework for assessment of clinical competence[8] (*see* Figure 18.1). The lowest level of assessment addresses a student's factual knowledge – what they *know*. The next level assesses competence – what a student *knows how* to do, followed by performance, or when a student *shows how* they complete a task. The final level is *does*, which focuses on action in practice rather than in an artificial test situation. Valid, reliable assessment at this level is the ultimate goal as it gives an accurate reflection of competence in real situations. Aptitude at all levels is however essential for overall competence and assessment must therefore cover all aspects of competence.[9]

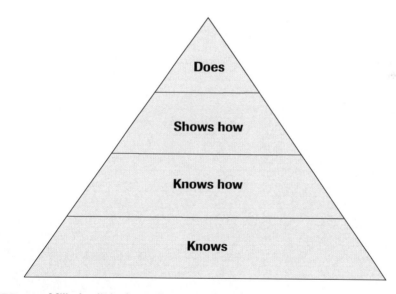

FIGURE 18.1 Miller's clinical competence pyramid

Medical schools utilise a variety of assessment methods to determine competence. These are tailored to the nature of different subjects in addition to the importance of areas of knowledge. Crucial knowledge or expertise may be assessed at a number of stages, whereby a certain level must be achieved to attain competence to pass and are therefore considered core. Additional material or transferable skills may only be gauged through formative assessment or less rigorous testing.

Grab the students by the tests and their hearts and minds will follow.

Swanson & Case 1997[10]

Assessment has been demonstrated to drive learning[10] and there must therefore be consideration of the impact of assessment choice on knowledge acquisition. Competence is content-specific and proficiency in one subject area is not predictive of ability in another. Therefore, assessment must be wide-ranging, covering all necessary skills for safe patient care. It must also be appropriate to the facets of competence being assessed, which include attitudes and communication in addition to skills and knowledge acquisition.

Assessment drives learning and in turn is responsible for the learning experience. Assessment should therefore be appropriate, enhancing the obtainment of clinical competencies. If assessment is not judged as appropriate, it may have a negative impact on learning experiences. For example, all students are required to undertake special study modules (SSMs) to develop learning skills and cultivate areas of interest outside the core curriculum.[11] SSMs are often assessed utilising standardised pro forma based on generic, transferable skills to account for the diverse projects undertaken.[12] However, whilst SSMs generally receive positive feedback, drive towards the assessment aspect potentially distracts from the learning experience, negating some of the positive effects it can have.[13] This provides an example of how striving for a reliable, valid assessment can stifle learning – and thus the assessment itself is restricting the acquisition of knowledge that it is attempting to test. Therefore, assessment must be as congruent to what is planned, taught to and learnt by students in order to achieve most benefit and be fit for purpose (Figure 18.2).

Achieving an appropriate balance between core and additional subjects and the degree to which they are assessed is therefore a challenge. Essential core topics must be included, but if overemphasised can stifle the acquisition of dynamic skills and abilities gained through alternative study. Conversely, overassessing non-core material may not only reduce knowledge of core material but may have a negative impact on the actual knowledge gained.

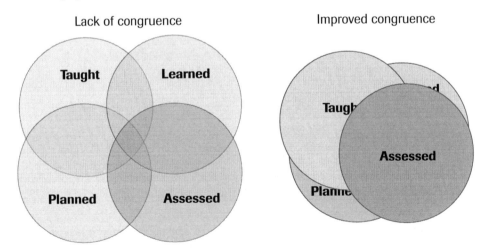

FIGURE 18.2 Relationship between assessment and taught, learnt and planned curriculum (from Fowell *et al.* 1999[12]). Optimising congruence between facets

HEALTH PROMOTION: ASSESSMENT AND INCONSISTENCIES

What is the standard required for each year during the undergraduate phase and what is the standard required for qualification is less easy to define within schools and between schools. With regard to this emerging discipline of health promotion there are substantial challenges. Boursicot, *et al.* (2004) tested six OSCE stations in five medical schools with final year students and found variability with all six stations but most variability was demonstrated with a smoking cessation OCSE station.[14] The reason for this was the variability in emphasis placed on smoking cessation teaching in the different schools.

What is to be examined within the broad field of health promotion and how best to examine is still part of the debate. Roddy *et al.*, for example, would expect medical students to have basic brief intervention skills for smoking cessation[15] but the capacity to teach this will vary and some would argue as to whether the qualifying doctor needs this skill. Behaviour-change skills in clinical one-to-one settings may seem reasonable skills to have for qualifying health professionals, being able to use evidence-based approaches with patients and or make suitable referrals. However such approaches are not universally practised by health professionals, the evidence is challenged and students may have inconsistent, contradictory or no experience of best practice during their student placements.[16,17] Even students who have had focused teaching on smoking cessation may not appreciate the transferability of these techniques to other behaviour-change situations.

Whilst the general practice setting in the UK has enhanced its health-promotion activity – this being linked to the Quality and Outcomes Framework and financial reward – their engagement with NICE guidance for weight management, for example, is suboptimum[18] and given that 15% of medical education in UK medical schools is based in general practice, students will not observe best practice.[19] Yet within their formal teaching sessions, lecture notes and other learning activities they will be expected to know why obesity is a risk factor for health, critique the evidence and the epidemiology as well as be aware of intervention options. There will be a theory–practice gap and under the pressure of examinations student may perform poorly. For medical educators and assessors there is a dilemma – could a student 'fail' because of a health promotion-related assessment? Hopefully not, and hence health promotion, like other challenging fields that are now core in curricula such as ethics, communication skills and professionalism need to ensure assessment approaches are a mix of examination and in-course assessment. This recognises and accepts that there is a dynamic process of change.

ASSESSMENT OPTIONS FOR HEALTH PROMOTION

Being pragmatic is essential given the amount of assessment students have and indeed the GMC's advice in *Tomorrow's Doctors* against excessive assessment.[20] Yet students are also pragmatists and if they judge the time spent working on a topic to be valuable and relevant to their success in examinations they will engage; if not, they will do the minimum necessary. Such efficiency is strategically beneficial to the student's health and well-being. It is therefore to important to link the health promotion content to relevant other teaching, using integrated and maximised assessment options with clarity about learning outcomes. Assessment falls into two main strands: in-course assessment, which may be formative and formal, summative examinations. Examples of the types of assessment instruments often used in these strands are given in Table 18.1.

TABLE 18.1 Examples of assessment options for in-course and formal examinations

In-course assessment	Formal examination
Presentation	Objective structured clinical examination
Poster	Computer-marked question papers
Essay/dissertation/report	Short answer written examination
Production – e.g. leaflet/DVD	
Portfolio	

In-course assessment at various stages of the students' undergraduate programme enables discrete learning events to be assessed.

Presentations are useful throughout undergraduate programmes and may also be beneficial to the assessors. For example students may present their evaluation of a local campaign to increase vaccination uptake to a primary care team. This would enable students to do a local needs assessment and epidemiological studies and explore factors influencing parents' decisions about vaccination. The work may also involve students considering or applying for ethics committee approval. The presentation is assessed but constructive feedback from assessors enables students to identify ongoing learning needs.

However, assessors, unless they are specialists in public health and health promotion, may be less familiar with the health promotion field and specifically evaluation methodology, than the students, given the students have engaged with the discipline. The assessors may be impressed with the quality of the presentation and the students' style but overall they may focus on the students' knowledge about herd immunity rather than their ability to evaluate the intervention campaign. It will be necessary therefore to provide clear guidelines and criteria for assessors and students. A minimum standard has to be reached as defined by the scoring criteria: all students may pass if they reach this standard but some may fail; ongoing quality assurance processes around examinations must ensure the tests are reliable and fair.

A *poster* as part of an information campaign or reporting back on a public health elective is a popular approach given that, like a presentation, criteria for assessors can be devised. Validity of the assessment can be enhanced in that all posters may then form a display for a short period of time, open to faculty and students alike. Skills needed to produce good posters have many benefits for students including learning to be succinct and how to present research at conferences.

A piece of *discursive written work* provides students with the opportunity to critique evidence and to source evidence about health promotion intervention, which will require a wider reading base and searching strategy than a purely scientific assignment. Developing an argument and exploring strengths and weaknesses associated with health promotion theory, evidence and implementation will enable students to use these skills with confidence. How much guidance students need will vary depending on the stage and the topic they are addressing. Students will put considerable effort into their work and anticipate that their assessors will also invest appropriate time in marking their work, as well as providing additional and constructive feedback. The standard-setting for such assessments is time-consuming and there is also a need to define – and make clear to all stakeholders – the range of marks that can be acceptable.

Whilst written work of this type for special study modules is often the preferred option, *essays* written for core curricular assessment may be limited given that many schools have large student cohorts. The capacity to use essays as part of the in-course assessment is highly variable from faculty to faculty and given the need for second marking and possibly moderators, it is unlikely that many schools will be able to undertake such approaches.

Producing a *leaflet* or other health-promoting resource has been part of assessment for a wider project or assignment such as malarial prevention leaflets for a public health elective, or a sexual health services pamphlet for a primary care attachment. Producing the leaflet will require students to have researched the issues concerned, the local needs, health literacy[21] as well as format, design and how to pilot such a simple but valuable resource. They will be able to then critique other information resources and their limitations. As with other in-course assessments, the assessors with need to be provided with clear marking framework and guidelines.

A *portfolio* about a large area of work such as the preparation for an elective can have within it discrete or integrated aspects of public health and health promotion. For example, the elective subject portfolio at King's College School of Medicine is mandatory for students in their penultimate year. They will explore the public health of the country and regions they intend to visit and the public health priorities and challenges, what the social and modifiable determinants of health are and how healthcare is provided, regardless of whether they are visiting a developed or developing country. In another section they will consider their own health and well-being, as they prepare for the elective and their early days post qualification: for example, what preventative steps they need to take such as immunisations, what personal health issues they would like to address such as taking more exercise and where to get reliable sources of health advice. A third option in the portfolio is to do a public health or health promotion research project whilst doing the elective. The portfolio would include the research question(s) or areas, the methods, the ethical approval and the plans. Such students would seek additional supervision for this.

It is not surprising that there has been increased attention and concern about how well equipped students are to deal with the plethora of health promotion issues they will encounter when newly qualified. Whilst the in-course approaches to assessing health promotion knowledge and skills are preferable to demonstrate student attainment, subjectivity inevitably mars the overall reliability of such approaches. Within increasingly larger student cohorts the capacity to handle in-course assessment is also a limiting factor.

Formal examinations however have become streamlined, with increased confidence in the reliability. Marking is still subject to human error and variability, but computer marking has substantially reduced the error margins and the time frame for managing high-stakes examinations. The challenges for these approaches to assessing health promotion are twofold: first, writing the stations and questions based on the specific defined learning outcomes whereby students have access to lecture notes and teaching materials as well as clinical skills practice for revision; and second, producing the learning materials that are based on facts and skills that are widely accepted and evidence-based.

Writing *OSCE station scenarios* could include a health promotion aspect such as smoking and antenatal screening, use of inhalers and smoking advice, breaking bad news regarding newly diagnosed diabetes or HIV and behaviour change. These might be relevant for final year OSCE stations. For more junior students the station may be solely about skill such as motivational interviewing about a specific behaviour change, or assisting with informed choice such as contraception advice or childhood immunisations. It will need to be clear to the student and the examiner what skills are to be demonstrated.

Writing *multiple-choice questions for computer marking* is challenging. Well-written items will test application of knowledge and critical – for example, diagnostic – skills, not just recall of knowledge. The need to reduce the likelihood of 'a good guess' but to avoid ambiguity is quite a challenge and questions need to be piloted. Like the OSCE the health promotion element may form the central part of the question or may be embedded in another 'topic'. For example, an elderly man with chronic obstructive pulmonary disease is smoking 10–15 cigarettes daily and the question is 'what is the success rate for smoking cessation?' A choice of five options is offered on the answer paper based on recent findings that were highlighted at mandatory symposia during respiratory rotation, or an elderly care placement. The question could be one of a series related to the management of such patients.

The contested nature of health promotion restricts the knowledge-type question that usually appears in written computer-marked papers.

LINKING ASSESSMENT TO BEST PRACTICE

Increasingly NICE guidance and *British Medical Journal* learning modules are harvesting best evidence relating to health promotion and public health issues, enabling examination questions to be drawn from a recognised and respected source, and one that teachers can be aware of to refer to when working with students in clinical practice.

These newer developments enable medical educators, assessors, teachers and practitioners to be lifelong learners and therefore role models for students. As noted in other parts of this book, many health professionals who are now teachers will have had limited formal education around the topic of health promotion, and public health has been marginal in curricula for some time. As this changes, not only do curricula have to reflect best practice in health promotion for current health professional undergraduate programmes, but also teachers and assessors must put in place assessment that is robust, relevant and acceptable to all the various protagonists.

REFERENCES

1 Schuwirth LWT, van der Vleuten CPM. *How to Design a Useful Test: the principles of assessment.* Edinburgh: Association for the Study of Medical Education; 2006. Available at: www.asme.org.uk/publications/understanding-medical-education.html (accessed 7 November 2009).
2 Harden RM, Gleeson FA. Assessment of clinical competence using an objective structured clinical examination (OSCE). *Med Educ.* 1979; **13**(1): 41–54.
3 Boursicot KAM, Roberts TE, Burdick WP. *OSCEs and Other Assessments of Clinical Competence.* Edinburgh: Association for the Study of Medical Education; 2007.
4 Davis MH. OSCE: the Dundee experience. *Med Teach.* 2003; **25**(3): 255–61.
5 Newble D. Techniques for measuring clinical competence: objective structured clinical examinations. *Med Educ.* 2004; **38**(2): 199–203.
6 General Medical Council. *Undergraduate Education.* Available at: www.gmc-uk.org/education/undergraduate.asp (accessed 7 November 2009).

7 General Medical Council. *Quality Assurance of Undergraduate Education.* Available at: www.gmc-uk.org/education/undergraduate/undergraduate_qa.asp (accessed 7 November 2009).

8 Miller GE. The assessment of clinical skills/competence/performance. *Acad Med.* 1990; **65**(9 Suppl.): S63–7.

9 Wass V, van der Vleuten CPM, Shatzer J, *et al.* Assessment of clinical competence. *Lancet.* 2001; **357**: 945–9.

10 Swanson D, Case S. Assessment in basic health science instruction: directions for practice and research. *Adv Health Sci Educ.* 1997; **2**(1): 71–84.

11 General Medical Council. *Tomorrow's Doctors.* London: General Medical Council; 1993.

12 Fowell S, Southgate L, Bligh J. Evaluating assessment: the missing link? *Med Educ.* 1999; **33**(4): 276–81.

13 Yates MS, Drewery S, Murdoch-Eaton D. Alternative learning environments: what do they contribute to professional development? *Med Teach.* 2002; **24**(6): 609–15.

14 Boursicot KAM, Roberts TE, Pell G. Standard setting for clinical competence at graduation from medical school: is it possible to achieve consensus? Presentation to the annual general meeting of the Association for the Study of Medical Education; Liverpool; 2004.

15 Roddy E, Rubin P, Britton J. A study of smoking and smoking cessation on the curricula of UK medical schools. *Tob Control.* 2004 (March); **13**(*et al.*Lough M, Brown M. An exploration of the knowledge, attitudes and practice of members of the primary care team in relation to smoking and smoking cessation in later life. *Prim Health Care Res Dev.* 2007; **8**(1): 68–79.

16 Kerr S, Watson H, Tolson D, *et al.* An exploration of the knowledge, attitudes and practice of members of the primary care team in relation to smoking and smoking cessation in later life. *Prim Health Care Res Dev.* 2007; **8**(1): 68–79.

17 Vogt F, Hall S, Marteau TM. General practitioners' and family physicians' negative beliefs and attitudes towards discussing smoking cessation with patients: a systematic review. *Addiction.* 2005; **100**(10): 1423–31.

18 National Institute for Health and Clinical Excellence. *Obesity: the prevention, identification, assessment and management of overweight and obesity in adults and children: NICE guideline 43.* London: NICE; 2006. http://guidance.nice.org.uk/CG43

19 Marteau T, Dieppe P, Foy R, *et al.* Behavioural medicine: changing our behaviour. *BMJ.* 2006; **332**(7539): 437–8.

20 General Medical Council. *Tomorrow's Doctors.* 2nd ed. London: General Medical Council; 2003.

21 Colledge A, Car J, Donnelly A, *et al.* Health information for patients: time to look beyond patient information leaflets. *J Roy Soc Med.* 2008; **101**(9): 447–53.

CHAPTER 19

Assessing health promotion learning outcomes: what is assessable?

Nisha Mehta and Ann Wylie

WHY IS HEALTH PROMOTION ASSESSMENT IMPORTANT AND CHALLENGING?

Emerging epidemics of chronic diseases and unhealthy lifestyles are important public health challenges in the new millennium. At the same time, a shift in the health agenda from a focus on 'making disease better' to 'maintaining health' has led to what has been described as a 'social turn', in which consideration of the socioeconomic, cultural and political forces which underpin the determinants of health are of paramount importance to the healthcare professions.[1] Since the World Health Organization (WHO) 1986 Ottawa Charter helped establish health promotion as an academic discipline,[2] the language of health promotion subsequently became familiar to both central policy makers and front-line healthcare professionals, and in 1993 the UK's General Medical Council (GMC) emphasised the importance of these subjects within the curriculum and committed all medical schools to rewarding students for their knowledge of community-based care, health promotion and public health.[3] The rationale behind the implementation of health promotion in curricula has been discussed in detail in earlier chapters. In this chapter, we describe and critically evaluate methods of assessment of health promotion in the undergraduate medical curriculum, illustrating our analysis with case studies from two medical schools which have made significant progress in raising the profile of health promotion within their own curricula.

In spite of clear guidance from the GMC, a commitment to health promotion by the World Federation for Medical Education in the Edinburgh Declaration, 1988[4] and a great deal of goodwill from many UK medical schools, it remains the case that implementation of successful health promotion teaching and assessment in undergraduate curricula has been far from uniformly successful. In 2002 the GMC reported that although the majority of medical schools had implemented the key recommendations contained in *Tomorrow's Doctors*, satisfactory health promotion teaching and assessment in curricula was still lacking in many instances.[5] There are several reasons for this, not least that the contested definition of this relatively new eclectic discipline, with an emerging epistemology, makes it difficult to create a core curriculum in the subject, leaving it vulnerable to exclusion from overcrowded curricula.[6] The best method of assessment of such a disparate and poorly defined subject remains a vexed question for medical educationalists. Furthermore, there are insufficient teachers who are suitably qualified or willing to teach health promotion.[7] These problems are root causes of the GMC observation about the relative lack of progress in health promotion teaching and assessment in many UK medical schools.

APPROACHES TO ASSESSMENT

Health promotion, such that it does currently exist within curricula, has been implemented as either a 'vertical theme' taught in an opportunistic manner at suitable points throughout the course, or offered in the form of one or more stand-alone modules within courses.[6] Opportunistic teaching may be effective, and has been shown to be assessable in objective marking using the objective structured clinical examination (OSCE) with good results. Roseby, *et al.* delivered a health promotion adolescent smoking cessation seminar to a group of Year 5 medical students in their paediatrics rotation and compared them to a control group who did not receive the seminar. The intervention cohort were significantly more likely (p=0.0001) to ask about smoking during a subsequent OSCE station with a 15-year-old patient with poorly controlled asthma. They were also significantly more likely (p=0.0004) to offer smoking cessation advice in the examination.[8]

It would seem that opportunistic health promotion teaching has merit, but it does not necessarily provide students with the tools to be able to apply the principles of health promotion to any given scenario. Indeed, this approach runs the risk of the student remembering to discuss smoking with patients during forthcoming assessments, but without fully comprehending the health promotion implications of this long after the learning from the seminar has faded. Even for those students who retain the main learning objectives and skills, the danger is that they relate it to that specific scenario or very similar rather than seeing it as applicable in a wider context. Final-year students at King's College London (KCL) recently reported that they could remember their smoking cessation seminar from Year 3 but were less sure about how to apply the generic principles of brief intervention and motivational interviewing for other health-risk behaviour modification. Of course the teaching may be very effective but reliance on simplistic evaluation, using OSCE assessment to link cause and effect, is of limited value.

For many reasons the OSCE has become a standard feature in medical and health professional assessment and as such should also include elements of health promotion assessment, but additional assessment approaches are also necessary either to wholly assess health promotion or to assess health promotion within other aspects of student examinations.

For this reason, when considering assessment approaches, it is prudent to ask why we are asking students to learn about health promotion. In a vocational and overcrowded course, what professional skills and attitudes do we wish to impart and assess? It seems that a stand-alone approach to health promotion within curricula may be preferable to ensure satisfactory engagement with what are novel and often difficult concepts and definitions. A brief overview of the approach to teaching and assessment taken by two different medical schools that have successfully established health promotion as an obvious and integral part of the curriculum is helpful for a discussion about assessment approaches. Our observations and conclusions are informed by qualitative data from individual semi-structured interviews with senior medical students from these universities.

KING'S COLLEGE LONDON AND HEALTH PROMOTION ASSESSMENT

At KCL, health promotion teaching and assessment aims are to give students 'the knowledge and skills to promote healthy behaviour change in their patients through the use of evidence-based interventions; and an awareness of the range, impact, and potential of community health promotion interventions, and some knowledge of how they can be used as part of patient care.[7] Health promotion teaching at KCL consists of core lectures and symposia, a community study and skills acquisition in clinical attachments supplemented by a variety of optional special study modules (SSMs) throughout the course that offer students the opportunity to explore the subject in greater depth. The structure of the course is such that all students will have some exposure to health promotion through compulsory elements, but there are ample opportunities for those who are interested to pursue the topic further under enthusiastic and committed supervision from medical school staff or staff at local specialist health promotion agencies such as Health First.[9]

A range of assessment approaches for core curriculum are used and described below but given the number of students (about 420 in each cohort) and the need to avoid excessive assessment, the health promotion elements are, where possible, linked to computer-marked assessment methods.

1 The first-year students have questions related to their 'What is good health' symposium integrated into written computer-marked papers. Multiple-choice questions (MCQs), extended matching questions (EMQs) and single best answer (SBAs) questions are used. They test factual knowledge related to the lecture notes and presentation, such as health data and definitions of health.
2 A similar approach is used in Phase 3 following a seminar related to a therapeutics strand. The seminar looks at non-pharmacological interventions in a clinical context for behavioural change and motivational interviewing. The sessions use a multi-media teaching pack and role play, and are directly related to the clinical rotations students will have had. Weight reduction, smoking cessation and alcohol awareness are used in the role-play scenarios. There are between five and six questions integrated into two three-hour written papers and focus is on skill to identify evidence of effectiveness on interventions (MCQs), when to intervene (EMQ) and what strategies are appropriate (SBAs).
3 In Phase 4 the health promotion content is greater and forms part of three elements on the phase programme. The community study is the only longitudinal study the students have where they follow a patient from late pregnancy to the third month of the child's life. The students do a presentation in pairs of the 'case' together with about six to seven pairs of students at the end of the year, in a community setting with their assigned seminar leader. This assesses their abilities to appreciate the complex interplay of psychosocial and health factors on the health experiences of women and their families, including contraception choices, place of birth, antenatal health issues and concerns such as vaginal bleeding and smoking, postnatal issues, family dynamics, income and work/childcare issues, infant feeding, infant healthcare and immunisation decisions. By presenting with other pairs of students, they are able to appreciate the need to consider each woman's experiences as unique, they

reflect on their developing communication skills in sensitive areas and the value of other agencies in the contribution to health and well-being.

At the same time students are assigned to a health promotion coordinator who facilitates students in pairs or small groups in doing a review of a community-based health promotion intervention. Students do a presentation of this review to their GP practice team, with the additional underlying brief to consider the probable impact of the intervention on the practice population. The assessment enables the student to demonstrate their ability to critique health promotion evidence and evaluation.

As part of the SSM but also part of core curriculum students do an elective portfolio, which covers various aspects of their planned elective which they do at the start of their final year. This is marked by their clinical advisor, who will have about eight assigned advisees, with a random selection being blind second-marked. A section on personal health, well-being and safety, about 1000 words, is required. Personal and sensitive information is not required although if students do want to give details they may. Usually we want students to demonstrate they have looked critically at their own health and health-related behaviour, the antecedents to any health-damaging behaviour and realistic plans for improvement. They dominate the section, however, with the pragmatics related to their forthcoming elective such as protection against disease, safety issues, emergency options such as needle-stick injury, money, access to help, the public health situation and Foreign and Commonwealth Office guidance. Students are given guidance and lecture notes, symposia and tutorials as needed. End-of-year OSCEs will have health promotion elements in two or four stations of a 22-station OSCE.

4   In the final year, students during their GP placement of eight weeks will demonstrate their abilities to clinically manage and appropriately refer patients, integrating and using the health promotion skills and knowledge base they have acquired. They may also do a health promotion focused SSM whilst in GP placement, but this is optional. The GP completes a formative and summative assessment with the student on all aspects of the GP placement including their applied health promotion activities. There are similar arrangements for the final-year OSCE as in Phase 4.

The in-course assessment in Phase 4, the two presentations and the portfolio, must be satisfactory for students to progress, although worth a small percentage of the whole. With written papers and OSCEs student could fail the health promotion elements but still progress. In practice, however, those students who are border-line or fail based on in-course assessment are usually struggling in summative assessments, and so far the situation has not arisen whereby a student has failed to progress because of failure in the health promotion aspects only.

Constant data analysis reviews are done on summative assessments to look at the reliability of questions and examiners. It would also be unusual for significant numbers of students to fail any of the health promotion elements but indeed a normal distribution of marks is one of the indicators of the reliability of the questions used.

These mixed methods of assessment are also pragmatic for the faculty, placing the responsibilities for assessment across a wide number of people without excessive work for a few, but the guidance – to students and assessors – enables assessors to work with predetermined and tested frameworks. As we know, integrated curricula need integrated assessment approaches. Finally, student feedback enables those who feel any aspect of their assessments to be unfair or had mitigating circumstances can raise this with assessment committees themselves or through the student committee. To our knowledge there has only been one student who failed all Phase 3 papers, who also questioned the health promotion-related questions, but no further action was taken.

Assessment of optional SSMs includes dissertations and vivas for library projects, and essays and presentations for practical projects, often carrying out detailed evaluation of health promotion interventions. These are always second-marked and it goes without saying that the teaching and assessment format of SSMs is an excellent way to achieve the aims of the course by giving students the time and space to consider the subject in depth using dedicated SSM time which is separate from the core curriculum. Students who have chosen these options speak highly of their experiences and usually do well, but each year a small number gain minimal pass marks and occasionally there are failures.

An advantage of this approach to teaching and assessment is that although the components of the course are 'stand-alone', they nevertheless form part of a vertical theme running through a 'spiral' curriculum, in which concepts introduced in early years are subsequently developed later in the course, with the assessment incorporating lessons learned in earlier years. Thus, with each exposure, students are increasingly familiar with the subject matter and by the time of their GP rotation in their final year, are able to actively hone their new skills whilst simultaneously being assessed. Practical application of health promotion is an invaluable learning tool and combining it with simultaneous assessment is an excellent way to cement the learning experience. Another advantage of repeated exposure is that any student at any point of the course is able to study the subject further due to the number of SSMs on offer.

Thanks to the efforts of proactive and approachable teaching staff who maintain a high profile through regular emails, lectures and campus notices, it is widely acknowledged within the student body that research and elective opportunities in health promotion are available at the Department of General Practice. Thus the 'compulsory' and 'assessed' elements of the course are, for interested students, merely a 'taster' of a far more comprehensive exposure to the topic that they are easily able to gain during their undergraduate years. For these students, the assessment is not the most important outcome, and an approach in which students are encouraged to move to academic independence allows them a sense of ownership over this part of the course which provides a refreshing contrast to many other aspects of life as a medical student. The net result of this is genuine engagement with the subject, and ultimately a more successful health promotion learning experience.

Relative to other courses, the written assessment burden in health promotion at KCL seems, according to students, deliberately light. This effort to follow the GMC guidelines to reduce the assessment burden in overcrowded curricula is commendable and, as discussed, gives students space for clinical creativity and academic enquiry and is something to be encouraged. However, one drawback of this approach is that those students who are not interested in health promotion find it relatively easy to get through the course without particularly engaging with the teaching on offer. Lack of curriculum space means that for students who choose not to take advantage of optional 'extras', there may not be enough health promotion in the core curriculum to register on their radar. For example, the community study is carried out in pairs, and although each student is required to help with the assessed presentation, it remains the case that a minority of students contribute relatively little to the project, which itself contributes relatively little (5%) to the overall mark for the year. There are also many students whose level of effort is commendable, but for whom the learning experience does not necessarily fall squarely within the territory of health promotion as an academic discipline. Presentations are marked by a wide variety of people, including GPs, some of whom simply do not have the specialist knowledge of the subject to be able to ensure specific learning outcomes are met and discussed on the assessment day (e.g. engagement with theoretical models of health promotion). Although it may logistically be easier said than done, perhaps exchanging one of the many other pieces of written coursework in the curriculum for at least one individual piece of writing solely dedicated to health promotion would go some way towards ameliorating this situation.

The assessments, like the curriculum, are constantly reviewed and modified.

EDINBURGH UNIVERSITY AND HEALTH PROMOTION ASSESSMENT

Health promotion enjoys significant space in the Edinburgh undergraduate medical curriculum. First-year students are given 15 hours of dedicated lectures and tutorials, supplemented by a community practical involving interviews with an older person and GP tutorials, in which students are expected to consider health promotion in a written report. The content of the course is also assessed in depth during end-of-year written examinations using the short answer question (SAQ) format. Health promotion is revisited in Year 3 during a workshop and seminar, although with no formal follow-up assessment at this point, and there is no further formal teaching or assessment at any point in Year 4 and Year 5, although the subject is covered during GP tutorials, communications skills sessions and elsewhere in an opportunistic, ad hoc manner and material from the course may be covered in the final examinations.

We asked senior medical students at Edinburgh University 'What do you think of the way health promotion is assessed in your course?' The feeling amongst three Year 5 students just about to sit their final examinations was that the social sciences part of the course (in which health promotion material is located during Year 1) was too long ago to be useful or relevant to them, and the learning outcomes not directly relevant to their finals. Indeed they did not even distinguish health promotion as distinct from the other elements of their Year 1 'Health and Society' course. Four out of five Years 3 and 4 students unanimously commented that the SAQ examination format in Year 1 was 'a bit artificial' and 'not something that you should be examined on formally: just because I memorised lists and theory then, it does not mean that I can remember it now'. They all argued that an in-course assessment would have been a more useful way of learning and cementing the knowledge that was viewed as potentially valuable and interesting to them. However, the Year 1 community study was not felt to be relevant to health promotion by any of the students, suggesting that a piece of coursework more specifically related to health promotion may be indicated at this stage. All Year 3 and 4 students were in agreement about the value of considering health promotion as part of portfolio case report assessments during the clinical years, and they all believed that consideration of such issues informed their performance in OSCEs during these years.

CONCLUSIONS

Analysis of the KCL and Edinburgh medical curricula, which contain established health promotion courses has identified case-based assessment as an effective method of cementing learning. Some form of in-depth, written coursework has also emerged as a favoured method of assessment. When senior medical students are asked to reflect on their experiences of health promotion assessment, a theme across both medical schools is a desire to engage properly with the subject matter, and to be rewarded for doing so through assessment, rather than to be asked to learn lists, or to negotiate relatively minor health promotion 'hurdles' in order to progress through the course. KCL students who have completed health promotion SSMs feel privileged to have contributed something to the community with their work. This sentiment was echoed by two Edinburgh students who favoured being given the option to complete a detailed health promotion project in place of their student selected component (SSC) in Year 4: 'it would be good to feel like you are doing something useful – you spend so much time in medicine standing around and annoying people!'

Similar observations have been made in Australia where students at Monash Medical School complete self-selected health promotion intervention evaluations in their second year, which form a major part of their core curriculum. Students on this course are very positive about their learning experiences, and valued the challenge of the assessment format, which takes the form of a poster presentation and written report.[10] Monash has prioritised this work, enabling faculty to have the time and resources for assessment. UK medical schools may be able to learn from the Monash model. As well as acknowledging the contribution to deeper learning that project work can provide, assessment also has to be within a faculty's resources. From the experience of working with Monash colleagues, the task of marking projects from all Year 2 students is significant and would not be possible, given the student numbers, at some UK medical schools. Equally, assessment approaches at one medical school, such as Monash, which does not have SSM curriculum time, may have limited practical application in other medical school curricula.

The lessons learnt from our experiences about health promotion and assessment are that we need to be willing to share information about assessment approaches, the limitations and advantages, the practical aspects and the links to theory and best practice within education. This is needed for many aspects of modern integrated medical curricula assessment but is especially relevant for a field such as health promotion, with its emerging epistemology and undefined parameters.

REFERENCES

1 Cribb A. The diffusion of the health agenda and the fundamental need for partnership in medical education. *Med Educ.* 2000; 34(11): 916–20.

2 World Health Organization. *Ottawa Charter for Health Promotion.* Geneva: World Health Organization; 1986.

3 General Medical Council. *Tomorrow's Doctors.* London: General Medical Council; 1993.

4 World Federation on Medical Education. *World Conference on Medical Education: Edinburgh report.* Edinburgh: World Federation on Medical Education; 1988.

5 Christopher DF, Harte K, George CF. The implementation of *Tomorrow's Doctors. Med Educ.* 2002; 36(3): 282–8.

6 Wylie A. *Health Promotion and Medical Education: an exploration of the epistemology and the challenge.* London: King's College; 2003.

7 Wylie A, Thompson S. Establishing health promotion in the modern medical curriculum: a case study. *Med Teach.* 2007; **29**(8): 766–71.

8 Roseby R, Marks MK, Conn J, *et al.* Improving medical student performance in adolescent anti-smoking health promotion. *Med Educ.* 2003; **37**(8): 704–8.

9 National Health Service. *Health First 1992–2008.* Available at: www.healthfirst.org.uk/index. htm (accessed 7 November 2009).

10 Jones KV, Hsu H. Health promotion projects: skill and attitude learning for medical students. *Med Educ.* 1999; **33**(8): 585–91.

CHAPTER 20

Does health promotion teaching make a difference to students, teachers, patients and populations? Where is the evidence?

Nisha Mehta, Aliya Kassam and Ann Wylie

DO WE NEED TO DEMONSTRATE DIFFERENCES?

As we reach the penultimate chapter of this book we have explored the *raison d'être* for health promotion (HP) in curricula and equally we have shared the challenges of establishing and sustaining evidence-based quality health promotion curriculum content.

Making this happen requires tenacity, persistence and champions as well as the cooperation of many other protagonists. Such effort for a topic that could easily be marginalised, is still considered by some as no more than common sense and is contested, has to be justified. The move to learning outcomes in curriculum design enables learning to be assessed, to establish that learners have the knowledge, the skills and attitudes required for examination success which is essential.[1] However, showing students have knowledge and factual recall and are able to do the right thing in an objective structured clinical examination (OSCE) is demonstrating just that. We extrapolate that these assessments are possibly indicators of how they will practise and apply these skills and whether there will be a difference for themselves, their teachers, patients and populations. Assessment has limitations but if the curriculum as a whole is fit for purpose then newly qualified doctors and health professionals, given favourable working environments and opportunities, should be health-promoting practitioners within the context of their clinical remit and have the background knowledge to see beyond the proximal as expected, for example, in the UK by the regulatory body for doctors.[2,3] We must remember, however, that any demonstrable health-promoting practices in the workplace would be difficult to attribute to isolated aspects of curricula. The cumulative impact of policies, campaigns, remuneration directives (where financial incentives play a role in health promotion action, such as GPs' incomes being enhanced by doing specific HP work), evidence base and public expectations all impact on professional practice. However we can look at a possible link to the curriculum in the example below.

By referring yet again to smoking we should expect the health professional who is a smoker to be aware of:

➤ the health risks this poses for them, to be able to contemplate change and access cessation services and support should they be ready to change

➤ their own smoking behaviour antecedents, the likelihood of discomfort and relapse should they attempt to quit and what action they can take to ameliorate this

➤ the risks they and all smokers may pose to others

➤ policy directives to reduce smoking prevalence, for their benefit and that of the wider public

➤ the burden of disease associated with smoking on the individual, families, public health, health services and the economy

➤ their role as a clinician in supporting patients who smoke with appropriate intervention based on evidence and current guidelines.

The above are difficult to measure once the professional is in the workplace: there were no baseline data before curricula changed; policy and practice have been evolving; and the variables associated with smoking behaviour cannot be easily controlled. Yet research questions could be formulated and asked, not only to ascertain if the professionals in question were aware of the above, but also if they were aware because of their education.

Teachers are also being exposed to specific health promotion content and many current clinical teachers would have had little or no formal involvement with this field during their training. Being used to more scientific topics many have had to invest time in their own learning to become more familiar with the discipline, especially with theory and evidence. Whilst many in general practice settings have been involved in applied health promotion, possibly also with postgraduate training, this is often limited to behavioural-change techniques, information- and advice-giving and referral to specialist nurses and services. Whilst clinical teachers may invest in their own professional development primarily for the satisfaction of teaching, we have yet to establish empirically what impact, if any, health promotion teaching is having on practice.

There is, however, a convincing argument that if our newly qualified health professionals have health promotion skills and their education involved teachers who are also clinical practitioners, that within clinical practice there will be a greater and more consistent evidence-based approach to health promotion, thus having an impact on population health. For those in clinical practice who also take a wider role in community and public health issues, they should be well equipped to critique evidence and engage with policy-making decisions. This chapter considers some of the evidence and indices that may support this argument. Ultimately this assessment is less focused on the student and their ability to perform under examination conditions, but more on the possible impact of contemporary medical education and the potential to promote health in practice, justifying the efforts and investment of a few.

WHAT IS THE IMPACT OF HEALTH PROMOTION TEACHING ON STUDENTS?

Students' own health, levels of morbidity and prevalence of risk-taking behaviour are variable, with limited and conflicting data making it difficult to generalise. That said, there are reasons to be concerned about the health of medical students as reported in Chapter 13.

The moral questions we have touched on centre on the parameters of responsibility for promoting medical students' own health and well-being within curricula.

There is an expectation that the faculties and universities have care and welfare responsibilities, but apart from meeting the defined curriculum outcomes, should there be an explicit and deliberate input to the curriculum to acknowledge these health-related concerns? Should we see the population of medical students and other health professional students such as dentists and nurses as a public health risk to themselves and others? It is beyond the scope of this chapter and book to take these questions much further, but to some extent there is an underlying presumption that health promotion teaching will have a positive impact on student health as an expected outcome. But if students seem to be more proactive in the future with regard to managing their own health or indeed if current student cohorts become proactive and reduce the prevalence of risk-taking behaviour when newly qualified, can that be attributable to the curriculum?

Monash Medical School and King's College London School of Medicine (KCL) have been conducting a longitudinal study on their respective senior students about the impact of health promotion teaching, with results expected to be reported in 2009. Early data analysis suggests that students frequently engage in health-promoting activities to maintain and improve their own health and have greater awareness of responsibility for their own health as well as an awareness of where and how to access resources. However, they also report high levels of alcohol use and risk-taking sexual activity. Is this part of student life and will it resolve, is it part of social norms, is it cause for concern? For some medical educators this is a taboo area whilst for others this would seem to be a failure – as medical students and future practitioners, this suggests a lack of congruence between the risk-taking behaviour and their duties as a doctor. Currently this is a debate that is probably confined to committees and corridors, common rooms and staffrooms, students and counsellors and occasionally the public. There is, however, an explicit requirement for new doctors to take steps to maintain their own health.[3] By implication the undergraduate curriculum presumably has a responsibility in this regard.

As noted in Chapter 18, students generally perform well in health promotion-related assessment and demonstrate appropriate skills for clinical practice following teaching.[4] It is no surprise that assessment drives learning. Health promotion teaching can arouse intellectual curiosity and enable students to pursue self-directed and elective projects in this field. Several senior students have now embarked on public health and health promotion special study modules (SSMs) and electives whereby they have designed a project or arranged to work alongside an existing project, have applied for ethics committee approval, have conducted small-scale studies and have presented findings at conferences with a view to preparing papers for publication. Many are involved in humanitarian work and well briefed in local and national public health issues and policies in the countries where they are based. At KCL some students have also been successful in being awarded highly sought-after bursaries and grants.

It is these students that report a direct link with the health promotion curriculum content and their interest in taking it further and although many will not ultimately specialise in public health they will be the potential champions of the future for health promotion as an integral part of health professional education and practice. They have found, in many cases, that their teachers have been good role models as well as being inspirational. Full of enthusiasm and confidence they assume they will be able to dedicate time, when junior doctors, to do health promotion work, although for some this will be difficult. The range of activity that these students have been involved in is eclectic as is health promotion itself and include prisoner health and smoking cessation provision, mentoring in schools in deprived inner-city areas, community services for people with sickle-cell disease, the health of medical students, preventing childhood obesity, use of natural family planning methods in various settings, such as poorer communities, and for subfertility diagnosis and early management, malaria prevention, Cuba's health system and smoking prevalence, sexual health and alcohol consumption, to name a few. For all of these students health promotion practice when qualified is likely to be as normal as good communication skills.

WHAT IS THE IMPACT OF HEALTH PROMOTION TEACHING ON TEACHERS?

Medical educationalists, medical teachers and facilitators are terms that are sometimes used interchangeably but for the purpose of this book they are distinguished.

➤ *Medical educationalists* are those with a significant remit within medical education, such as curriculum design and assessment. They may have higher qualifications in education and may have a clinical specialty or other specialty associated with healthcare, health policy or health management, for example.

➤ *Medical teachers* are those with a remit to do front-line teaching, in any format, to deliver curriculum content, whether or not they have be involved in its development. They will have pedagogy skills, which could be as basic as 'how to teach' level or may have a higher degree in education and be educationalists as well. They will usually be practising clinicians familiar with the topic being taught. Teaching will be a complementary aspect of their clinical or healthcare role rather than their mainstream work.

➤ *Facilitators* may be as above but in their role as a facilitator they enable learning rather than proactively teach, as in problem-based learning (PBL). They will have guidance and briefing notes for the session which typically is small-group format. Their expertise is in facilitation rather than a topic but they will be familiar with the topic and may or may not have a clinical and healthcare role.

To date we have limited data about the impact of teaching health promotion on teachers and their own subsequent clinical practice and whilst many small-scale studies are under way, most of those teaching health promotion have come from the primary care and general practice fields where they are already more likely to have been engaged in health promotion activity and hence are favourable to teaching and facilitating such sessions.

By working with a selected group of 10 experienced medical teachers, Wylie at KCL developed a multimedia teaching pack for teaching behavioural change. Designing and piloting this with those whose everyday practice involved helping patients change their health-related behaviour was essential if the pack was going to have credibility with teachers and students, but equally its content had to reflect best evidence. At the early stages it was noted that many teachers weren't sure about best practice in behavioural change approaches but 'did it their way' or followed government guidelines with limited awareness of the underpinning theories. Initially some of these teachers felt that students didn't need to appreciate underpinning theory and evidence, but through discussion and having been signposted to some references about behavioural change there was agreement that this evidence should be part of the teaching material.[5] Many said they were impressed and could see how their own practice was limited, but planned to improve their own practice with regard to behavioural change and brief intervention before the next group of students came to their practices.

After the material was used for the first time by all the teachers, focus groups were held to review the acceptability of the sessions and the multimedia packs. Without exception all the teachers claimed to have shared with the students how this had enabled them to reflect on and improve their clinical practice, which in turn they felt was encouraging for students to hear. During the sessions many students were feeding back about their observations in clinical settings, indicating they had seen little in the way of consistent good practice with patients who smoked, were overweight or drank excessive alcohol. They were concerned about their knowledge and skill base in forthcoming assessment and these sessions had clarified in the students' minds not just that smoking cessation advice should be given but also how.

Those medical teachers who were also involved in assessment of health promotion elements have reported favourably, not only on their experience but also on the opportunity to reflect and review and, in some circumstances, to modify their own practices.

However, these are a minority of teachers and many students go on clinical placement where the teachers are first and foremost clinicians, and currently there is ample evidence to suggest that health promotion training has been limited – which in turn suggests these clinical practitioners are less likely to be good role models for students or indeed able to teach elements of health promotion.

The attitude of the clinicians towards health promotion delivery for patients plays a role in whether patients receive health promotion and therefore whether it works. Some GPs lack confidence in their training and ability to encourage changes in smoking behaviour, diet or level of physical activity. This could be linked to their limited experiences and exposure to health promotion during their own medical education, their attitudes or both.

Steptoe, et al. examined attitudes to cardiovascular health promotion among GPs and practice nurses.[6] The majority of GPs and practice nurses supported the idea that practice nurses are the most appropriate professional to deliver health promotion. This could be problematic because the GP is seen more often than the practice nurse and medical students are more likely to observe the doctor. Even if the GP makes a referral to the practice nurse, there is still a need for the GP to initiate a health promotion intervention. Practice nurses were more likely to endorse lifestyle counselling than GPs were. Lifestyle counselling, however, was seen as most effective for managing hypertension and high cholesterol but ineffective for obesity and physical activity. Significantly more practice nurses than GPs regarded the detection of high cholesterol, obesity or lack of physical activity to be part of their daily work and identified hypertension and smoking as important aspects of their work. Those GPs and practice nurses who felt they did not have time for health promotion had a more negative view of lifestyle counselling than those who did not. The authors concluded:

> It is recognized that health promotion involves more than the provision of simple information and advice, but GPs and practice nurses lack confidence in lifestyle

counselling skills. The attitudes of health professionals are crucial to the implementation of prevention strategies and require regular review.[6]

A survey of attitudes to and involvement in health promotion and lifestyle counselling conducted in the UK found that health promotion or preventive medicine took up approximately 16% of total general practice clinical time. Although 75% of GPs placed health promotion at 'somewhat' or 'very high' in their overall clinical priorities, there was a large difference in the proportion of GPs who reported being prepared to counsel patients on lifestyle issues and those who indicated they felt confident in actually helping patients change these behaviours. For example, 83% of GPs felt 'prepared' or 'very prepared' to counsel patients about alcohol consumption, yet only 21% felt they were 'effective' or 'very effective' in helping patients reduce the amount of alcohol they consumed. It is recommended that additional information, training and support are required by GPs to help them deliver health promotion.

Brotons, *et al.* examined the views of GPs in Europe on prevention and health promotion in clinical practice.[7] They observed that more than half of the GPs surveyed were reluctant to help patients to reduce smoking, decrease alcohol consumption and maintain a normal weight. It is important to note, however, that such surveys are based on self-reporting by GPs and reflect what GPs *should* do. Objective information such as that ascertained through auditing patient charts would reveal more objectively what GPs *actually* do in practice. There are gaps between GPs' knowledge and evidence-based health promotion practices. Training, either in medical education or through continuing professional development, needs to be devised to address these gaps and inconsistencies. What may be more concerning is the recent evidence in the UK about smoking cessation referral inconsistencies, thereby denying some patients access to free local evidence-based smoking cessation services.[8,9]

Curricuum is aimed at students but if health promotion elements are to be taught by clinical practitioners there is an opportunity, maybe an imperative, to supplement their continuing professional development with skills and knowledge for health promotion practice and teaching. As health promotion becomes established through the curriculum of health professionals there is an expectation that this will impact on the professional practice of teachers.

WHAT IS THE IMPACT OF HEALTH PROMOTION TEACHING ON PATIENTS AND POPULATION?

In Chapter 2 we considered the limited evidence base for health promotion *per se*, but given the combined increased efforts of professional guidelines, teaching students about behaviour-change techniques and incentives for those engaging with health promotion, we are now in a position to begin to examine the effect of this on patients and populations.

Clinicians often have heavy workloads and cannot carry out public health interventions themselves to promote healthy behaviours in the population. It is therefore important for health promotion in a clinical setting to be supported by a wide-ranging strategy through which patients can be targeted for matters concerning their health. This is where health education programmes and health promotion campaigns are useful and necessary. Support from health authorities, charities and other medical organisations are important for successful educational programmes when delivering health promotion. Additionally, well focused mass media campaigns can generate more impact.

How does one measure whether a health promotion campaign is effective? A difference in prevalence of unhealthy behaviours may seem the most obvious way of determining whether a health promotion campaign has been successful. But campaigns deemed successful may not have a measurable population-level effect.[10]

Success is based on evaluations that measure a full range of variables where the aims of the campaign have been to increase awareness and proximal variables such as social norms. The success is linked to the symbiotic relationship between the aims of a campaign and supportive complementary local provision. Carefully constructed and implemented campaigns, especially if appropriately targeted and resourced, with methodologically sound evaluation strategies, have been able to demonstrate improved sexual health-related behaviour.[11]

A WORK IN PROGRESS

Health promotion activity in teaching, in clinical practice and in community- and population-based strategic interventions has been shown to be effective in modifying health-related behaviours. Yet there is much still to be done.

As research demonstrates the effectiveness of health promotion activity, healthcare professionals will need to consider what is generalisable, transferable and applicable in their context. The large-scale, multisite 'DESMOND' programme (diabetes education and self-management programme for people with newly diagnosed type 2 diabetes), for example, resulted in significant and sustained improvements for patients, using a structured group education programme. There were improvements in weight loss, smoking status, physical activity and depression.[12] Such findings need to be given considerable attention of course, but what is important with this work is that it builds on evidence that educational programmes with a theoretical basis and using cognitive reframing are associated with improved outcomes. The philosophy was based on patient empowerment and incorporated theories such as self-efficacy and behavioural change.

Health promotion in medical education and health professional curricula will constantly evolve once it is established. What this study suggests, however, is that there are basic principles, theories and skills that can be included in curriculum content at undergraduate level.

Students themselves may be the first beneficiaries of quality health promotion teaching in curricula, enabling them to maintain and improve their health. They may become a critical mass within the healthcare workforce with the skills and competence to implement and evaluate evidence-based health promotion. GPs and other health professionals involved in health promotion teaching may feel more confident to improve their own health promotion practice. Patients and the populations at large may anticipate and expect more proactive health promotion activity to enable them to improve their health and well-being.

Tools and strategies to monitor health promotion practice from when it is introduced in medical education and throughout a clinician's career need to be developed. Chart audits, for example, could be conducted on a regular basis to ensure health promotion is part of the doctors' work. It is also important to monitor doctors' attitudes towards health promotion, which may be influenced by how well the effectiveness evidence is disseminated. This can be achieved by ongoing medical education both during and after medical school. Patient surveys can also help to determine what their health promotion needs are, as individuals and within their communities. Support for clinicians to develop and maintain their confidence in lifestyle counselling as well as more complex health promotion activities is of paramount importance, and this could be done in partnership with medical educators.

REFERENCES

1 Harden R, Crosby JR, Davis MH, *et al.* AMEE Guide No. 14: Outcome-based education: Part 5 – From competency to meta-competency; a model for the specification of learning outcomes. *Med Teach.* 1999; **21**(6): 546–52.

2 General Medical Council. *Tomorrow's Doctors.* 2nd ed. London: General Medical Council; 2003.

3 General Medical Council. *The New Doctor.* Available at: www.gmc-uk.org/education/postgraduate/new_doctor.asp (accessed 7 November 2009).

4 Roseby R, Marks MK, Conn J, *et al.* Improving medical student performance in adolescent anti-smoking health promotion. *Med Educ.* 2003; **37**(8): 704–8.

5 Marteau T, Dieppe P, Foy R, *et al.* Behavioural medicine: changing our behaviour. *BMJ.* 2006; **332**(7539): 437–8.

6 Steptoe A, Doherty S, Kendrick T, *et al.* Attitudes to cardiovascular health promotion among GPs and practice nurses. *Fam Pract.* 1999 (April); **16**(2): 158–63.

7 Brotons C, Björkelund C, Bulc M, *et al.* Prevention and health promotion in clinical practice: the views of general practitioners in Europe. *Prev Med.* 2005; **40**(5): 595–601.

8 Vogt F, Hall S, Marteau TM. General practitioners' and family physicians' negative beliefs and attitudes towards discussing smoking cessation with patients: a systematic review. *Addiction.* 2005; **100**(10): 1423–31.

9 Hilton S, Doherty S, Kendrick T, *et al.* Promotion of healthy behaviour among adults at increased risk of coronary heart disease in general practice: methodology and baseline data from the Change of Heart study. *Health Educat J.* 1999; **58**(1): 3–16.

10 Cavell N, Bauman A. Changing the way people think about health-enhancing physical activity: do mass media campaigns have a role? *J Sports Sci.* 2004; **22**(8): 771–90.

11 Zimmerman RS, Palmgreen PM, Noar SM, *et al.* Effects of a televised two-city safer sex mass media campaign targeting high-sensation-seeking and impulsive-decision-making young adults. *Health Educ Behav.* 2007 (October); **34**(5): 810–26.

12 Davies MJ, Heller S, Skinner TC, *et al.* Effectiveness of the diabetes education and self management for ongoing and newly diagnosed (DESMOND) programme for people with newly diagnosed type 2 diabetes: cluster randomised controlled trial. *BMJ.* 2008; **336**(7643): 491–5.

CHAPTER 21

Future challenges: emerging knowledge, changing health issues and continuing uncertainties

Nisha Mehta and Alan Maryon Davis

As we have seen, the field of health promotion is not static. It is constantly changing with each emerging public health issue and each new approach to influencing policy, practice and behaviour. In teaching health promotion skills and competencies, we need to be aware of these new challenges. We have to understand how they might impact on what we teach and the way that we teach it. And we have to ensure that our teaching is truly fit for purpose.

In this chapter we consider the main changes occurring in the field of health promotion and look at ways in which current teaching and learning might have to adapt in order to properly prepare practitioners to face future challenges.

As we move into the twenty-first century, we are beginning to see the shape of things to come for health promotion. The main trends fall into four broad categories:

➤ changes in public health issues, challenges or threats
➤ changes in health systems and services
➤ new health promotion tools
➤ the evolving international agenda – health as a global movement.

CHANGES IN PUBLIC HEALTH ISSUES

In developed countries like the UK, a number of public health issues are emerging as priorities for action. These include (in no particular order):

➤ obesity, with an emphasis on preventing child obesity
➤ alcohol misuse, especially binge drinking among young people
➤ unplanned teenage pregnancy
➤ chlamydia infection and subfertility
➤ resurgence of HIV
➤ high blood pressure linked to excessive intake of salt
➤ passive smoking by children
➤ depression linked to social isolation

➤ healthcare-associated infections
➤ living with long-term conditions
➤ migrant (including asylum seeker) health
➤ threat of pandemic influenza and other globalised infectious diseases
➤ health consequences of climate change.

Health promotion comprises a key element in the armoury for tackling each of these issues – whether in terms of reducing risk, improving well-being, signposting services or increasing access to those services. There are also often cross-benefits of particular behaviour changes. For example, encouraging the use of condoms will help to reduce the risk of chlamydia, HIV and unplanned pregnancy. So too will discouraging binge drinking – so often associated with unsafe sex. Encouraging active travel will not only help reduce people's waistlines, but also their carbon footprint and hence slow global warming.

COMBATING OBESITY

Obesity provides an excellent case study in how health promotion is changing. As well as premature death from obesity-related causes such as coronary heart disease and various cancers, obesity can cause many years of chronic disease. The burden of obesity-related illnesses on healthcare budgets is already considerable, and is predicted to increase to cripplingly high levels throughout the world over the next few decades – the so-called 'obesity time-bomb'.

The key behavioural goals are much the same as ever – to encourage people to become more physically active and eat healthier diets – 'move a little more and eat a little less'. But the ways in which the messages are put across is changing through more sophisticated approaches to social marketing, increasing use of the new digital media and harnessing the muscle of the commercial sector – particularly the food industry.

But encouraging the public to make lifestyle changes is just one element of a comprehensive strategy. The 'Three Es' model calls for action on three broad fronts – encouragement, empowerment and environment.[1]

- *Encouragement* is motivating people to adopt a healthier lifestyle – eating more fruit and vegetables and becoming more active. Many health campaigns are all about encouragement. So too is one-to-one diet and exercise advice from a doctor or other health professional. But encouragement is rarely effective without empowerment.

- *Empowerment* is helping people to gain the life skills, confidence, control and freedom to make healthy choices. Much of basic education is about empowerment. So too is teaching cooking skills, working with particular community groups and helping people get access to useful advice and information. But empowerment and encouragement also need a healthful environment.

- *Environment* is shorthand for ensuring that the physical, social, cultural and economic backdrop in which people live, work and play is conducive to health – in other words, healthy public policy. Examples with regard to obesity include increasing access to affordable fruit and vegetables, easy-to-understand nutritional labelling and safe places to walk and cycle.

From a more international perspective, the main changes in public health issues and challenges include:

➤ the widening gap between rich and poor – both within and between nations
➤ globalisation of infectious diseases
➤ the steady rise of chronic diseases.

The widening gap between rich and poor – both within and between nations

In spite of recent events which have rocked the foundations of the financial world, we still have a global economy in which world leaders fundamentally believe in market forces and free trade and in which foreign aid is less fashionable than 'fair trade'. The UN Millennium Development Goals are far from being met, and life expectancy in sub-Saharan Africa continues to fall with malnutrition, maternal mortality and infectious diseases at the helm of these trends.

Globalisation of infectious diseases

Changing migrant populations have globalised infectious diseases such as multi-drug resistant TB and HIV strains, which are prevalent in deprived parts of inner-city London as well as sub-Saharan Africa. At the same time, middle-class sectors of society, which benefit from booming economies, drive consumerism in which natural resources are used up at an unsustainable rate, and in which uncontrolled emissions of greenhouse gases contribute to 'climate chaos' and the devastating floods, heatwaves and outbreaks of vector-borne diseases which result. The World Health Organization (WHO) estimates that over 150 000 excess deaths occur annually due to climate change, compared to their baseline figures of 1961–90.

The steady rise of chronic diseases

According to the WHO report, *The Global Burden of Disease: 2004 update*,[2] non-communicable diseases – notably diabetes, hypertension, coronary heart disease, stroke, chronic obstructive pulmonary disease (COPD) and lung cancer – will cause 75% of all deaths by 2030, up from 60% in 2004. Total deaths from tobacco use are rising sharply and will reach 8.3 million in 2030, up from 5.4 million in 2004.

Global patterns of free trade not only have consequences for malnourished populations, but also they have conversely fuelled the rise in diet-related chronic diseases. Although patterns of trade and consequences for diet are poorly understood, Rayner, *et al.* have considered the complex issues underlying the rise in diet-related chronic diseases, and make a compelling case that links global patterns of trade with obesity, diabetes, cardiovascular diseases, cancer, dental disease and osteoporosis. They argue that as food imports exceed exports in developed countries the 'traditional' food chain that relies on locally grown and sourced produce becomes less important. Processed food and supermarket forces lead to an increased emphasis on cheap convenient meals, whilst liberal advertising laws simultaneously effect a shift in societal and cultural expectations in the national diet. For example, Coca Cola and PepsiCo spent more on advertising and promotion than the WHO's entire annual budget in 2004.[3] Commentators identify a time lag between the identification of public health problems and an effective response for them and call for a swift response from health promotion.

CHANGES IN HEALTH SYSTEMS AND SERVICES

Shift towards primary care

The UK has had a well-developed, universally available primary care system since the birth of the National Health Service (NHS) in 1948. It is in primary care – general medical practice, general dental practice, community pharmacy and optometry – that most patient contacts take place. As well as diagnosing and treating minor illnesses and acting as 'gatekeepers' to investigation and treatment in the hospital setting, GPs have an important part to play in promoting health, reducing risk and facilitating early diagnosis.

But despite this crucial multifaceted role, the lion's share of NHS resources has always gone to the secondary care sector. Highly labour-intensive, high-tech hospitals have always soaked up most of the NHS budget. However, things are changing – and government policy as set out in the White Paper, *Our Health, Our Care, Our Say*[4] has set out a clear policy of shifting resources from secondary into primary care. This will help to tip the balance towards prevention and health promotion.

Emphasis on self-care

Alongside the steady build-up of primary care services is an increasing emphasis on self-care, not only for minor self-limiting illnesses, but also for long-term conditions. With steadily increasing life expectancy, the population is ageing. GPs, hospital doctors, nurses and other health professionals can expect to deal with an ever higher proportion of older patients with a wide range of chronic disorders and disabilities. They will need health promotion skills in order to help patients live optimally with their chronic condition and contribute to their own care.

Focus on quality of services

The NHS in England has recently been dominated by the so-called 'quality agenda', encapsulated in Lord Darzi's report[5] and its subsequent directives. Again there is a strong emphasis on promotion of health and prevention of disease as well as diagnosis and care. A new vascular risk reduction programme aims to maximise control of cardiovascular risk factors in primary care and link check-ups and healthy lifestyles advice more firmly into the Quality and Outcomes Framework for incentivising practices.[6] Similar initiatives are being rolled out in other parts of the UK.

Consumerism and the internet

The consumer movement has been gathering pace in the UK since the 1960s and has permeated most of the developed world. Patients increasingly see themselves as consumers of health services, with the rights they would expect as a consumer of any other service. These include the right to be involved in planning and developing the services they use. Successive governments have reaffirmed these rights to patient and public involvement – most recently enshrined in the NHS Constitution.[7]

A prerequisite for effective patient and public involvement is an appropriately informed group of people representing patients or the public. Providing such information in an accessible form is an important aspect of health promotion and one in which doctors and other health professionals, by explaining complex procedures or services and interpreting acronyms and jargon, can be especially helpful. It is all part of empowering individuals and groups to use their best efforts for the collective good.

It is estimated that by 2012 three-quarters of British homes will have broadband access and this phenomenal growth in the 'information highway' is having a profound effect on people's ability to access information about health and healthcare. The government's main health portal, NHS Choices[8] is among the most frequently visited websites in the UK. But there are thousands of other health websites – many providing information of dubious veracity. Doctors and other health professionals will need to be aware of the main reliable web sources and be able to guide their patients in gathering useful information via the internet. New media such as SMS texting and podcasting will become increasingly important tools for health professionals to communicate directly with patients.

Development of public health genetics

As we get ever better at mapping the human genome and manipulating specific genes, a new preventive service is beginning to unfold. The clinical consequences of being able to predict an individual's vulnerability to a range of diseases and disorders with greatly enhanced accuracy will lead to new demands in terms of conveying information and advice, particularly about lifestyles and prevention. Tomorrow's doctors will need to know how best to communicate such things to their patients.

Emerging markets in health and healthcare

In most countries there is no socialised health service funded out of taxation. Instead there is usually a private fee-for-service system, often combined with insurance, voluntary or compulsory. Healthcare is a marketplace – and so too is health insurance.

In the UK, the NHS is free for the end user at the point of need. But in England NHS healthcare services are increasingly being provided by the commercial sector under contract to the NHS. Patients are offered a choice of providers, some of which might be commercial. Part of a health professional's health promotion role might be to advise and assist patients in steering their way through the information they are given about the merits (or demerits) of different providers in the developing UK healthcare marketplace.

Local government role in well-being

Section 2 of the Local Government Act 2000 offered the so-called 'Well-being Power' to local authorities in England and Wales encouraging them to be inventive in promoting the economic, social and environmental well-being of their areas. In many cases this has been interpreted as including cultural well-being and the promotion or improvement of the health of residents and visitors.[9]

This has coincided with the policy of creating non-statutory 'local strategic partnerships' (LSPs), involving local authorities, local NHS bodies, the voluntary sector, chambers of commerce, schools, police, residents' associations and others in a multi-agency process for tackling high-priority local issues, including health challenges. The resulting 'local area agreements' (LAAs) are the blueprints for local partnership action for such issues as teenage pregnancy, childhood obesity, binge drinking and social disorder, crime and mental ill-health, respiratory health and housing and many others. They are a key vehicle for health promotion at the local level in England.[9] Similar approaches have been adopted in Scotland, Wales and Northern Ireland.

Such multi-agency partnerships for health promotion were a key recommendation of the Bangkok Charter for Health Promotion in a Globalized World,[10] and the principle has been reaffirmed in subsequent major international reports on public health and health promotion.

Cross-government working at national level

Another change, which has become increasingly important in recent years, has been the move towards closer cross-government collaboration around major public health issues – more 'joined-up' government working. Examples include national strategies to deal with obesity (jointly issued by the Department of Health and Department of Children, Schools and Families)[11] and alcohol.[12]

A cross-government approach is a recurrent theme in international reports on health promotion and tackling health inequalities – a recent example being the report of the WHO Commission on Social Determinants of Health – *Closing the Gap in a Generation.*[13]

THE EVOLVING INTERNATIONAL AGENDA: HEALTH AS A GLOBAL MOVEMENT

The Ottawa Charter for Health Promotion[14] outlined an approach to tackling the main health promotion challenges of the mid-1980s. At that time the world was a very different place – infectious diseases appeared to be declining, the HIV/AIDS epidemic was yet to take hold, global poverty and the health impacts of climate change were less topical issues than they are today and chronic diseases were viewed as the next big public health problem.[15] Consequently, the key tenets of the Ottawa Charter focused on:

➤ building healthy public policy
➤ strengthening community action
➤ developing personal skills
➤ creating supportive environments
➤ reorienting health services.

In the intervening years, health promotion, not only in terms of its principles and practice, but also as an academic discipline, was established with varying degrees of success in health systems and medical (and other health professional) curricula around the world. Jackson, *et al.* use case studies of health promotion interventions to argue that the tenets of the Ottawa Charter have worked best when applied in combination, and suggest that such combined action will continue to be 'relevant and important in addressing the emerging health challenges of the 21st century'.[16]

However, the discipline of health promotion is constantly evolving and the Ottawa Charter has since been augmented by several subsequent milestones. One such was the Bangkok Charter for Health Promotion in a Globalized World.[10] This WHO-sponsored charter acknowledged that the new challenges facing societies since 1986 include:

➤ increasing inequalities within and between countries
➤ new patterns of consumption and communication
➤ commercialisation
➤ global environmental change
➤ urbanisation.

The Bangkok Charter pointed out that migration, often prompted by food insecurity or ethnic clashes, can lead to marginalisation, hardship and poor health or healthcare. It also cited the particular issues concerning the place of women in some societies leading to disadvantage and inequalities for women and their children.

On the positive side, the charter suggested that new information technologies, such as mobile phones, cheap computers and the internet are allowing enhanced sharing of information and improved communications. It also pointed to encouraging evidence that health is increasingly being placed at the centre of development – the Millennium Development Goals playing an important part in this respect.

The Bangkok Charter reaffirmed the key role of health promotion in helping people to enjoy the fundamental human right of achieving the highest attainable standard of health and well-being for themselves and their families. The charter defined health promotion as:

> ... the process of enabling people to increase control over their health and its determinants, and thereby improve their health. It is a core function of public health and contributes to the work of tackling communicable and non-communicable diseases and other threats to health.[10]

The charter advocated five specific actions to take health promotion forward in the new more globalised world:
➤ advocate for health based on human rights and solidarity
➤ invest in sustainable policies, actions and infrastructure to address the determinants of health
➤ build capacity for policy development, leadership, health promotion practice, knowledge transfer and research and health literacy
➤ regulate and legislate to ensure a high level of protection from harm and enable equal opportunity for health and well-being for all people
➤ partner and build alliances with public, private, non-governmental and international organisations and civil society to create sustainable actions.[10]

The Bangkok Charter called for a world in which health promotion considerations inform all elements of domestic and foreign policy and international relations. This principle has been echoed by many others who argue that the future of health promotion lies in sustained funding, governmental support and multidisciplinary awareness and intersectoral collaboration – more so than ever before.[1,3–5]

In 2008, the WHO-sponsored Commission on Social Determinants of Health issued its final report aimed at national, regional and local governments, professionals, academics, major corporations and civil society.[13] The Commission focused on the fundamental issue of poverty from the angle of inequity and social injustice and outlined three key approaches to promoting health through improving the social determinants of ill-health and inequity.
➤ Improve the conditions of daily life – the circumstances in which people are born, grow, live, work and age.
➤ Tackle the inequitable distribution of power, money and resources – the structural drivers of those conditions of daily life – globally, nationally and locally.
➤ Measure the problem, evaluate action, expand the knowledge base, develop a workforce that is trained in the social determinants of health and raise public awareness about the social determinants of health.[13]

Among its key recommendations was a call to develop a strong public sector that is committed to reducing inequity, has the strategies to do so, and is adequately financed. This would also require strengthened support for civil society, an accountable private sector and people across society to invest in health-promoting collective action.

Another recommendation was to ensure that health inequity is measured, within countries and globally. Globally, nationally, regionally and locally, health equity surveillance systems for routine monitoring of health inequity and the social determinants of health should be established and maintained, and should evaluate the health equity impact of policy and action.

A third key recommendation was to ensure that, at all levels and in all settings, there is sufficient organisational capacity and an appropriate skill-base to act effectively on health inequity. This requires investment in the training of policy-makers, health practitioners and the public in issues around social determinants of health. It also requires a stronger focus on social determinants in public health research.

Needless to say, these recommendations have major implications for the education and training of doctors and other health professionals with particular regard to public health and health promotion.

Also in 2008, the WHO's world health report, *Primary health care: now more than ever*,[17] published 30 years after The Alma-Ata Declaration, focused on the shortcomings of health systems around the world and reaffirmed the main conclusion of Alma-Ata that resources need to be shifted 'upstream' towards health promotion, prevention (primary and secondary) and primary healthcare. One of the report's key criticisms was that resources tend to favour 'high-tech' curative services based in major hospitals, neglecting the potential of health promotion and risk reduction to prevent up to 70% of the disease burden.

HOW WILL CURRENT CURRICULAR HEALTH PROMOTION APPROACHES PREPARE PROFESSIONALS FOR THE FUTURE?

In 1993, The General Medical Council (GMC) committed UK medical schools to 'increase commitment to learning in the community, health promotion and public health'.[18] The GMC also instructed medical schools to 'reduce the burden of factual information'. Nevertheless, curricula remain overcrowded and assessment is focused on acquisition of factual knowledge. The medical student must know *what* to think in any given clinical scenario. This is clearly essential to ensure the training of safe, competent doctors.[18]

In comparison, other degree courses, most notably the arts, are focused on teaching academically transferable skills, including reasoning, argument, critical evaluation and analysis. The student graduates with an intuitive understanding of *how* to think, but with little or no practical knowledge. Graduate medical students are quick to pick up on the fundamental differences between the two degrees. Many students (graduates and nongraduates alike) express their frustration about the lack of space in the curriculum for development of these analytical faculties. Some find an outlet in an intercalated BSc, others through the occasional inspirational special study module, and yet others through research carried out in their own time.

DOES CURRENT TEACHING OF HEALTH PROMOTION NEED TO CHANGE?

Existing methods of teaching health promotion in curricula have been discussed in detail elsewhere in this book. Many approaches have been successfully implemented and evaluated and could usefully continue to be used as a method of engaging students with the evolving issues in health promotion that we have identified in this chapter. However, success in teaching and assessment has not been uniform, either within or between curricula, and health promotion techniques do not necessarily stay with all students in the same way as the 'holy grail' of factual knowledge. Some students do not see the relevance of health promotion, especially when it is presented in a didactic and theoretical way and/or during the preclinical years of the course. In a course with multiple competing demands, and in which there is an identifiable need to teach students *how* – rather than *what* – to think, it must be possible to meet this need whilst simultaneously bringing health promotion to life for every student.

An excellent way to address both of these issues simultaneously would be to follow the Monash Medical Course model, and allocate students a significant period of time within the later years of the curriculum to focus on the analysis, evaluation and poster presentation of a given health promotion intervention. Students report a sense of pride in their achievement during this substantial part of the course.[19] Learning about health promotion through a practical exercise, and subsequently forcing their observations through the rigour of a theoretical model, would achieve multiple goals of cementing health promotion lessons in the learning of students whilst allowing them time to engage with a sociologically or anthropologically oriented discipline and to benefit from all that this style of learning has to offer.

HEALTH PROMOTION: A SUFFICIENTLY ROBUST DISCIPLINE?

This method of teaching could also be used to address the vexed question of whether the discipline is, or will ever be, sufficiently robust to persuade practitioners of its merits. Existing evidence for the success of the Ottawa Charter objectives is sparse, and evidence-based health promotion remains an elusive goal.[16] Giving students the time and space to critically evaluate the project they have studied will allow them to draw wider conclusions about the discipline and will draw future generations of doctors into the debate. An honest approach to the difficulties inherent in this broad discipline is likely to be rewarded with a genuine engagement on the part of the students. An approach that favours rote learning of theory and methodology with no real practical application or room for critical debate risks being forgotten at best, and fostering resentment at worst.

EMBRACING THE NEW HEALTH PROMOTION TOOLS

The acquisition and application of IT skills within the field of health promotion may play an increasingly important role in future curricula. Electronically stored personal health records will improve health promotion in the same way that all other aspects of care will benefit from greater continuity.[20] The bridging of the gap between primary and secondary care records should encourage those working in the hospital setting to engage more with illness prevention and health education. In future, informatics may transform the doctor–patient relationship, for example through tailored communications at specific times to facilitate compliance and encourage attendance for screening checks.[21] Students should be exposed to these changes, and should be encouraged to consider possible ways in which they could use informatics in their own future practice.

Use of the internet by patients will be an increasing challenge for future practitioners, who will need to be able to recommend and direct their 'information-rich' patients to sites and groups that will benefit them (e.g. podcasts, internet support groups, chat rooms or interactive websites). They will also need to be aware of the dangers of poor computer literacy and possible negative health outcomes (e.g. internet use for information seeking about controversial topics such as eating disorders or abortion). These will become basic skills that will add significantly to the health promotion armoury of any practitioner, but which must not be left out of future curricula.

THE ROLE OF THE DOCTOR

In 2008 the UK medical profession, represented through a range of national bodies, produced a consensus statement on the role of the doctor. The statement not only emphasised the importance of preventive advice for individual patients, but also recognised a wider population role:

> All doctors have a role in the maintenance and promotion of population health, through evidence-based practice. Some will enhance the health of the population through taking on roles in health education or research, service improvement and re-design, in public health and through health advocacy. Notwithstanding the primacy of the individual doctor-patient relationship, the doctor must appreciate the needs of the patient in the context of the wider health needs of the population.[22]

This clear recognition of the doctor's role extending beyond the clinic or consulting room will have important consequences for medical education and training. Similar statements have been made for the education and training of nurses, midwives and allied health professionals.[23]

All of our observations point to the fact that multidisciplinary input is crucial to the future success of the discipline. If medical curricula are to keep pace with the changes in health promotion, the doctors of tomorrow need to be prepared for a very different world. Cribb identifies some useful steps for medical educators to achieve this goal, arguing persuasively that multidisciplinary collaboration is needed in educating medical students, an effort which should be supported by an active network of academic and professional links:

> The contemporary world of healthcare requires that doctors see themselves as only one voice in a societal 'conversation' about health and healthcare, and that when they fail to see themselves as situated in this way they are failing to understand the world they inhabit.[24]

Certainly it is not only essential for medical students and doctors to understand that they are just one part of the health promotion team or workforce, but also that they can bring a particularly valuable set of skills and competencies to bear. Doctors enjoy a high level of trust by the public, fellow practitioners and policy-makers. They often find themselves in positions of influence and can shape important agendas. In the UK they may be involved in shaping clinical services including preventive services, perhaps as a contribution to commissioning or service planning. GPs, for example, might participate in 'practice-based commissioning' of services such as health visiting, midwifery services, community dietetics or exercise referral, many of which have a significant health promotion element to them. Clearly it is important that such doctors are sufficiently well versed in the principles and practice of health promotion.

In many overseas countries, doctors are even more likely to be in senior positions in the health system, and less likely to have any training in the key principles and skills of health promotion or even public health. An important element of capacity building and leadership development must therefore be to educate and train doctors in these crucial disciplines.

CONCLUSION

It is imperative that future health promotion practice in the twenty-first century continues to build on the successful principles of the Ottawa Charter, but that it also considers the many changes that have occurred in the health promotion environment since then, including the profound health impacts of globalisation, urbanisation, health system imbalance, inequity and social injustice. At the same time, those involved in teaching health promotion and public health must raise awareness of these issues in curricula in a way that will enable future healthcare professionals to engage confidently, competently and effectively with the emerging challenges and not risk being left behind as the world changes around them.

REFERENCES

1 Maryon-Davis A. Weight management in primary care: how can it be made more effective? *Proc Nutr Soc.* 2005; **64**(1): 97–103.
2 World Health Organization. *The Global Burden of Disease* (2004 update). Geneva: World Health Organization; 2004.
3 Rayner G, Hawkes C, Lang T, *et al.* Trade liberalization and diet transition: a public health response. *Health Promot Int.* 2006; **21**(Suppl. 1): 67–74.
4 Department of Health. *Our Health, Our Care, Our Say.* London: Department of Health; 2006.
5 Lord Darzi. *High Quality Care for All: NHS next stage review: final report.* London: Department of Health; 2008.
6 National electronic Library for Medicines (NeLM). *Update on Primary Care Cardiovascular Quality and Outcomes Framework.* Available at: www.nelm.nhs.uk/en/NeLM-Area/News/490422/490638/490643 (accessed 8 November 2009).
7 NHS Consortium website. Available at: www.nhsconsortium.com (accessed 8 November 2009).
8 NHS Choices website. Available at: www.nhs.uk/Pages/HomePage.aspx (accessed 8 November 2009).
9 Department for Communities and Local Government. *Practical Use of the Well-being Power.* London: Department for Communities and Local Government; 2008. Available at: www.communities.gov.uk/publications/localgovernment/practicalwellbeingpower (accessed 8 November 2009).
10 World Health Organization. *Bangkok Charter for Health Promotion in a Globalized World.* Geneva: World Health Organization; 2005.

11 Department of Health. *Healthy Weight, Healthy Lives: a cross government strategy for England*. London: Department of Health; 2008.

12 Department of Health, Home Office, Department for Education and Skills, Department for Culture. *Safe, Sensible, Social: the next steps in the National Alcohol Strategy*. London: The Stationery Office; 2007.

13 Commission on Social Determinants of Health. *Closing the Gap in a Generation: health equality through action on the social determinants of health. The final report of the WHO Commission on Social Determinants of Health*. Geneva: World Health Organization; 2008.

14 World Health Organization. *Ottawa Charter for Health Promotion*. Geneva: World Health Organization; 1986.

15 McMichael AJ, Butler CD. Emerging health issues: the widening challenge for population health promotion. *Health Promot Int*. 2006; **21**(Suppl. 1): 15–24.

16 Jackson SF, Perkins F, Khandor E, *et al*. Integrated health promotion strategies: a contribution to tackling current and future health challenges. *Health Promot Int*. 2006; **21**(Suppl. 1): 75–83.

17 World Health Organization. *The World Health Report 2008. Primary health care: now more than ever*. Geneva: World Health Organization; 2008.

18 General Medical Council. *Tomorrow's Doctors*. London: General Medical Council; 1993.

19 Jones KV, Hsu-Hage B. Health promotion projects: skill and attitude learning for medical students. *Med Educ*. 1999; **33**: 585–91.

20 Department of Health. *NHS Connecting for Health*. Available at: www.connectingforhealth.nhs.uk (accessed 8 November 2009).

21 Kukafka R. Public health informatics: the nature of the field and its relevance to health promotion practice. *Health Promot Pract*. 2005; **6**(1): 23–8.

22 Medical Schools Council. *The Role of the Doctor*. Available at: www.medschools.ac.uk/AboutUs/Projects/Pages/The-Role-of-the-Doctor.aspx (accessed 8 November 2009).

23 Department of Health. *Framing the Nursing and Midwifery Contribution: driving up the quality of care*. London: Department of Health; 2008.

24 Cribb A. The diffusion of the health agenda and the fundamental need for partnership in medical education. *Med Educ*. 2000; **34**(11): 916–20.

Index